Innovations in Gastrointestinal Endoscopy

Prateek Sharma • Nageshwar Reddy
Editors

Innovations in Gastrointestinal Endoscopy

Springer

Editors
Prateek Sharma
Division of Gastroenterology and Hepatology
University of Kansas School of Medicine
VA Medical Center
Kansas City, MO
USA

Nageshwar Reddy
Department of Gastroenterology
Asian Institute of Gastroenterology
Hyderabad, Andhra Pradesh
India

ISBN 978-981-15-9246-1 ISBN 978-981-15-9247-8 (eBook)
https://doi.org/10.1007/978-981-15-9247-8

This Springer imprint is published by the registered company Springer Nature Singapore Pte Ltd.
The registered company address is: 152 Beach Road, #21-01/04 Gateway East, Singapore 189721, Singapore

I would also like to dedicate this book to the memory of my father, Professor SN Sharma, Professor Emeritus of Plastic Surgery at Baroda Medical College who has been a source of inspiration for me and always taught me to follow my passion

Prateek Sharma

Preface

Despite the COVID-19 pandemic that has hit the world, global endoscopy has continued to innovate and provide cutting-edge patient care.

We are delighted to present this compilation of chapters by leaders and masters in the field of gastrointestinal endoscopy. We hope that this book will add to the medical knowledge of gastroenterology and endoscopy practitioners, educators, trainees and endoscopy personnel who strive to provide the best care for their patients. By providing this book in the 'old fashioned' print format, we aim to reach even the remotest places where 'digital print' may be difficult to obtain. Both of us will work with the gastrointestinal and endoscopy societies and other stakeholders worldwide and attempt to provide access to this state-of-the-art innovative procedure book including images, figures and tables to the developing countries to foster education, research and innovation in every part of the world. Finally, we are indeed indebted to our colleagues, friends and experts who have selflessly devoted their valuable time and efforts to make this a reality.

Kansas City, MO — Prateek Sharma
Hyderabad, Andhra Pradesh, India — Nageshwar Reddy

Contents

About the Editors

Prateek Sharma graduated from Baroda Medical College in India and completed his Gastroenterology and Advanced Gastroenterology fellowship from the University of Arizona, Tucson, Arizona. He is a Professor of Medicine and Director of Fellowship Training at the University of Kansas School of Medicine and Veterans Affairs Medical Center, Kansas City, Missouri. He has been at the forefront in improving diagnosis and management of GI diseases and cancer, specifically in advanced imaging and endoscopic treatments. He is a world-renowned physician, teacher, and educator.

Dr. Sharma has been interviewed by the *Wall Street Journal* and *Newsweek*. He has over 400 publications, including original articles and book chapters, and is regularly invited to present at major national and international meetings. In addition, he has co-edited several important books. Dr. Sharma has and continues to publish in several high-profile national and international journals, including the *New England Journal of Medicine, Annals of Internal Medicine, Gastrointestinal Endos copy, Gastroenterology,* and *American Journal of Gastroenterology.* Dr. Sharma is currently a Governing Board Member of the American Society for Gastrointestinal Endoscopy and President of the International Society for Diseases of the Esophagus and has held numerous positions at World Gastroenterology Organization(WGO), American Gastroenterological Association (AGA), and American College of Gastroenterology (ACG).

Nageshwar Reddy Duvvur graduated from Kurnool Medical College and completed his gastroenterology fellowship from Post Graduate Institute of Medical Education and Research, Chandigarh, India. He is currently the Chairman of Asian Institute of Gastroenterology, Hyderabad, India, and was the Professor of Gastroenterology at Guntur Medical College, Guntur. He has around 600 peer-review-published papers and given numerous named orations. He is past president of World Endoscopy Organization. He has been a visiting faculty for over 200 international endoscopy workshops and forum member of Asian Endoscopy Masters Forum. He was awarded the highest civilian award "Padma Bhushan" from the Government of India. He won many awards which include Dhanwantri Award in 2004, Master Endoscopist Award from American Society for Gastrointestinal Endoscopy (ASGE) in 2009, International Service Award

American Society of Gastroenterology (DDW Crystal Awards) in 2011. Master of World Gastroenterology Organization Award from World Gastroenterology Organization in 2014. ASGE President's Award—American Society of Gastroenterology (DDW Crystal Awards) in 2020. Fellow of American Gastroenterological Association (FAGA) Award in 2020. Fellow of Japan Gastroen terological Endoscopy Society (JGES) Award in 2020. Master of ASGE from American Society for Gastrointestinal Endoscopy (MASGE) Award in 2020.

Gastric Peroral Endoscopic Myotomy: G-POEM

1

M. Barthet and J. M. Gonzalez

1.1 Introduction and Background

Gastroparesis is a functional motility disorder that dramatically affects the quality of life of patients, and for which the therapeutic options have always been limited [1–3]. This leads patients to difficult situations, including severe consequences on their nutritional as well as their psychological conditions. Indeed, besides the medical treatments, which seems poorly effective over the time, associated with adverse events and tachyphylaxia [4–6], the different interventional therapies have also been disappointing. The endoscopic approaches include intra-pyloric injection of botulinum toxin, which did not demonstrate real efficacy in two recent randomized studies [7–12] despite a 51.4% efficacy in a single-center retrospective series with 179 patients [13]. Endoscopic stenting has also been assessed in nonrandomized series with an efficacy reaching 75% clinical response in case series [14, 15]. Nevertheless, endoscopic stenting is associated with a high rate of stent migration [14, 15]. The surgical laparoscopic pyloroplasty suggested some efficacy reaching 60% of clinical response but remained a technically complicated and invasive procedure for a functional disease [16, 17]. More recently, the gastric electrical stimulation with surgical implantation was evaluated in randomized studies; however, the outcomes in terms of efficacy were low, mainly on symptoms of chronic vomiting [18–22].

Physiopathological pathways are complex, leading to the conclusion that mechanical management alone could not be sufficient [23]. Pathophysiology of gastroparesis combines dysfunction of smooth muscle, enteric and extrinsic autonomic nerves, and alterations of the interstitial cells of Cajal which are the pacemaker of the stomach wall [23]. Therefore at least, gastroparesis is related to a mechanical muscle anomaly and electric intrinsic disorder. Etiologies are mainly represented by

M. Barthet (✉) · J. M. Gonzalez
Department of Gastroenterology, Aix Marseille Université, APHM,
Service de Gastro-entérologie, Hôpital Nord, Marseille, France
e-mail: marc.barthet@ap-hm.fr

P. Sharma, N. Reddy (eds.), *Innovations in Gastrointestinal Endoscopy*,
https://doi.org/10.1007/978-981-15-9247-8_1

diabetes, postoperative issues, autoimmune disorder, and finally could be idiopathic in more than one-third of the case [24–26].

1.2 Gastroparesis Assessment and Grading: How to Assess?

Because clinical symptoms of gastroparesis are confused and nonspecific, the diagnosis of gastroparesis should require both clinical assessment using the GCSI score and quantification using gastric emptying scintigraphy (GES) [24–26].

The diagnosis of gastroparesis should be suspected in patients with nonspecific symptoms, widely reported in clinical practice. These symptoms include, according to a 0–5 scale, nausea, vomiting, retching, stomach fullness, being not to be able to finish a normal meal, excessive satiety, loss of appetite, bloating, and abdominal distension [27].

As these symptoms are nonspecific, it requires imaging or quantifiable measurement. GES could confirm the diagnosis of gastroparesis and should be performed to follow the patient after endoscopic procedure. Results of GES should include half gastric emptying time (mn) and residual % at 1, 2, 3, 4 h, and their normal values have been validated [28–31]. Another alternative could be the use of antroduodenal manometry which is still confidential or breath tests 13C-spirulina [23]. The sensitivity reaches 89% in two series with an 80% specificity rate [32]. The gastric emptying breath test agrees with GES in 73–97% of the time [23, 33].

However, until now in almost G-POEM series, the results of G-POEM are assessed by clinical evaluation (GCSI score) and functional imaging evaluation based upon GES [25, 26, 34–36].

1.3 Endoscopic Procedure: How to Do?

The technique gastric peroral endoscopic myotomy (G-POEM) was firstly proposed in 2014, looking to interesting results of laparoscopy and the lack of other options [16, 17, 37, 38]. It resulted from physiologic study conducted many years ago by Mearing et al. [39] who showed that gastric hypomotility was not exclusively involved in gastroparesis, but also an antro-pyloric hyper tonicity with a defect of gastric clearance. The G-POEM has been indeed firstly performed in the USA [37], and right after in Europe [38] with promising results. Since then, many series have been published [24–26, 34–36], reaching an acute efficacy around 80% (range 61–85%), which is the best outcome achieved for this disease to date. However, these preliminary results were provided with short-term follow-up less than 6 months.

Technically, G-POEM is based upon submucosal tunnelization as described by H. Inoue for endoscopic treatment of achalasia [40]. G-POEM is a submucosal pyloromyotomy (Figs. 1.1, 1.2, 1.3, 1.4, 1.5, 1.6, 1.7, and 1.8). The mucosal entrance is done at 5 cm from the pylorus, in a 5-o'clock position that allow to push the endoscope in a right direction toward the pylorus, alongside the greater curve of the

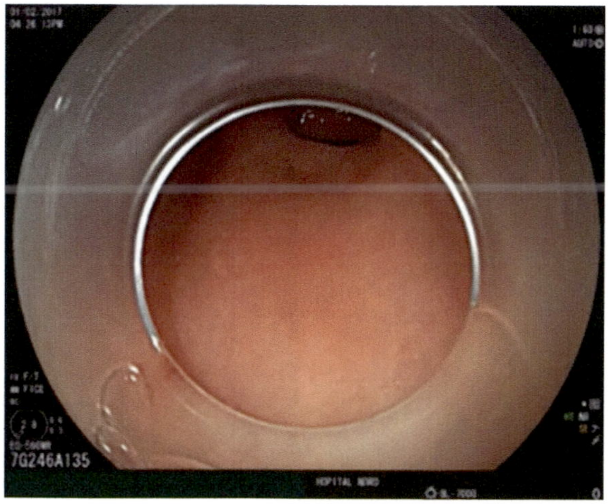

Fig. 1.1 Site of mucosal entrance (5 o'clock greater curve)

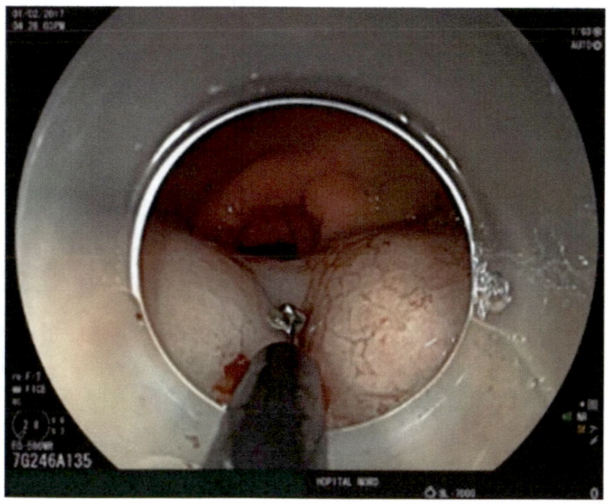

Fig. 1.2 Mucosal incision after submucosal lifting

stomach. During the tunnel progression, it is preferable to go regularly outside of the submucosal tunnel in order to check the adequate orientation of the tunnel. After careful submucosal dissection, the pyloric sphincter then appears as a white arch that should be precisely made free from surrounding structures avoiding mucosal injury before endoscopic section. Pyloric sphincter section should be performed within the whole thickness of the muscle and extended toward a 2 cm length antral myotomy. Then the mucosal entrance is closed using clipping method.

The procedure is feasible most of the time in less than 1 h (mean 48 mn in our monocenter studies including 26 patients), without serious per-procedural events, mostly bleeding that should be prevented by prophylactic coagulation of submucosal vessels [41]. Idiopathic cause is usually associated with submucosal intense fibrosis that could bother the creation of the tunnel [25]. The reproducibility is high

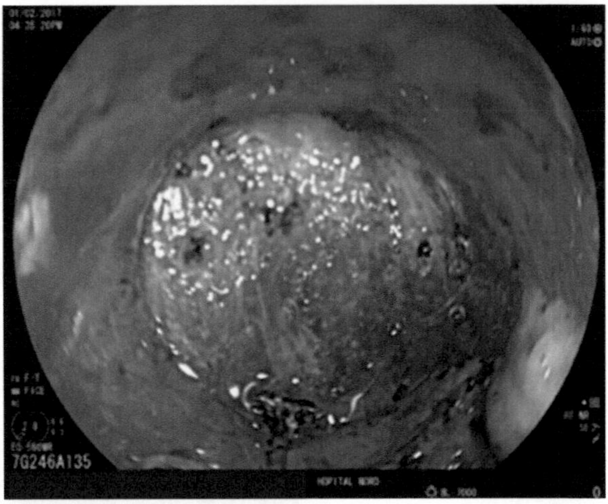

Fig. 1.3 Submucosal dissection

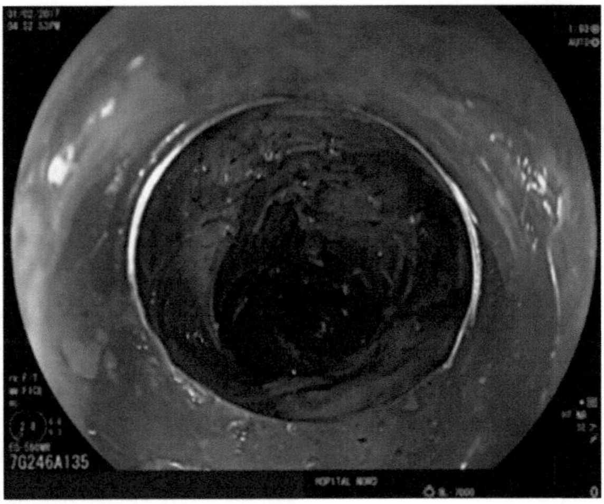

Fig. 1.4 Submucosal tunnel

since the operator achieve the specific aspect of pyloric arch when the pylorus is reached, as soon as the tunnel access is performed at 5 o'clock from the pylorus [25, 41].

1.4 Results of G-POEM

The pyloromyotomy according to the G-POEM technique is a new therapeutic approach that reinforces the concept of submucosal intra-mural endoscopy [40, 42]. It also provides a new way to treat patients with severe gastric motility disorders, which considerably affect their quality of life.

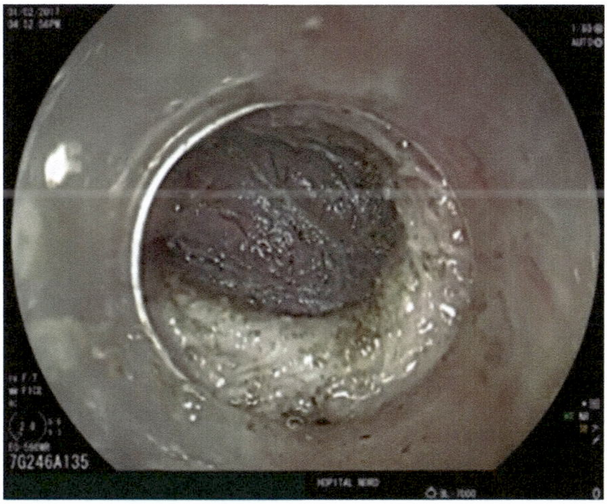

Fig. 1.5 Pyloric arch

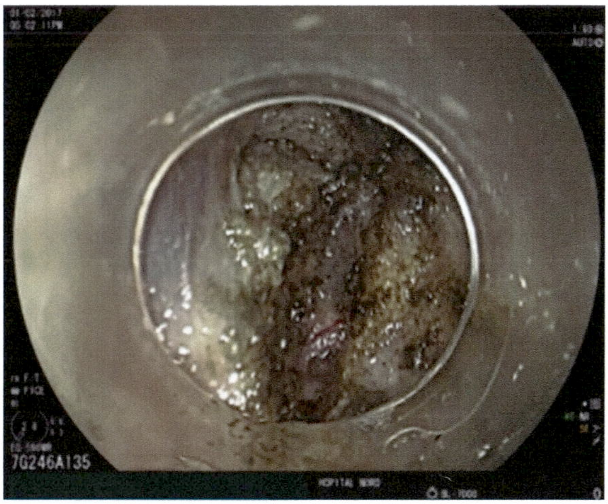

Fig. 1.6 Pyloromyotomy

When looking at the literature, there are seven series without overlap, reporting the results of G-POEM (Table 1.1). They included a total of 196 patients, 2 being prospective and 5 retrospective [24–26, 36, 43–45]. The mean procedural time in these series was 69 min ranging from 39 to 99 mn. Pooled analysis shows a constant technical success (100%), with a clinical success rate (based on the GCSI) reaching 82%. In all the series evaluating the GCSI score before and after the procedure, a statistically significant improvement was shown [24–26, 36, 43–45]. A significant GES improvement considering half gastric emptying time occurred in 72% of the cases [24–26, 34–36]. Mean time decreased from 222 to 143 mn in a recent multi-center study [26]. The average percentage of residues at 4 h decreased significantly in 5 series with a – 22.3% difference in mean values [24–26, 36, 45]. However, there were some limitations because most of them were retrospective studies, the

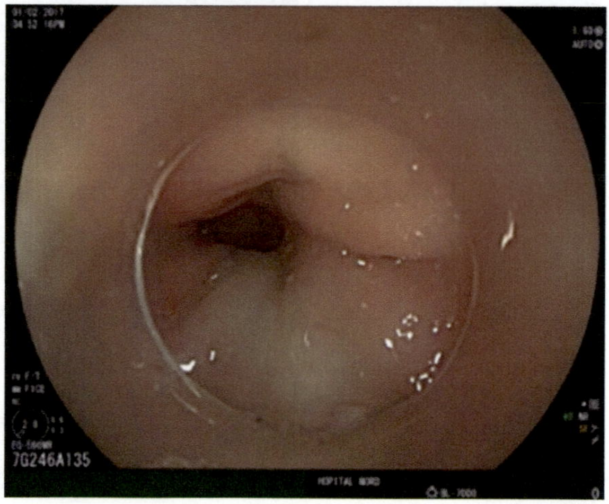

Fig. 1.7 Endoluminal view of the reopened pylorus with the blue submucosal visible under the mucosa

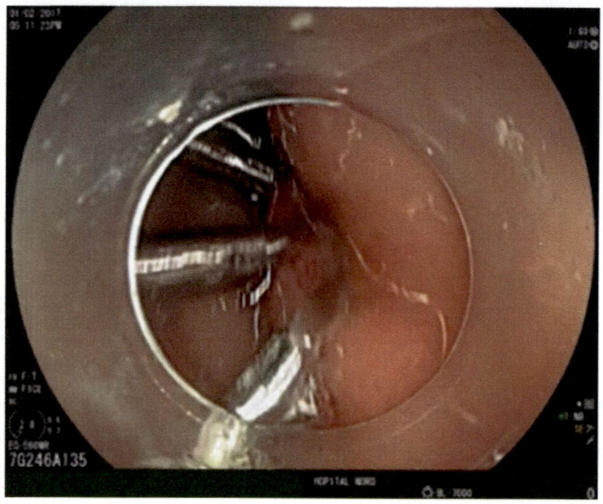

Fig. 1.8 Mucosal closure

follow-up remaining short in time (less than 6 months) and etiologies not always given. Therefore, both clinical assessment with GCSI score and scintigraphic evaluation with GES seem to be improved in short-term follow-up by G-POEM. Questions about the homogeneity of these results at 1-year follow-up need to be solved.

In a large monocenter study providing homogenous results with a median follow-up of 10.4 months, the clinical success rate was 79% at 3 months and 69% at 6 months, with a significant decreasing of the mean GCSI compared to preoperative (3.3 ± 0.9 vs. 1 ± 1.2 and 1.1 ± 0.9, respectively) [24]. The GES ($n = 23$) normalized in 70% of cases, with a significant improvement of the mean half emptying time and retention at 2 h, and discordance in 21% of the cases [24].

The most recent multicenter series reported results coming from USA, Venezuelan, and French centers including 33 patients with a 11.5-months follow-up

Table 1.1 Main series about G-POEM

	Number of patients	Etiology (diabetes/idiopathic/surgery)	Clinical efficacy	GES	Adverse events
Kashab et al. [25]	30	36%/23%/40%	86%	47%	6.6%
Gonzalez et al. [24]	29	34%/52%/17%	79%	75%	10.2%
Kahaleh et al. [26]	33	21%/36%/36%	85%	222–143 mn	6%
Rodriguez et al. [43]	47	25%/57%/17%	GCSI score decrease, 4.6–3.3	80%	0%
Mekaroonka et al. [44]	30	40%/40%/16%	80%	NA	3%
Malik et al. [45]	13	7%/30%/61%	73%	66%	7%
Xue et al. [36]	14	42%/42%/7%	61%	83%	0%

[26]. G-POEM was technically successful in all the cases with an 85% rate of clinical success. Mean GES improved significantly from 222.4 to 143.16 mn ($p < 0.001$). Two minor complications occurred (one bleeding and one ulceration). The mean procedure duration was 77.6 mn (37–255 mn).

1.5 Are Long-Term Results Yet Available?

Most of the series presented results with a short-term evaluation ranging between 3 and 6 months except two series with 10.4 and 11.5 months, respectively [24, 26]. In the former which is a monocenter study, the efficacy at 3 months was 79%, which is consistent with the remaining literature [24]. The mid-term efficacy at 6 months was 69%, showing a slight decrease despite it is still promising for the patients, especially in such disorder where no serious therapeutic alternatives is available. Only two patients out of 29 had a recurrence between 3 and 6 months, one suffering from severe diabetes with terminal renal insufficiency. Regarding the scintigraphic evaluation, the discordance rate was 21%; in all the cases but one, it was in favor of a clinical improvement despite not reaching a normal values GES. This could be explained by the sensitivity of this examination which is known not to be complete [28, 29], even if an abnormal result is correlated with the severity [30]. Interestingly, all the discordances were observed in case of idiopathic gastroparesis. In the Kahaleh's multicenter study, the results at 1 year showed an 85% significant clinical improvement with a significant decrease of GCSI score from 3.3 to 0.8 at 11.5 months [26].

1.6 Is There Any Predictive Factor for Efficacy?

Predictive factors for success or failure of the procedure seem to be mainly related on the etiologies. In the overview of the literature including 7 series with 196 patients (without overlap), the etiologies were idiopathic in 43% of the cases, 26% postoperative, and 28% related to diabetes (Table 1.1). In a large monocenter series with a 10.4-months follow-up, clinical response occurred in 92% for idiopathic, 80% for postoperative, and 57% for diabetes [24]. In this series, with univariate analysis, the female gender and the diabetes were significantly associated with failure, while in the meantime, the idiopathic and postoperative etiologies were predictive of success. The hypothesis concerning diabetes is that the motility disorder does not only affect the stomach, but is also extended to the small bowel, leading to worse outcomes. However, in multivariate analysis, these trends were not statistically confirmed, probably because of the insufficient sample in each group [24]. Interestingly, when looking at the literature focused on gastric electrical stimulation, it appears that the efficacy is significantly higher in patients with vomiting, and mainly in those with diabetes. Oppositely, the outcomes were disappointing, with around 70% failure, in idiopathic diseases [18, 19]. This could be a very promising field of study, in order to propose to the patients a personalized therapeutic approach depending on the etiology, and also the predominant symptoms. This could also open the door to a combined approach in order to increase the efficacy.

1.7 What Are the Expected Complications?

In the 7 series of the literature including 196 patients (Table 1.1), only 12 complications (6.1%) occurred [24–26, 36, 43–45]. Capnoperitoneum was the most frequent adverse event, easily managed with needle decompression and exsufflation. Peptic ulcer, bleeding, pulmonary embolism, abscess, and stricture were also reported. The complication rate in a large monocenter series with 29 patients included one case of bleeding and one case of abscess (6.9%) [24]. The complication rate in the most recent multicenter study including five different centers was 6% with one ulcer and one case of mild bleeding [26].

1.8 Future, Questions and Ongoing Development

Comparative studies and randomized series are required. One randomized series comparing G-POEM to intra-pyloric injection of botulin toxin is going on and results are waited. One recent retrospective study compared the results of laparoscopic pyloroplasty (LP) to G-POEM [46]. Patients undergoing LP had longer hospital stay, operative time, and increased blood loss. They had also more complications, whereas clinical improvement looking to GCSI score and gastric emptying were similar [46].

Questions about the procedural aspects include the length of the myotomy associated with the pylorotomy, the realization of multiradial incision of the pyloric sphincter. The technique of G-POEM is not yet standardized since it is a very recent endoscopic procedure, first cases being published in 2014 [37, 38].

As the results of G-POEM are not complete with a loss of efficacy with time, one could wonder about the association with gastric electric stimulation, i.e., gastric pacemaker. It seems that patients with failure of previous gastric pacemaker surgically implanted had better results than others [24]. It could be postulated that results in patients with diabetes could be improved by the association G-POEM–gastric pacemaker.

Finally, is there any medical treatment that could be an alternative or could be associated with G-POEM in order to achieve full efficacy? A randomized study has evaluated the results of relamoreline in the management of gastroparesis in diabetics with promising results [47]. Four of five symptoms of the GCSI score were significantly improved despite vomiting was not. Significant improvement of gastric emptying assessed by breath tests 13C-spirulina was also observed [47]. None is known about the role of relamoreline to select patients for G-POEM, to improve disappointing G-POEM results or to be associated with G-POEM for instance in patients with diabetes.

In conclusion, the G-POEM is safe and effective for treating refractory gastroparesis, with an acute and mid-term efficacy very promising. There is a trend to lower outcome for female gender and diabetes. Association with electric pacemaker stimulation could be a door for improving unsatisfactory results or in diabetes. It is now time for going ahead on prospective randomized studies to confirm these results, as well as largest sample for more accurate sub-group analyses.

References

1. Hasler WL. Gastroparesis: symptoms, evaluation, and treatment. Gastroenterol Clin N Am. 2007;36:619–47, ix
2. Parkman HP, Hasler WL, Fisher RS. American Gastroenterological Association technical review on the diagnosis and treatment of gastroparesis. Gastroenterology. 2004;127:1592–622.
3. Soykan I, Sivri B, Sarosiek I, et al. Demography, clinical characteristics, psychological and abuse profiles, treatment, and long-term follow-up of patients with gastroparesis. Dig Dis Sci. 1998;43:2398–404.
4. Rao AS, Camilleri M. Review article: metoclopramide and tardive dyskinesia. Aliment Pharmacol Ther. 2010;31:11–9.
5. Maganti K, Onyemere K, Jones MP. Oral erythromycin and symptomatic relief of gastroparesis: a systematic review. Am J Gastroenterol. 2003;98:259–63.
6. Dumitrascu DL, Weinbeck M. Domperidone versus metoclopramide in the treatment of diabetic gastroparesis. Am J Gastroenterol. 2000;95:316–7.
7. Arts J, Holvoet L, Caenepeel P, et al. Clinical trial: a randomized-controlled crossover study of intrapyloric injection of botulinum toxin in gastroparesis. Aliment Pharmacol Ther. 2007;26:1251–8.
8. Ezzeddine D, Jit R, Katz N, et al. Pyloric injection of botulinum toxin for treatment of diabetic gastroparesis. Gastrointest Endosc. 2002;55:920–3.

9. Bromer MQ, Friedenberg F, Miller LS, et al. Endoscopic pyloric injection of botulinum toxin A for the treatment of refractory gastroparesis. Gastrointest Endosc. 2005;61:833–9.
10. Miller LS, Szych GA, Kantor SB, et al. Treatment of idiopathic gastroparesis with injection of botulinum toxin into the pyloric sphincter muscle. Am J Gastroenterol. 2002;97:1653–60.
11. Friedenberg FK, Palit A, Parkman HP, et al. Botulinum toxin A for the treatment of delayed gastric emptying. Am J Gastroenterol. 2008;103:416–23.
12. Ukleja A, Tandon K, Shah K, et al. Endoscopic botox injections in therapy of refractory gastroparesis. World J Gastrointest Endosc. 2015;7:790–8.
13. Coleski R, Anderson MA, Hasler WL. Factors associated with symptom response to pyloric injection of botulinum toxin in a large series of gastroparesis patients. Dig Dis Sci. 2009;54:2634–42.
14. Clarke JO, Sharaiha RZ, Kord Valeshabad A, et al. Through-the-scope transpyloric stent placement improves symptoms and gastric emptying in patients with gastroparesis. Endoscopy. 2013;45(Suppl 2):E189–90.
15. Kashab MA, Besharati S, Ngamruengphong S, et al. Refractory gastroparesis can be successfully managed with endoscopic transpyloric stent placement and fixation. Gastrointest Endosc. 2015;82:1106–9.
16. Toro JP, Lytle NW, Patel AD, et al. Efficacy of laparoscopic pyloroplasty for the treatment of gastroparesis. J Am Coll Surg. 2014;218:652–60.
17. Hibbard ML, Dunst CM, Swanström LL. Laparoscopic and endoscopic pyloroplasty for gastroparesis results in sustained symptom improvement. J Gastrointest Surg. 2011;15:1513–9.
18. Abell T, McCallum R, Hocking M, et al. Gastric electrical stimulation for medically refractory gastroparesis. Gastroenterology. 2003;125:421–8.
19. van der Voort IR, Becker JC, Dietl KH, et al. Gastric electrical stimulation results in improved metabolic control in diabetic patients suffering from gastroparesis. Exp Clin Endocrinol Diabetes. 2005;113:38–42.
20. Levinthal DJ, Bielefeldt K. Systematic review and meta-analysis: gastric electrical stimulation for gastroparesis. Auton Neurosci. 2017;202:45–55.
21. Richmond B, Chong B, Modak A, et al. Gastric electrical stimulation for refractory gastroparesis: predictors of response and redefining a successful outcome. Am Surg. 2015;81:467–71.
22. Lal N, Livemore S, Dunne D, et al. Gastric electrical stimulation with the Enterra system: a systematic review. Gastroenterol Res Pract. 2015;2015:762972.
23. Camilleri M. Novel diet, drugs, and gastric interventions for gastroparesis. Clin Gastroenterol Hepatol. 2016;14:1072–80.
24. Gonzalez JM, Benezech A, Vitton V, et al. G-POEM with antro-pyloromyotomy for the treatment of refractory paresis: mid-term, follow-up and factors predicting outcome. Aliment Pharmacol Ther. 2017;46:364–70.
25. Kashab MA, Ngamruengphong S, Carr-Locke D, et al. Gastric per-oral endoscopic myotomy for refactory paresis: results from the first multicenter study on pyloric myotomy (with video). Gastrointest Endosc. 2017;85:123–8.
26. Kahaleh M, Gonzalez JM, Xu MM, et al. Gastric peroral endoscopic myotomy for the treatment of refractory gastroparesis: a multicenter international experience. Endoscopy. 2018;50(11):1053–8. Epub ahead of print
27. Revicki DA, Camilleri M, Kuo B, et al. Development and content validity of a gastroparesis cardinal symptom index daily diary. Aliment Pharmacol Ther. 2009;30(6):670–80.
28. Coleski R, Baker JR, Hasler WL. Endoscopic gastric food retention in relation to scintigraphic gastric emptying delays and clinical factors. Dig Dis Sci. 2016;61:2593–601.
29. Sachdeva P, Malhotra N, Pathikonda M, et al. Gastric emptying of solids and liquids for evaluation for gastroparesis. Dig Dis Sci. 2011;56:1138–46.
30. DiBaise JK, Patel N, Noelting J, et al. The relationship among gastroparetic symptoms, quality of life, and gastric emptying in patients referred for gastric emptying testing. Neurogastroenterol Motil. 2016;28:234–42.

31. Camilleri M, Iturrino J, Bharucha AE, et al. Performance characteristics of scintigraphic measurement of gastric emptying of solids in healthy participants. Neurogastroenterol Motil. 2012;24:1076–e562.
32. Szarka LA, Camilleri M. Methods for measurement of gastric motility. Am J Phys. 2009;296:G461–75.
33. Kuo B, Viazis N, Bahadur S. Non invasive simultaneous measurement of intra-liminal pH and pressure: assessment of gastric emptying and upper GI manometry in healthy subjects. Neurogastroenterol Motil. 2004;16:666.
34. Shlomovitz E, Pescarus R, Cassera MA, et al. Early human experience with per-oral endoscopic pyloromyotomy (POP). Surg Endosc. 2015;29:543–51.
35. Dacha S, Mekaroonkamol P, Li L, et al. Oucomes and quality-of-life assessment after gastric per-oral endscopic pyloromyotomy (with video). Gastrointest Endosc. 2017;86:282–9.
36. Xue H, Fan H, Meng X, et al. Fluoroscopy-guided gastric per-oral endoscopic pyloromyotomy (G-POEM): a more reliable and efficient method for treatment of refractory gastroparesis. Surg Endosc. 2017;31:4617–24.
37. Khashab MA, Stein E, Clarke JO, et al. Gastric peroral endoscopic myotomy for refractory gastroparesis: first human endoscopic pyloromyotomy (with video). Gastrointest Endosc. 2013;78:764–8.
38. Gonzalez J-M, Vanbiervliet G, Vitton V, et al. First European human gastric peroral endoscopic myotomy, for treatment of refractory gastroparesis. Endoscopy. 2015;47(Suppl 1):E135–6.
39. Mearin F, Camilleri M, Malagelada JR. Pyloric dysfunction in diabetics with recurrent nausea and vomiting. Gastroenterology. 1986;90:1919–25.
40. Inoue H, Minami H, Kobayashi Y, et al. Peroral endoscopic myotomy (POEM) for esophageal achalasia. Endoscopy. 2010;42:265–71.
41. Gonzalez JM, Lestelle V, Benezech A, et al. Gastric per-oral endoscopic myotomy with antro-pylormyotomy in the treatment of refractory gastroparesis: clinical experience with follow-up and scintigraphic evaluation (with video). Gastrointest Endosc. 2017;85:123–8.
42. Wang X-Y, Xu M-D, Yao L-Q, et al. Submucosal tunneling endoscopic resection for submucosal tumors of the esophagogastric junction originating from the muscularis propria layer: a feasibility study (with videos). Surg Endosc. 2014;28:1971–7.
43. Rodriguez JH, Haskins IN, Strong AT, et al. Per oral endoscopic pyloromyotomy for refractory gastroparesis: initial results from a single institution. Surg Endosc. 2017;31:5381–8.
44. Mekaroonkamol P, Dacha S, Wang L, et al. Gastric peroral endoscopic pylormyotomy reduces symptoms, increases quality-of-life, and reduces health care usage for patients with gastroparesis. Clin Gastroenterol Hepatol. 2018;17(1):82–9.
45. Malik Z, Kataria R, Modayil R, et al. Gastric per-oral endoscopic myotomy (G POEM) for the treatment of refractory gastroparesis: early experience. Dig Dis Sci. 2018;63(9):2405–12.
46. Landreneau JP, Strong AT, El-Hayek K, et al. Laparoscopic pyloroplasty versus endoscopic per-oral pyloromyotomy for the treatment of gastroparesis. Surg Endosc. 2019;33(3):773–81. Epub ahead of print
47. Camilleri M, McCallum RW, Tack J, et al. Efficacy and safety of relamorelin in diabetics with symptoms of gastroparesis: a randomized, placebo-controlled study. Gastroenterology. 2017;153:1240–50.

2 EUS-Guided Gastroenterostomy

Takao Itoi

2.1 Emerging Endoscopic Ultrasonography-Guided Gastroenterostomy

Endoscopic ultrasonography (EUS)-guided gastroenterostomy (EUS-GE) [1–3] (Fig. 2.1) emerged as an alternative treatment for malignant gastric outlet obstruction (MGOO), which has been traditionally treated by surgical or endoscopic metal stenting [4, 5]. EUS-GE is a novel technique that is minimally invasive and has a long patency with less re-intervention than current techniques.

EUS-GE was first proposed by Fritscher-Ravens et al., who tested the technique in animal models and cadavers [6, 7]. However, as the technique was complicated owing to the use of special devices (button type) and the need for endoscope exchange, it was not clinically adopted. In 2012, Binmoeller and Shah described successful EUS-GE in an animal model using a lumen-apposing metal stent (LAMS) that can attach the gastric and enteric walls and was shown to be an ideal device for EUS-GE [8]. Since LAMSs allow adhesion between two organs like a surgical anastomosis, the clinical application of EUS-GE became reality.

2.2 Technical Indication of EUS-GE [9]

There are some indications and contraindications of EUS-GE. One such indication is that the targeted site within the duodenum or jejunum is adjacent to the stomach. Preprocedural CT and MRI should be used to select the puncture site; the coronal view is often the most helpful. The anastomotic site is usually the body of the stomach; therefore, in patients with gastric or pancreatic cancer, care should be taken in case of tumor invasion into the gastric wall. Similarly, if the tumor extends into the

T. Itoi (✉)
Department of Gastroenterology and Hepatology, Tokyo Medical University, Tokyo, Japan
e-mail: itoi@tokyo-med.ac.jp

P. Sharma, N. Reddy (eds.), *Innovations in Gastrointestinal Endoscopy*,
https://doi.org/10.1007/978-981-15-9247-8_2

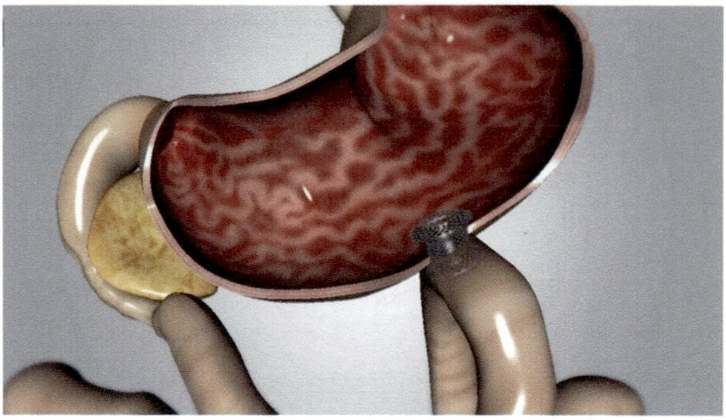

Fig. 2.1 Endoscopic ultrasonography (EUS)-guided gastroenterostomy

body of the stomach, the fourth portion of the duodenum, or the proximal jejunum around the ligament of Treitz, EUS-GE may be contraindicated. Although EUS-GE may be possible if there is a small volume of ascites, it should be avoided if there is a large volume of ascites because of the poor fixation of the jejunum owing to small bowel floating phenomenon. Patients with MGOO usually have a large amount of gastric residue, which may preclude successful EUS-GE and cause serious adverse events. Therefore, refraining from food or adhering to a low-residue diet until the scheduled EUS-GE may be ideal. However, if there is gastric residue, the residue should be removed before performing EUS-GE using a snare catheter, basket catheter, or net catheter.

2.3 History of Lumen-Apposing Metal Stents

In 2011, Binmoeller and Shah [10] introduced a LAMS (AXIOS™ stent, Xlumena, CA, USA) that can attach two organs under EUS guidance, as in surgical anastomosis. This LAMS consists of a fully covered metal stent with bilateral anchor flanges. Fully expanded, the anchor flange diameter is twice that of the "saddle" section. The stent anchors distribute pressure evenly on the luminal wall and securely anchor the stent, which prevents migration. The proximal and distal anchor flanges also securely hold the wall of targeted cavity to the gastric wall, which serves to prevent detachment. Therefore, this novel LAMS can be used for interventional EUS, cystogastrostomy, gallbladder drainage, biliary drainage, and even gastrojejunostomy. EUS-GE, which can lead to failed EUS-GE with adverse events.

The AXIOS-EC™ stent, often referred to as "Hot AXIOS," was developed later (Fig. 2.2) and includes an electrocautery-enhanced delivery system. This system allows placement of the stent without needle puncture or guidewire placement, which decreases the likelihood of missing the target during interventional EUS.

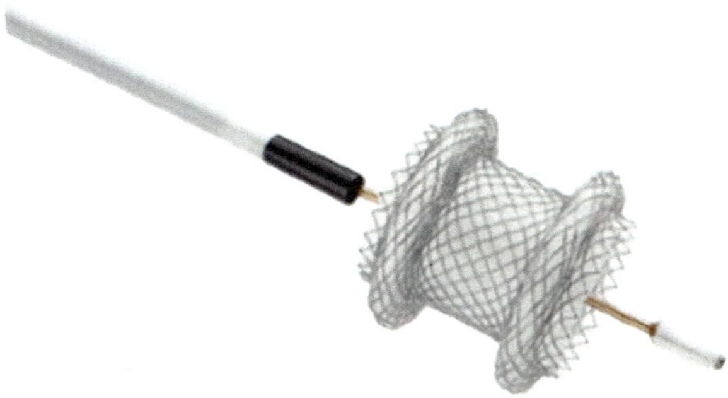

Fig. 2.2 Electrocautery-enhanced delivery system (AXIOS-EC™ stent)

2.4 EUS-GE Techniques [1–3, 9]

Recently, several investigators have developed unique and novel techniques in combination with LAMSs for EUS-GE, namely direct EUS-GE, assisted EUS-GE, and EUS-guided balloon-occluded gastrojejunostomy bypass (EPASS).

2.4.1 Direct EUS-GE Technique

The direct EUS-GE technique entails the direct puncture of a small bowel loop adjacent to the stomach using a 22-guage needle, after which the duodenum and jejunum are distended by saline injection. After transgastric puncture using a 19-gauge fine-needle aspiration (FNA) needle, enterography is performed, and a wire is passed through the needle into the small bowel. The GE tract is dilated over the wire, and the LAMS is placed. The GE tract dilation diameter is gauged to ensure the anastomotic LAMS delivery system can be introduced. Overly aggressive dilation should be avoided as it can lead to luminal leakage during the exchange and prior to stent deployment.

2.4.2 Assisted EUS-GE Technique

The assisted EUS-GE technique uses insertion of a retrieval/dilating balloon, nasobiliary drain, or ultraslim endoscope around the duodenal-jejunal flexure. Of these, retrieval/dilating balloon-assisted EUS-GE is the preferred technique [1, 2]. Balloon-assisted EUS-GE involves the transoral passage of a balloon catheter over a wire placed into the small bowel. The balloon is filled with fluid (contrast fluid or water) while in the duodenum or jejunum. The fluid-filled balloon is localized transgastrically by EUS after the echoendoscope is passed alongside the balloon. The balloon is then punctured with a 19-gauge FNA needle, which serves to indicate the correct positioning of the needle tip within the small bowel lumen. A guidewire is advanced through the FNA needle, and the LAMS is placed. Intravenous glucagon is administered as needed to decrease small bowel peristalsis. When nasobiliary drains are placed, contrast material is injected into the duodenum and jejunum to distend and identify the duodenal or jejunal loop both endosonographically and fluoroscopically.

In ultraslim endoscope-assisted EUS-GE, a small caliber endoscope is passed perorally or through an existing gastrostomy site into the stomach and then beyond the stricture. Saline is injected through the ultraslim scope to distend the bowel lumen. The echoendoscope is then advanced into the stomach, alongside the ultraslim endoscope if the ultraslim scope was introduced perorally. A guidewire is then advanced through the needle and coiled within the bowel lumen. If possible, forceps introduced through the ultraslim scope are used to grasp the guidewire for traction as an internal rendezvous technique. A fistulous tract is created, and the LAMS is deployed.

2.4.3 **EPASS** (Figs. 2.3 and 2.4)

EPASS was first described in our animal study [11]. A special double-balloon enteric tube (Tokyo Medical University type, Create Medic Co., Ltd., Yokohama, Japan) is used for this procedure. This type of balloon allows for saline to be delivered directly in the drainage lumen of the enteric tube between the two inflated balloons.

A standard upper GI endoscope is advanced into the third portion of the duodenum. A guidewire is then advanced as far as possible beyond the duodenum and jejunum loop, and the endoscope is removed, leaving the guidewire in place. An overtube can be used to facilitate passage of the preinflated balloon catheter to avoid

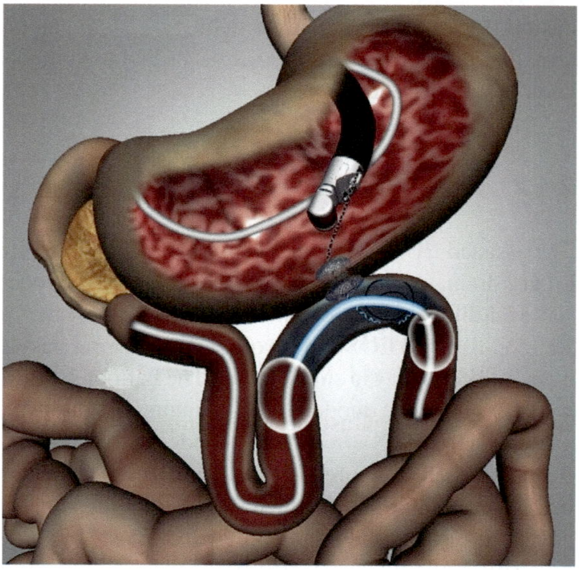

Fig. 2.3 Schema of endoscopic ultrasonography-guided balloon-occluded gastrojejunostomy bypass (EPASS) procedure

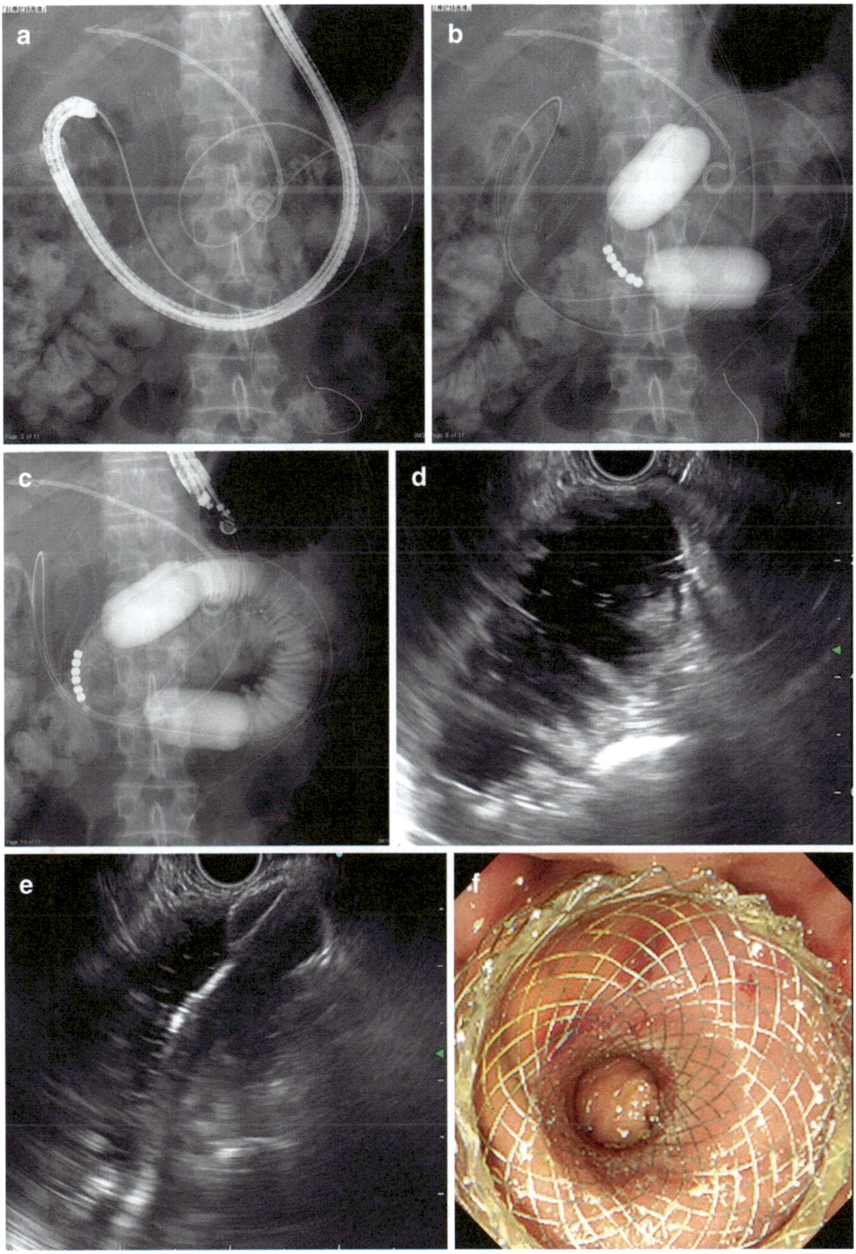

Fig. 2.4 Endoscopic ultrasonography (EUS)-guided balloon-occluded gastrojejunostomy bypass (EPASS) procedure. (**a**) First, a guidewire is inserted with a catheter under a standard upper GI endoscope. (**b**) A double-balloon catheter is advanced across the stomach over the wire and the balloons are inflated. (**c**) Saline with contrast agent is injected into the jejunum between the two balloons. Then, the EUS endoscope is advanced into the stomach. (**d**) EUS depicts the distended jejunum, and a cautery-enhanced lumen-apposing metal stent is advanced into the jejunum. (**e**) The distal flange is deployed under EUS guidance and pulled back toward the gastric wall as an anchor. (**f**) Finally, the proximal flange is deployed under endoscopic guidance. (**g**) Post-procedural computed tomography scan showing a well-placed stent connecting the stomach and the jejunum

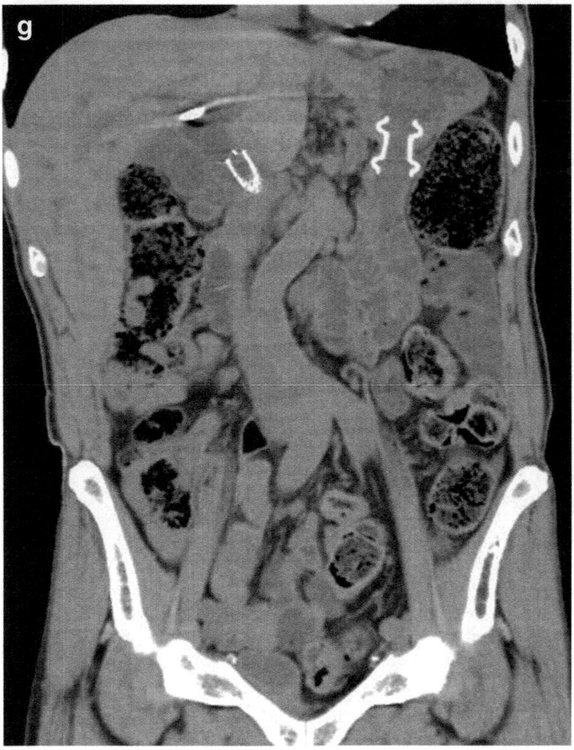

Fig. 2.4 (continued)

looping in the fornix of the stomach as it passes through the pyloric-duodenal stenosis. A double-balloon tube is inserted perorally over the guidewire in combination with a 0.89-inch dedicated guidewire for better torquability, and two balloons are placed in the duodenum and jejunum in an area adjacent to the stomach. Both balloons are filled with saline and contrast material, which holds the small intestine open. A sufficient amount of saline with contrast material is then introduced into the space between the two balloons to distend the small bowel lumen. An echoendoscope is advanced into the stomach to identify the distended duodenum or jejunum.

There are two EPASS procedures, namely the one-step procedure (freestyle technique) and the two-step procedure (standard technique). The freestyle technique is performed using direct electrocautery-enhanced tip delivery system insertion without needle puncture, whereas the standard technique involves a more standard procedure. For the standard technique, a 19-gauge FNA needle is used to puncture the duodenum or jejunum under EUS guidance. A guidewire is then inserted through the needle. When the AXIOS™ stent is used for EPASS, the needle is removed, and the gastrojejunostomy tract is dilated over the wire using a 6-Fr electrocautery dilator and a 6-mm dilating balloon. The delivery system is advanced over the guidewire into the duodenum or jejunum. When the AXIOS-EC™ stent is used, the delivery system is directly advanced over the guidewire into the duodenum or jejunum while applying current (usually Autocut mode, 100 W, Effect 4). For the freestyle technique, an electrocautery-enhanced tip delivery system using the

AXIOS-EC™ stent is directly advanced into the distended duodenum or jejunum while applying current. The stent is deployed across the GE tract under combined EUS, fluoroscopic, and endoscopic guidance. Finally, the deployed stent lumen is dilated to 10 mm with a dilating balloon.

2.5 Outcomes of EUS-GE for MGOO

Three relatively large (10 or more cases) case series of EUS-GE have shown a technical success rate of approximately 90%, regardless of the technique used [1–3], although two were retrospective studies [1, 2]. In these studies, a retrieval or dilating balloon was frequently used during assisted EUS-GE to help puncture the duodenum and jejunum. Among patients who received EPASS, the success rate of the one-step procedure was higher than that of the two-step procedure (100% vs 82%). Interestingly, almost all cases in which the stent was successfully placed showed clinical success within 25 min. Although no patients died, several developed adverse events, but none were serious. One failed case of balloon-assisted EUS-GE was converted to laparoscopic gastrojejunostomy. In two failed cases of EPASS, clinical improvement was achieved with conservative treatment. Interestingly, a recent large case series including benign GOO [12] had technical success in 94.2% of cases involving direct EUS-GE and 90.9% of cases involving balloon-assisted EUS-GE. The mean procedure time was shorter with the direct technique (35.7 ± 32.1 min vs 89.9 ± 33.3 min), and EPASS had the shortest mean procedure time (25.5 min) [3]. The clinical success rate was 92.3% for the direct technique and 90.9% for EPASS.

A recent comparative study between EUS-GE and endoscopic enteral stenting showed that EUS-GE may be ideal for MGOO, with comparable effectiveness and safety to endoscopic enteral stenting while being associated with lower symptom recurrence and reintervention [13]. Another comparative study [14] between EUS-GE and surgical GE showed that although the technical success rate was significantly higher in the SGJ group than in the EUS-GE group (100% vs. 87%), the clinical success rate was not different (90% vs. 87%). The rate of adverse events was lower in the EUS-GE group, but the difference was not statistically significant (16% vs. 25%). The mean time to reintervention was also similar (88 days vs. 121 days). An international study [15] comparing EUS-GE and laparoscopic GE (Lap-GE) revealed that technical success was achieved in 29 (100%) Lap-GE group patients and 23 (88%) EUS-GJ group patients. However, adverse events occurred in 41% ($n = 12$) of patients in the Lap-GE group and 12% ($n = 3$) of patients in the EUS-GE group.

If there are skilled endosonographers, three procedures, other than EUS-GE, are available for GOO treatment: endoscopic enteral stenting, open surgical GJ, and laparoscopic GJ. Although there are no highly evidenced comparative data, EUS-GE may be superior to endoscopic enteral stenting in terms of prolonged stent patency because of the shorter stent length (1 cm) and the fully covered metal stent, even though the anastomotic site is limited. Conversely, Lap-GE appears to be inferior to EUS-GE in terms of procedure time and invasiveness (pain score, etc.), and length of hospital stay. EUS-GE may be particularly unsuitable for patients with end-stage malignancies.

2.6 Future Clinical Application of EUS-GE

In general, the frequency of GOO in patients with benign diseases, e.g., acute pancreatitis, chronic pancreatitis, and duodenal ulcer, is extremely low. EUS-GE can be an option for the temporary treatment of GOO before the patient undergoes irreversible surgical intervention or unremovable duodenal stenting. A retrospective study of EUS-GE for benign diseases described that technical and clinical success were achieved in 96.2% and 84% of patients, respectively. Surprisingly, the rate of unplanned re-intervention was 4.8% [16].

Another clinical application is the treatment of afferent loop syndrome, which is mostly caused by recurrent stricture of primary cancer and leads to cholangitis and/or pancreatitis. Several case reports have reported on EUS-GE using LAMSs [17, 18] (Fig. 2.5). Theoretically, EUS-GE is reasonable for the treatment of afferent loop syndrome because of the so-called short cut technique between the stomach and the distended afferent loop.

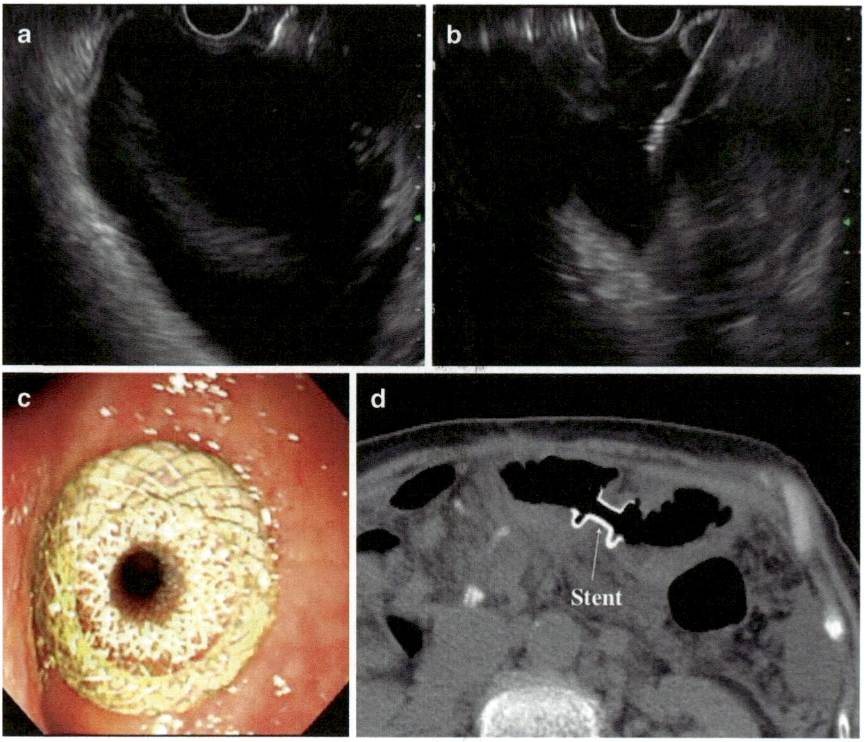

Fig. 2.5 Endoscopic ultrasonography-guided gastroenterostomy (EUS-GE) for afferent loop syndrome. (**a**) EUS is used to show the distended afferent loop, such as a pseudocyst. A cautery-enhanced lumen-apposing metal stent is advanced into the distended jejunum. (**b**) The distal flange is deployed under EUS guidance and pulled back toward the gastric wall as an anchor. (**c**) Finally, the proximal flange is deployed under endoscopic guidance. (**d**) Post-procedural computed tomography scan showing a well-placed stent connecting the stomach and the jejunum

References

1. Khashab MA, Kumbhari V, Grimm IS, Ngamruengphong S, Aguila G, El Zein M, et al. EUS-guided gastroenterostomy: the first U.S. clinical experience (with video). Gastrointest Endosc. 2015;82:932–8.
2. Tyberg A, Perez-Miranda M, Sanchez-Ocaña R, Peñas I, de la Serna C, Shah J, et al. Endoscopic ultrasound-guided gastrojejunostomy with a lumen-apposing metal stent: a multicenter, international experience. Endosc Int Open. 2016;4:E276–81.
3. Itoi T, Ishii K, Ikeuchi N, Sofuni A, Gotoda T, Moriyasu F, et al. Prospective evaluation of endoscopic ultrasonography-guided double-balloon-occluded gastrojejunostomy bypass (EPASS) for malignant gastric outlet obstruction. Gut. 2016;65:193–5.
4. Jeurnink SM, Steyerberg EW, van Hooft JE, van Eijck CH, Schwartz MP, Vleggaar FP, et al. Surgical gastrojejunostomy or endoscopic stent placement for the palliation of malignant gastric outlet obstruction (SUSTENT study): a multicenter randomized trial. Gastrointest Endosc. 2010;71:490–9.
5. Upchurch E, Ragusa M, Cirocchi R. Stent placement versus surgical palliation for adults with malignant gastric outlet obstruction. Cochrane Database Syst Rev. 2018;5:CD012506.
6. Fritscher-Ravens A, Mosse CA, Mills TN, Mukherjee D, Park PO, Swain P. A through-the-scope device for suturing and tissue approximation under EUS control. Gastrointest Endosc. 2002;56:737–42.
7. Fritscher-Ravens A, Mosse CA, Mukherjee D, Mills T, Park PO, Swain CP. Transluminal endosurgery: single lumen access anastomotic device for flexible endoscopy. Gastrointest Endosc. 2003;58:585–91.
8. Binmoeller KF, Shah JN. Endoscopic ultrasound-guided gastroenterostomy using novel tools designed for transluminal therapy: a porcine study. Endoscopy. 2012;44:499–503.
9. Itoi T, Baron TH, Khashab MA, Tsuchiya T, Irani S, Dhir V, et al. Technical review of endoscopic ultrasonography-guided gastroenterostomy in 2017. Dig Endosc. 2017;29:495–502.
10. Binmoeller KF, Shah J. A novel lumen-apposing stent for transluminal drainage of nonadherent extraintestinal fluid collections. Endoscopy. 2011;43:337–42.
11. Itoi T, Itokawa F, Uraoka T, Gotoda T, Horii J, Goto O, et al. Novel EUS-guided gastrojejunostomy technique using a new double-balloon enteric tube and lumen-apposing metal stent (with videos). Gastrointest Endosc. 2013;78:934–9.
12. Chen YI, Kunda R, Storm AC, Aridi HD, Thompson CC, Nieto J, et al. EUS-guided gastroenterostomy: a multicenter study comparing the direct and balloon-assisted techniques. Gastrointest Endosc. 2018;87:1215–21.
13. Chen YI, Itoi T, Baron TH, Nieto J, Haito-Chavez Y, Grimm IS, et al. EUS-guided gastroenterostomy is comparable to enteral stenting with fewer re-interventions in malignant gastric outlet obstruction. Surg Endosc. 2017;31:2946–52.
14. Khashab MA, Bukhari M, Baron TH, Nieto J, El Zein M, Chen YI, et al. International multicenter comparative trial of endoscopic ultrasonography-guided gastroenterostomy versus surgical gastrojejunostomy for the treatment of malignant gastric outlet obstruction. Endosc Int Open. 2017;5:E275–81.
15. Perez-Miranda M, Tyberg A, Poletto D, Toscano E, Gaidhane M, Desai AP, et al. EUS-guided gastrojejunostomy versus laparoscopic gastrojejunostomy: an international collaborative study. J Clin Gastroenterol. 2017;51:896–9.
16. Chen YI, James TW, Agarwal A, Baron TH, Itoi T, Kunda R, et al. EUS-guided gastroenterostomy in management of benign gastric outlet obstruction. Endosc Int Open. 2018;6:E363–8.
17. Ikeuchi N, Itoi T, Tsuchiya T, Nagakawa Y, Tsuchida A. One-step EUS-guided gastrojejunostomy with use of lumen-apposing metal stent for afferent loop syndrome treatment. Gastrointest Endosc. 2015;82:166.
18. Yamamoto K, Tsuchiya T, Tanaka R, Mitsuyoshi H, Mukai S, Nagakawa Y, et al. Afferent loop syndrome treated by endoscopic ultrasound-guided gastrojejunostomy, using a lumen-apposing metal stent with an electrocautery-enhanced delivery system. Endoscopy. 2017;49:E270–2.

The Pocket-Creation Method of Endoscopic Submucosal Dissection

3

Hironori Yamamoto, Yoshikazu Hayashi, Satoshi Shinozaki, and Alan Kawarai Lefor

3.1 Introduction

Achieving a cure is the most important consideration when treating neoplastic lesions. In order to reach this goal, both complete local excision of the tumor and complete control of metastases are required. Inability to control metastatic disease is a clear limitation of endoscopic treatment. Therefore, accurate assessment of the risk of lymph-node metastases is required when we consider expanding the indications for endoscopic resection of gastrointestinal (GI) tumors. Intramucosal GI tumors do not have any risk of lymph-node metastases. However, invasive cancers need consideration of lymph-node resection according to the risk of metastases. The risk of lymph-node metastases of submucosally invasive cancers can be reliably estimated by examining risk factors such as the depth of submucosal invasion, presence of lymphovascular invasion and histopathological type based on examination of a high-quality pathological specimen obtained by endoscopic resection. *En bloc* resection, negative margins, and a thick submucosa with minimum thermal damage are important factors when evaluating the quality of the resected specimen needed to make an accurate histopathological evaluation. Since most of the factors associated with an increased risk of lymph-node metastases are dependent on examination of the submucosal layer of the specimen (Fig. 3.1 (1)) [1, 2], a superficial tumor

H. Yamamoto (✉) · Y. Hayashi
Division of Gastroenterology, Department of Medicine, Jichi Medical University, Shimotsuke, Japan
e-mail: ireef@jichi.ac.jp

S. Shinozaki
Division of Gastroenterology, Department of Medicine, Jichi Medical University, Shimotsuke, Japan

Shinozaki Medical Clinic, Utsunomiya, Japan

A. K. Lefor
Department of Surgery, Jichi Medical University, Shimotsuke, Japan

P. Sharma, N. Reddy (eds.), *Innovations in Gastrointestinal Endoscopy*,
https://doi.org/10.1007/978-981-15-9247-8_3

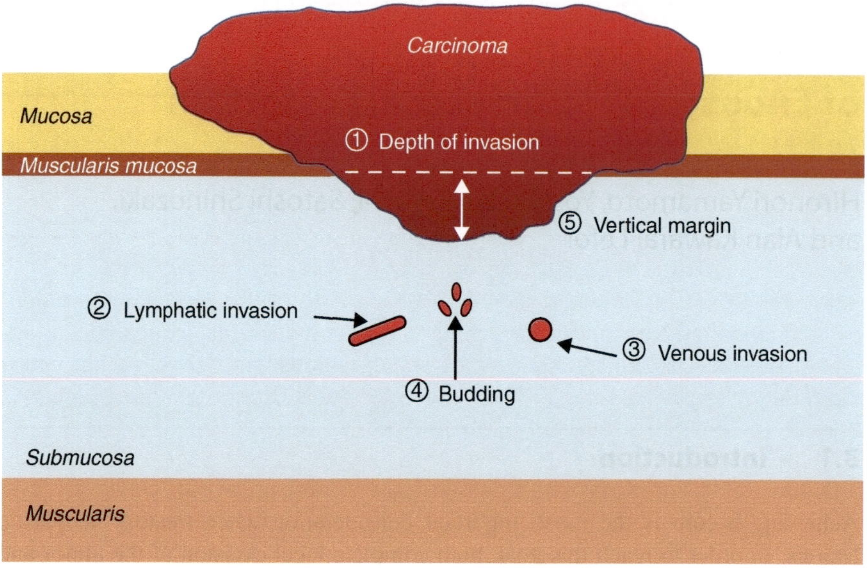

Fig. 3.1 Pathologic features in the submucosa that relate to the need for intestinal resection with lymph-node dissection: (1) Depth of invasion is 1000 μm or more; (2) Lymphatic invasion; (3) Venous invasion; (4) Budding grade is grade 2 or 3; and (5) Positive vertical margin. When at least one of the factors of (1)–(4) is positive regardless of a negative vertical margin, intestinal resection with lymph-node dissection is considered. When the vertical margin is positive, a salvage surgical resection is recommended

with a suspicion of submucosal invasive cancer must be resected *en bloc* with a thick submucosal layer to provide a high-quality pathological specimen. Ideally, even intramucosal tumors would be resected in an *en bloc* fashion with negative margins to avoid local recurrence after piecemeal resection [3].

It is technically difficult to resect a large superficial tumor with the conventional endoscopic mucosal resection (EMR) technique using a snare to obtain an *en bloc* specimen with negative margins when the tumor is greater than 2 cm in diameter or is accompanied by severe submucosal fibrosis even if the tumor is intramucosal. A considerable number of large superficial tumors or lesions in difficult locations are surgically resected even if they can be cured by complete local resection. However, endoscopic submucosal dissection (ESD), which is a more sophisticated technique than EMR, is now available to overcome the limitations of snare resection techniques and achieves an *en bloc* resection regardless of tumor size, shape, location [3, 4], or degree of submucosal fibrosis [5]. The use of ESD is more widespread in recent years because of an increased desire for less invasive curative treatment of superficial gastrointestinal tumors. However, it is believed by many that ESD is much more technically demanding than EMR and requires intensive training and experience to gain sufficient facility. We have established the pocket-creation method (PCM) as a strategical ESD method to obtain high-quality pathological specimens and secure safe and reliable ESD [5–9]. If you perform ESD using the

PCM, you can realize that ESD can be performed without significant difficulty in many cases. We strongly recommend the PCM for trainee endoscopists who want to develop skills in ESD from this point in time, as their standard ESD strategy.

3.2 Advantages of the Pocket-Creation Method

Although the PCM was developed to overcome difficulties associated with ESD for large sessile tumors, the PCM has many advantages in routinely performed ESD as well (Fig. 3.2) [10]. The PCM facilitates ESD by maintaining mucosal elevation, providing good traction and visualization in the submucosal layer, enabling a tangential approach in difficult circumstances and stabilization of the tip of the endoscope in the pocket regardless of motion due to normal cardio-pulmonary activity.

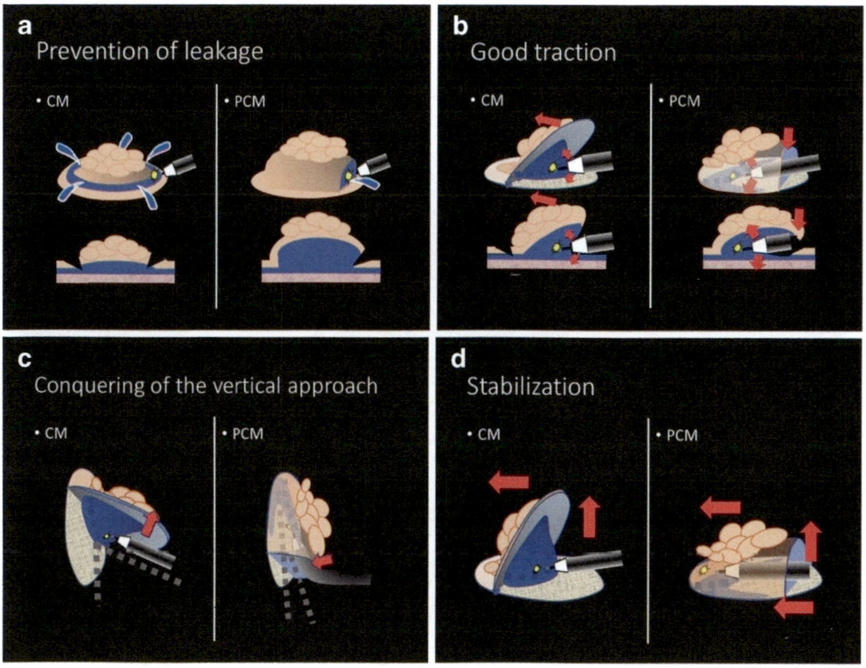

Fig. 3.2 Advantages of the pocket-creation method (PCM) compared with the conventional method (CM): (**a**) The PCM prevents leakage of the submucosal injection solution, which results in a prolonged thick submucosa; (**b**) The tip of the ST hood provides traction and countertraction stretching the submucosal tissue in the submucosal pocket; (**c**) The PCM changes the approach angle to the muscularis from a vertical approach to a tangential approach; and (**d**) The PCM stabilizes the endoscope tip by synchronizing the endoscope in the pocket to fluctuation of heartbeats and respiratory movements

3.3 Devices Suitable for the Pocket-Creation Method

A small-caliber-tip transparent (ST) hood (DH-33GR [11] or DH-34CR, Fujifilm, Tokyo, Japan) (Fig. 3.3) or a short-type ST hood (DH-28GR, DH-29CR, DH-30CR, Fujifilm) is suitable for the PCM. A lens cleaner such as Cleash® (Fujifilm) is applied to the surface of the endoscope lens, both inside and outside of the hood with the tip of a cotton swab to assure that the lens is clean just before the procedure. A 0.4% sodium hyaluronate solution (MucoUp®, Boston Scientific, Marlborough, MA) with 0.001% epinephrine and 0.002–0.004% indigocarmine is used for injection. A needle-type knife such as the Flushknife BT-S (Fujifilm) or Dualknife (Olympus, Tokyo, Japan) is used as the electric knife. The Flushknife BT-S is 2.5 mm or 1.5 mm long for stomach or colorectum, respectively. The Dualknife is 2.0 mm or 1.5 mm long for stomach or colorectum, respectively. The VIO-300D (ERBE Elektromedizin Ltd., Tübingen, Germany) is usually used as an electrosurgical generator in our hospital. The mucosal incision and submucosal dissection are performed using Endo cut I with effect 1, duration 4 and interval 1 mode and Swift coag with effect 4 and maximum 25–30 watts, respectively. Hot hemostasis forceps (HOYA Corporation, Tokyo, Japan) are used to control bleeding using Soft coag with effect 4 and 80 watts on the VIO-300D. An endoscope with an approximately 10 mm tip diameter is good for the ST hood (DH-33GR) and a water-irrigation channel such as EG-L580RD (Fujifilm), GIF-Q260J (Olympus) as a gastroscope,

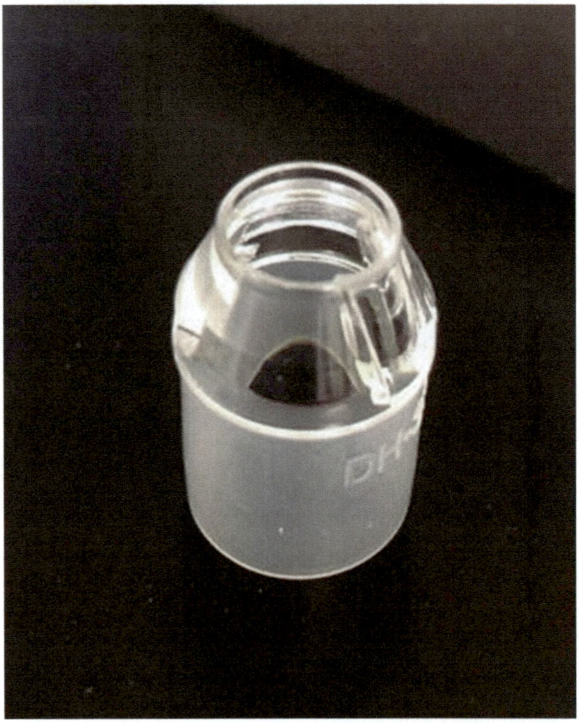

Fig. 3.3 A small-caliber-tip transparent (ST) hood (DH-33GR, Fujifilm, Tokyo, Japan) is suitable for the pocket-creation method of endoscopic submucosal dissection

EC-580RD (Fujifilm), EC-L600MP7 (Fujifilm), PCF-Q260J (Olympus), PCF-H290TI (Olympus) as a colonoscope or EI-580BT (Fujifilm) as a double-balloon endoscope (DBE) is suitable for the PCM. The DBE needs a BioShield irrigator® (US Endoscopy, Mentor, OH) because the DBE does not have a water-irrigation channel [12]. Balloon-assisted ESD using the DBE is useful for right-colon tumors with unstable endoscopic maneuverability or if total colonoscopy could not be completed using a conventional colonoscope [12, 13].

3.4 The Procedure for the Pocket-Creation Method

The procedure for the PCM is as follows. A solution containing 0.4% sodium hyaluronate is injected in the submucosal layer to create a submucosal cushion. The mucosal elevation created by the submucosal injection should be made from outside the edge of the tumor toward the center of the tumor. As an entrance to the submucosal pocket, an initial mucosal incision is made in normal mucosa at least 1 cm in front of the tumor. The incision should be limited to about 2 cm in length to make the pocket entrance narrow enough to keep the endoscope stable within the pocket (Fig. 3.4a). A few strokes of submucosal dissection just below the initial mucosal incision can easily make the entrance larger to let the endoscope tip with the ST-hood pass into the submucosal space (Fig. 3.4b). Aspirating intraluminal gas can loosen the mucosa around the incision, which facilitates insertion of the ST-hood tip. The surface of the muscularis can be identified through the translucent submucosal tissue through the ST hood. More solution is injected just above the muscularis to expand the deep portion of the submucosa (muscularis side) to elevate branches of blood vessels and fatty tissue which are dominant in the shallow portion of the submucosa (mucosal side), which facilitates subsequent submucosal dissection avoiding immediate bleeding and splashing of thermally aerosolized fat during the submucosal dissection. The submucosa is laterally dissected identifying a safe and appropriate dissection plane just above the muscularis looking at the surface of the muscularis. Submucosal dissection is best accomplished with a succession of short maneuvers. Traction is applied to the submucosal tissue in a safe direction about 1–2 mm with an electric knife tip first and then cut with short-duration coagulation, which creates a short distance of dissection with minimum thermal damage. A series of these short dissections is repeated along the surface of the muscularis, which results in a long precise dissection line. It is not necessary to dissect the submucosa with single long strokes of the electric knife. Holding the surface of the muscularis by the ST hood tip maintains a safe distance between the muscularis and the electric knife tip, protecting the muscularis from accidental damage which may result in a perforation. After the area below the tumor is dissected (Fig. 3.4c), we switch from pocket creation to opening the pocket. The pocket should be opened from the side where fluid would flow by gravity ("downhill") to take advantage of the traction caused by gravity (Fig. 3.4d). It is not necessary to stick to the "down" side in colorectal ESD because changing the patient's body position is usually possible during the procedure. An additional submucosal injection should be made at

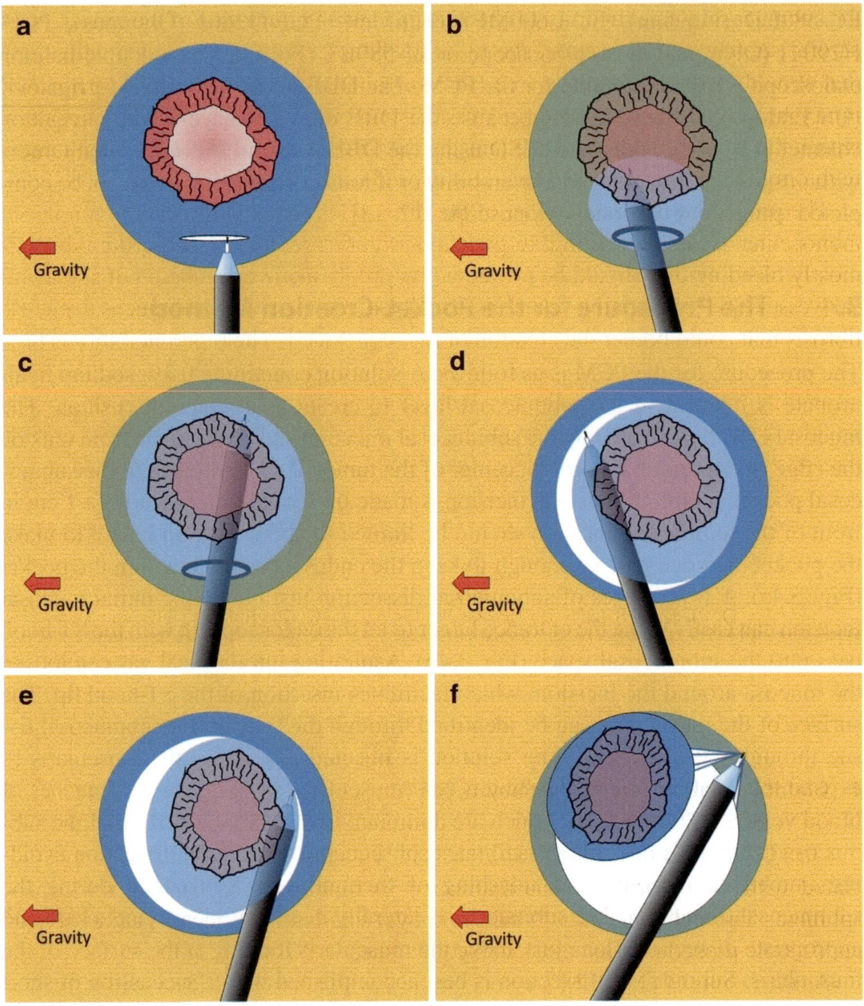

Fig. 3.4 The procedure for the pocket-creation method (PCM) of endoscopic submucosal dissection (ESD): (**a**) initial mucosal incision, (**b**) entering the pocket and dissecting the submucosa, (**c**) the area under the tumor is dissected, (**d**) opening the pocket on the side where fluid flows by gravity ("downhill"), (**e**) opening the pocket from another side and (**f**) *en bloc* resection is accomplished

the mucosal surface outside of the pocket. The elevated mucosa is incised about 1 cm in length in each dissection. The submucosa below the incision is subsequently hooked and cut with the electric knife tip from inside of the pocket toward the outside. The entire submucosa below the mucosal incision should be dissected completely. Next, the other side of the pocket is opened by repeating additional injections, mucosal incisions, and submucosal dissections. After opening the remaining area in the same manner (Fig. 3.4e), the *en bloc* resection has been accomplished (Fig. 3.4f).

There are some salient points to be emphasized regarding performance of the PCM. The mucosal elevation should be extended by injecting sodium hyaluronate to the edge of the previous mucosal elevation like arranging roof tiles to diminish the risk of injection in the muscularis (Fig. 3.5). During the submucosal dissection, blood vessels should not be accidentally punctured with the needle when the injection needle is inserted into the submucosa. Immediate bleeding from a punctured blood vessel may cause a submucosal hematoma which makes the submucosa appear opaque and thus interferes with identification of submucosal blood vessels and the muscularis through the submucosa. The PCM does not need a lot of insufflation to maintain the visual field during the ESD because the ST hood maintains the working field inside it. Therefore, we frequently aspirate gas from the lumen during the ESD by moving the tip of the endoscope out of the pocket. A lumen without insufflated gas stabilizes endoscopic maneuverability and changes the intestinal wall to a tangential direction (Fig. 3.6). A non-insufflated lumen loosens the intestinal mucosa and submucosa and maintains submucosal elevation by the injected solution. When the submucosal pocket is opened, the endoscope tip becomes unstable because the endoscope tip becomes free after being held by the submucosal pocket. It is important to keep the intestinal lumen collapsed by aspirating the gas as much as possible to secure stable maneuverability and to hook the mucosa and submucosa easily because they are loosened by aspiration. Opening the pocket is relatively difficult especially for those with less experience although the submucosal dissection can be easily performed in the pocket because the tip of the endoscope is stabilized in the pocket. A scissors-type knife, IT knife, and SafeknifeV may facilitate opening the pocket in an unstable situation.

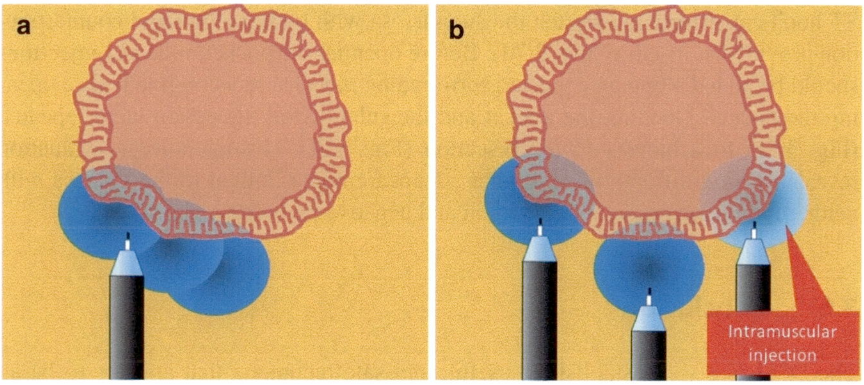

Fig. 3.5 Mucosal elevation: (**a**) a good example: mucosal elevation is extended by injecting to the edge of previous mucosal elevation to diminish the risk of injecting to the muscularis and (**b**) a bad example: mucosal elevations are done separately. This manner of injection increases the risk of intramuscular injection and makes recognition of the submucosa difficult during dissection which may result in intraprocedural perforation

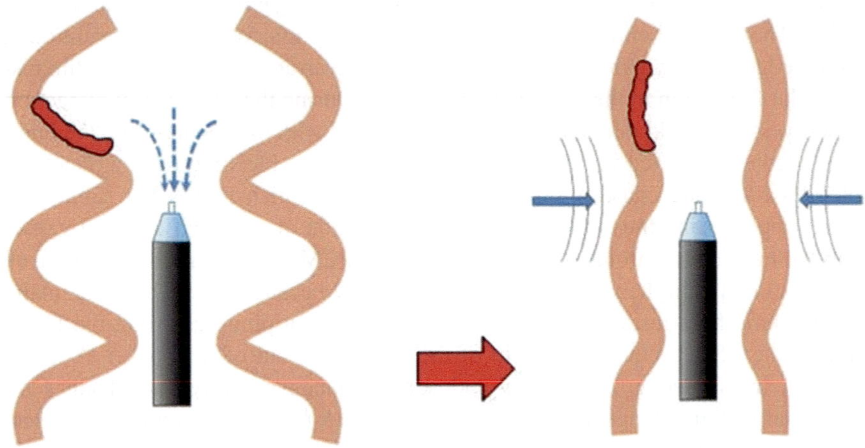

Fig. 3.6 Deflating the lumen by aspirating intraluminal gas makes the intestinal wall tangential. A tumor behind a fold can be changed to a tangential position

3.5 Case Presentation: The Pocket-Creation Method of ESD

A 77-year-old man presented with a laterally spreading tumor, non-granular, flat type in the sigmoid colon (Fig. 3.7a). A solution of 0.4% sodium hyaluronate was injected from the surrounding mucosa into the tissue below the tumor (Fig. 3.7b). After going into the submucosal pocket, additional submucosal injections were done just above the muscularis which can be seen through the submucosa to expand translucent lower portion of the submucosa (Fig. 3.7c). The submucosa was continuously dissected maintaining a safe distance between the electric knife tip and the muscularis while holding the surface of the muscularis using the ST hood. The ST hood can effectively stretch the submucosa with both traction and countertraction provided at its edge (Fig. 3.7d). Before opening the pocket, mucosal injections should be added along an expected surrounding mucosal incision line before opening the pocket. Opening the pocket and the submucosal dissection were repeated (Fig. 3.7e) to achieve *en bloc* resection (Fig. 3.7f). Histopathologic evaluation revealed a well-differentiated tubular adenocarcinoma limited to the mucosa with neither lymphatic nor venous invasion and negative pathologic margins.

3.6 Conclusion

The PCM is a well-established, useful, and safe technique that appears to be an effective strategy for ESD. Those with less experience in ESD should learn the PCM first as their standard ESD strategy. The PCM provides a shortcut to improving one's skill in performing ESD and allows one to step up to challenging lesions after obtaining skill in precise submucosal dissection through use of the PCM.

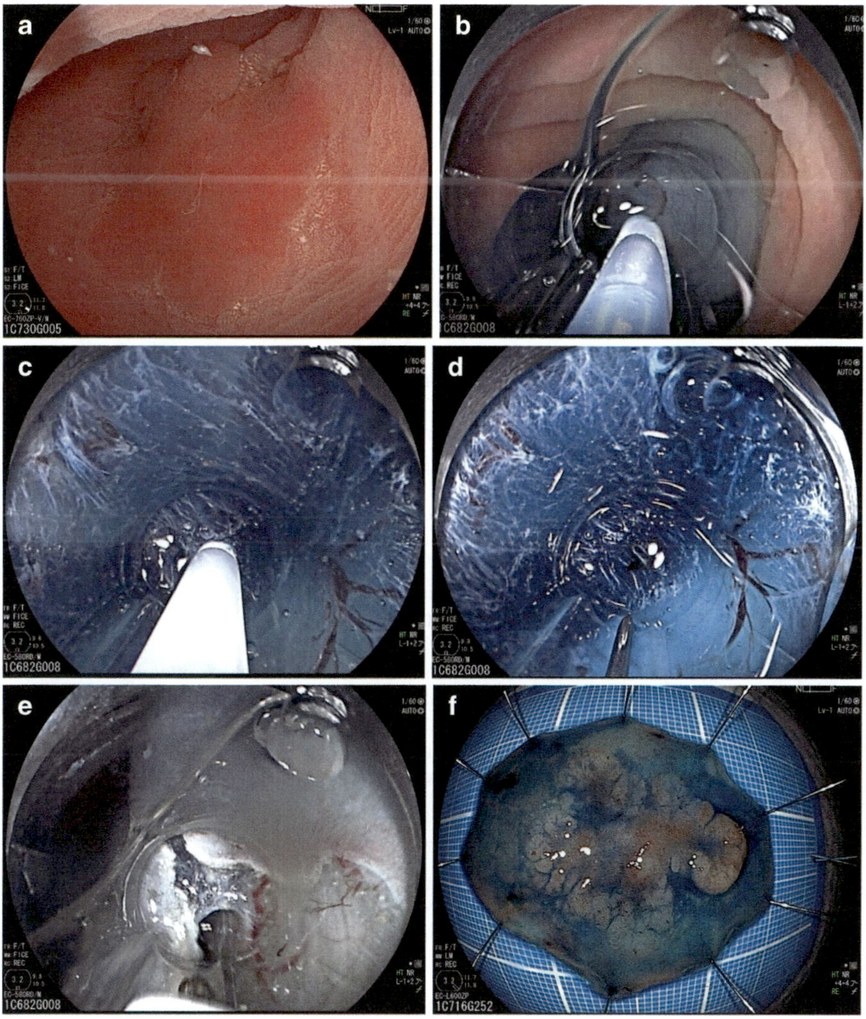

Fig. 3.7 Endoscopic submucosal dissection with the pocket-creation method for a laterally spreading tumor in the sigmoid colon: (**a**) a laterally spreading tumor—non-granular, (**b**) mucosal elevation, (**c**) a submucosal injection just above the muscularis, (**d**) clear visualization of the muscularis through the transparent hood, (**e**) opening the pocket, and (**f**) *en bloc* resection

References

1. Watanabe T, Itabashi M, Shimada Y, Tanaka S, Ito Y, Ajioka Y, et al. Japanese Society for Cancer of the Colon and Rectum (JSCCR) guidelines 2014 for treatment of colorectal cancer. Int J Clin Oncol. 2015;20(2):207–39.
2. Ono H, Yao K, Fujishiro M, Oda I, Nimura S, Yahagi N, et al. Guidelines for endoscopic submucosal dissection and endoscopic mucosal resection for early gastric cancer. Dig Endosc. 2016;28(1):3–15.

3. Hotta K, Saito Y, Matsuda T, Shinohara T, Oyama T. Local recurrence and surveillance after endoscopic resection of large colorectal tumors. Dig Endosc. 2010;22(Suppl 1):S63–8.
4. Hayashi Y, Shinozaki S, Sunada K, Sato H, Miura Y, Ino Y, et al. Efficacy and safety of endoscopic submucosal dissection for superficial colorectal tumors more than 50 mm in diameter. Gastrointest Endosc. 2016;83(3):602–7.
5. Sakamoto H, Hayashi Y, Miura Y, Shinozaki S, Takahashi H, Fukuda H, et al. Pocket-creation method facilitates endoscopic submucosal dissection of colorectal laterally spreading tumors, non-granular type. Endosc Int Open. 2017;5(2):E123–E9.
6. Hayashi Y, Sunada K, Takahashi H, Shinhata H, Lefor AT, Tanaka A, et al. Pocket-creation method of endoscopic submucosal dissection to achieve en bloc resection of giant colorectal subpedunculated neoplastic lesions. Endoscopy. 2014;46(Suppl 1 UCTN):E421–2.
7. Hayashi Y, Miura Y, Yamamoto H. Pocket-creation method for the safe, reliable, and efficient endoscopic submucosal dissection of colorectal lateral spreading tumors. Dig Endosc. 2015;27(4):534–5.
8. Miura Y, Hayashi Y, Lefor AK, Osawa H, Yamamoto H. The pocket-creation method of ESD for gastric neoplasms. Gastrointest Endosc. 2016;83(2):457–8.
9. Takezawa T, Hayashi Y, Shinozaki S, Sagara Y, Okada M, Kobayashi Y, et al. The pocket-creation method facilitates colonic endoscopic submucosal dissection. Gastrointest Endosc. 2019;89(5):1045–53.
10. Miura Y, Shinozaki S, Hayashi Y, Sakamoto H, Lefor AK, Yamamoto H. Duodenal endoscopic submucosal dissection is feasible using the pocket-creation method. Endoscopy. 2017;49(1):8–14.
11. Hayashi Y, Nomura T, Lee RF, Miura Y, Shinozaki S, Sunada K, et al. Introducing the next evolution of the small-caliber-tip transparent hood: enhancing the pocket-creation method by building on previous successes. Endoscopy. 2020;52(8):E297–9.
12. Yamashina T, Hayashi Y, Sakamoto H, Yano T, Miura Y, Shinozaki S, et al. Balloon-assisted endoscopy facilitates endoscopic submucosal dissection of difficult superficial proximal colon tumors. Endoscopy. 2018;50(8):800–8.
13. Hayashi Y, Sunada K, Yamamoto H. Prototype holder adequately supports the overtube in balloon-assisted endoscopic submucosal dissection. Dig Endosc. 2014;26(5):682.

Endoscopic Ultrasound (EUS)-Guided Biliary Drainage

4

Marc Giovannini

4.1 Introduction

Endoscopic biliary stenting is the method used most commonly to treat obstructive jaundice. In 3–12% of cases, selective cannulation of the major papilla fails and surgery or percutaneous biliary drainage is required. Percutaneous techniques of biliary drainage have a high rate of complication as bleeding or peritoneal bile leakage (20–30%), and the morbidity and the mortality of surgery for such palliative procedures are respectively of 35–50% and 10–15%. A new technique for biliary drainage using EUS- and EUS-guided puncture of the bile duct (common bile duct or left hepatic duct) is now possible. Using EUS guidance and dedicated accessories, it is now possible to create bilio-digestive anastomosis.

The aim of this chapter is:

1. to describe the material needed for such procedures;
2. to describe the technique of biliary duct drainage under EUS guidance;
3. to describe the place of these techniques today in comparison with ERCP.

4.2 Material

4.2.1 Interventional Echoendoscopes

Around 1990, the Pentax-Corporation developed an electronic convex curved linear array echoendoscope (FG32UA) with an imaging plane in the long axis of the device that overlaps with the instrumentation plane. This EUS scope, equipped with

M. Giovannini (✉)
Endoscopic Unit, Paoli–Calmettes Institute, Marseille, France
e-mail: giovanninim@ipc.unicancer.fr

P. Sharma, N. Reddy (eds.), *Innovations in Gastrointestinal Endoscopy*,
https://doi.org/10.1007/978-981-15-9247-8_4

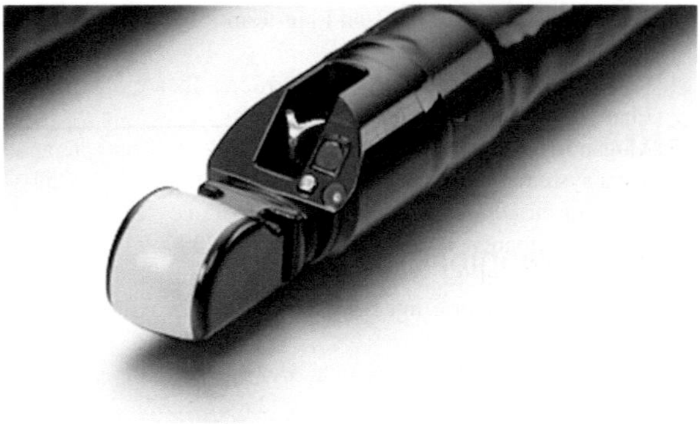

Fig. 4.1 New therapeutic EUS scope with large working channel (4.0 mm)

a 2.0-mm working channel, enabled fine-needle biopsy under EUS guidance (EUS FNA). However, the relatively small working channel of the FG 32UA was a drawback for pseudocyst drainage because it necessitated exchange of the EUS scope for a therapeutic duodenoscope to insert either a stent or nasocystic drain. To enable stent placement using an EUS scope, the EUS interventional echoendoscopes (FG 38X, EG 38UT, and EG 3870UTK) were developed by Pentax-Hitachi. The FG 38X has a working channel of 3.2 mm, which allows for the insertion of an 8.5-F stent or nasocystic drain. The EG38UTand EG3870UTK have a larger working channel of 3.8 mm, with an elevator that allows for the placement of a 10F stent [1–3]. More recently, a new generation of therapeutic EUS scope (EG38UJ10) is available with a 4.0-mm working channel (Fig. 4.1).

The Olympus Corporation has also developed convex array EUS scopes. GF-UCT160-OL5, offering a large working channel (3.7 mm). The UCT160-OL5 provides a 150° ultrasound scanning range when connected to the EU-C60 ultrasound center.

The fujinon corporation has also developed a therapeutic EUS scope. The EG-580UT, an ultrasound endoscope with Forceps Elevator Assist which enables convex scanning, was developed for therapeutic interventions. The endoscope has a large working channel of 3.8 mm and is equipped with an Albarran lever.

4.2.2 Needles and Accessories for Drainage

Using a 19G FNA needle (Wilson-Cook Corporation), a 0.035-inch guidewire can be inserted through the needle into the dilated bile duct. However, one of the main problems during these new techniques mainly hepaticogastrostomy is the difficulty manipulating the wire guide through the 19-gauge EUS needle. The main issue was "stripping" of the wire coating, which in turn created a risk of leaving a part of the wire coating in the patient and also the impossibility of continuing the procedure and inserting the stent. To solve this problem, we worked with Cook

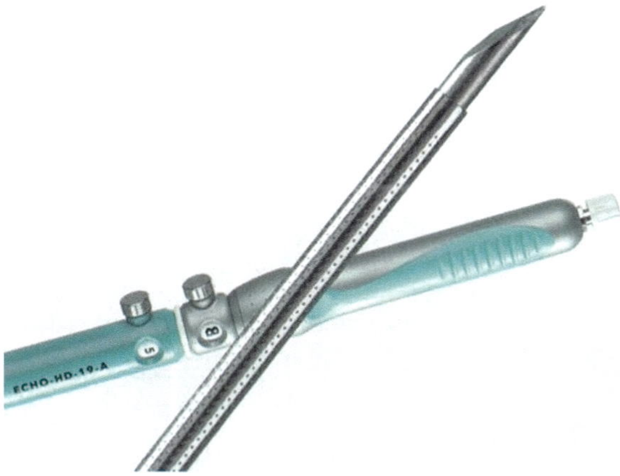

Fig. 4.2 EchoTip® Access Needle (Cook Medical, Wiston Salem, USA)

Medical to design a special needle called the EchoTip® Access Needle* (Fig. 4.2). This needle is original because the stylet is sharp, and it is relatively easy to insert the needle into the bile duct, the pancreatic duct, or a pseudocyst. When the stylet is withdrawn, the needle left in place is smooth and the manipulation of the wire guide is easy and the device is designed to decrease the possibility of the wire stripping.

4.3 Technique for Biliary Duct Drainage Under EUS Guidance

The proximity of the EUS device to the obstruction area results in a higher resolution than CT or MRI and EUS is a minimally invasive procedure with a lower complication rate compared with ERCP. EUS-guided cholangiography and pancreatography were first described by Wiersema et al. Subsequently, EUS-guided transmural biliary drainage was reported by Giovannini et al. as well as by Burmester [3–6].

Actually, biliary drainage using EUS- and EUS-guided puncture of the bile duct (common bile duct or left hepatic duct), and EUS-guided *rendezvous* techniques are available options in some reference centers. We classified the different approaches as follows:

(a) Intrahepatic approach (hepaticogastrostomy, puncture for *rendezvous* technique, and placement of a transhepatic anterograde self-expandable metal stent (SEMS)) [7, 8]
(b) Extrahepatic approach (choledoco-duodenostomy, puncture for *rendezvous* technique via main bile duct)

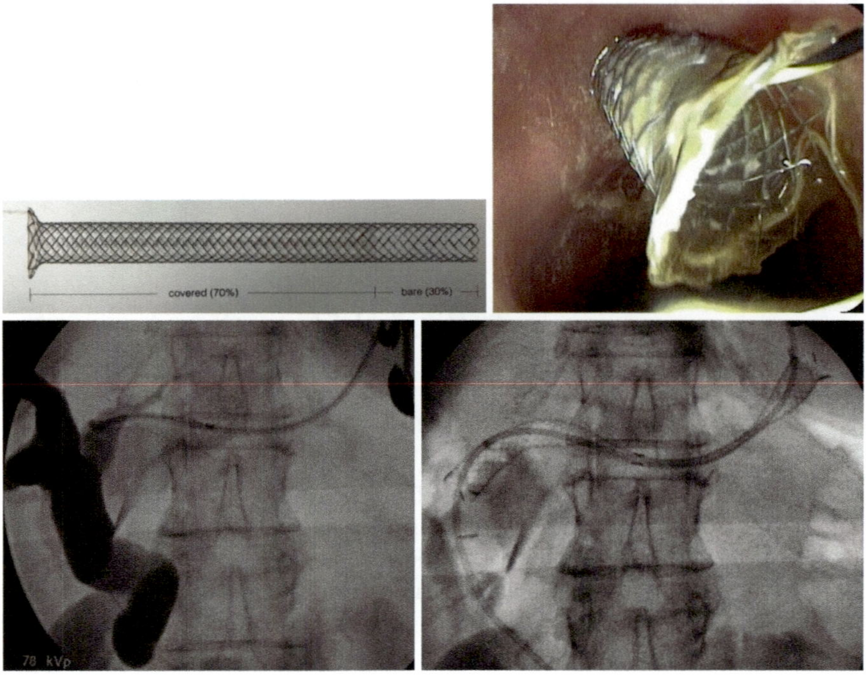

Fig. 4.3 Hepaticogastrostomy using a GIOBOR stent (Taewoong Medical, Seoul, South Korea)

4.4 Technique of Left HepaticoGastrostomy Under EUS Guidance (HGE) (Fig. 4.3)

EUS-guided hepaticogastrostomy was first reported by Burmester et al. [6] in 2003. The technique is also similar to EUS-guided drainage of pancreatic pseudocysts. By using an interventional echoendoscope, the dilated left hepatic duct (segment III) was well visualized. HGE was then performed under combined fluoroscopic and ultrasound guidance, with the tip of the echoendoscope positioned such that the inflated balloon was in the middle part of the small curvature of the stomach. A needle (19G, EchoTip® Access Needle, Cook Ireland Ltd., Limerick, Ireland) is inserted transgastrically into the distal part of the left hepatic duct, and contrast medium is injected for demonstration of dilated biliary ducts. The needle is exchanged over guidewire; a 6F cystostome is then used to enlarge the channel between the stomach and the left hepatic duct. The cystostome is introduced by using cutting current. After exchange over a guidewire (0.035-inch diameter), a dedicated hepaticogastrostomy stent is introduced, this stent is partially covered metallic stent (70% covered to prevent the bile leakage and 30% uncovered to prevent the migration, the uncovered part is introduced in the bile duct). We use the GIOBOR metallic stent (Taewoong-Medical Co, Seoul, South Korea) or the Hanaro

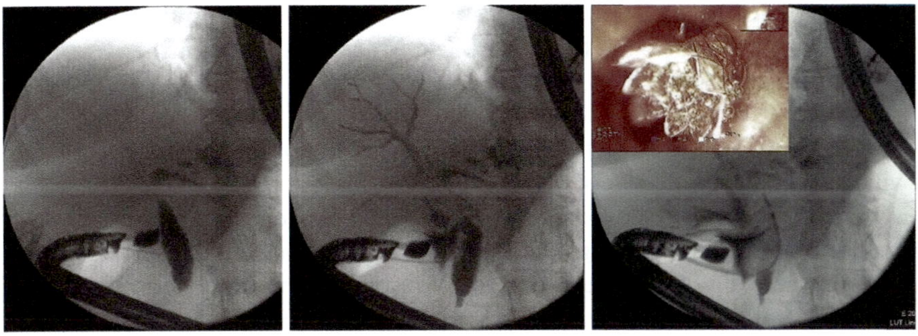

Fig. 4.4 EUS-choledoco-duodenostomy

stent (Mi-TECH Mi-TECH-Medical Co, Seoul, South Korea). Hepaticogastrostomy is sometimes combined with the placement of an additional plastic stent (7F, 10 cm double pigtail) to prevent the migration of the metallic stent.

4.4.1 EUS-Choledoco-Duodenostomy (Fig. 4.4)

A 19-G needle (EchoTip; Cook Endoscopy) is inserted trans-duodenally into the bile duct under EUS guidance. Bile is aspirated and contrast medium is injected into the bile duct for cholangiography. A 450-cm long, 0.035-inch guidewire is inserted through the 19-G needle into the bile duct. The choledochoduodenal fistula is dilated using a biliary catheter for dilation (Soehendra biliary dilator; Wilson-Cook), or a 6F cystostome (Endoflex, company). A fully covered self-expandable metallic stent is placed through the choledochoduodenostomy site into the extrahepatic bile duct. More recently, some series reported the use of LAMS (Hot Axios stent, 10 mm, Boston Scientific Co, USA) to create an anastomosis between the bile duct and the bulbus.

4.5 EUS-Guided Rendez-Vous Technique

After puncture of the left hepatic biliary system or in the bulb for extrahepatic approach using a 19-G needle (Echo–Tip19; Cook Endoscopy), a 0.035-inch hydrophilic guidewire (Tracer Metro Direct, Cook Endoscopy or Jagwire, Boston scientific, Paris, France) is inserted into the biliary duct and then rolled up inside the duodenum. Then, the echoendoscope was gently withdrawn, leaving the guidewire in place. Afterwards, a duodenoscope was inserted parallel to the guidewire and placed in the third duodenum, allowing for a retrograde approach. The guidewire was then caught with a standard snare through the working channel and after over-the-wire biliary sphincterotomy, stones removal or stent placement could be achieved as usual.

4.5.1 Endoscopic Ultrasonography-Guided Transhepatic Anterograde Self-Expandable Metal Stent (SEMS) Placement (Fig. 4.5)

EUS-guided puncture is performed transgastrically into the left intrahepatic duct with a 19-G Access needle (Cook Medical, Inc., Winston Salem, North Carolina, USA). The needle is removed after bile has been obtained and the cholangiogram has been acquired. A 0.035″ guidewire reached the jejunum, and Soehendra's dilators 6Fr and 7Fr (Cook Medical, Inc., Winston Salem, North Carolina, USA) advanced over the wire and a MaxForce 4-mm balloon (Boston Scientific, Galway, Ireland) could be employed to dilate the stenosis. Afterwards, EUS-guided anterograde stent placement via the transhepatic route can be accomplished. The stent is advanced through a therapeutic echoendoscope over the guidewire, and deployed across the stricture.

4.6 Place of the Bilio-Digestive Anastomosis Guided by EUS in Comparison with ERCP

ERCP is the gold-standard technique for the drainage of obstructive jaundice due to pancreatic cancer. Success rate of biliary stenting using ERCP is around 80–85%, but ERCP may fail to selectively cannulate the papilla or fail to reach the papilla at all, in the case of duodenal obstruction.

The percutaneous procedure is the accepted alternative, but these new techniques of biliary drainage using EUS guidance represent an additional alternative. Percutaneous techniques of biliary drainage (PTBD) have a high rate of complication as bleeding, or peritoneal bile leakage (20–30%) and the morbidity and the mortality of surgery for such palliative procedures are, respectively, of 35–50% and 10–15%. One previous study prospectively compared EUS-BD (choledochoduodenostomy (CD)) and PTBD. Twenty-five subjects were randomized (13 EUS-CD and 12 PTBD). All procedures were technically and clinically successful in both groups.

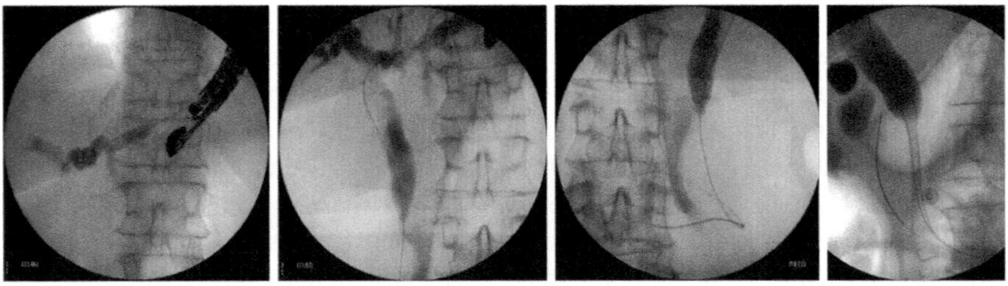

Fig. 4.5 Endoscopic ultrasonography-guided transhepatic anterograde self-expandable metal stent (SEMS) placement

After 7-day follow-up, there was a significant reduction in total bilirubin in both groups (EUS-CD, 16.4–3.3; $P = 0.002$ and PTBD, 17.2–3.8; $P = 0.01$), although no difference was noted comparing the two groups (EUS-CD to PTBD; 3.3 vs. 3.8; $P = 0.2$). There was no difference between groups in the rates of complications ($P = 0.44$, EUS-CD (2/13; 15.3%), PTBD (3/12; 25%)). Costs were also similar in both groups ($5673-EUS-CD vs. $7570-PTBD; $P = 0.39$). The authors concluded that EUS-CD can be an effective and safe alternative to PTBD with similar success, complication rate, cost, and quality of life [9].

The advantages of EUS-guided hepaticogastrostomy over PTBD include puncture of the biliary tree with real-time US when using color-Doppler information to limit the possibility of vascular injury, the lack of ascites in the interventional field when present in the peritoneum, and the lack of an external drain. There are some reports about that the extrahepatic approach has a greater chance of complication than the intrahepatic approach. However, Itoi et al. reported the limitations of intrahepatic approach as follows: (1) non-apposed gastric wall and the left liver lobe, with a certain displacement between the puncture site of the gastric wall and intrahepatic bile duct, resulting in possibility of procedure failure, (2) risk of mediastinitis with a transesophageal approach, (3) difficulty of puncture in case of liver cirrhosis, (4) risk of injuring the portal vein, and (5) necessitating the use of small-caliber stents or MS with a small-diameter delivery device.

To date, 42 studies with 1192 patients about EUS-BD have been reported. The cumulative technical success rate (TSR), functional success rate (FSR), and adverse-event rate are 94.71%, 91.66%, and 23.32%, respectively. The common adverse events associated with EUS-BD were as follows: bleeding (4.03%), bile leakage (4.03%), pneumoperitoneum (3.02%), stent migration (2.68%), cholangitis (2.43%), abdominal pain (1.51%), and peritonitis (1.26%) [10].

One meta-analysis that compared transduodenal (TD) and transgastric (TG) approaches for EUS-BD regarding efficacy and safety included ten studies. Compared with the TG approach, the TSR, FSR, and adverse-event rate of the TD approach had pooled odds ratios of 1.36 (95% CI, 0.66–2.81; $P > 0.05$), 0.84 (95% CI, 0.50–1.42; $P > 0.05$) and 0.61 (95% CI, 0.36–1.03; $P > 0.05$), respectively, which indicated no significant difference in the TSR, FSR, or adverse-event rate between groups [10].

4.6.1 What Stent Should Be Used?

From a clinical standpoint, the most relevant technical choice appears to be the type of stent. It is difficult to draw significant conclusions from the published reports, since no formal comparisons have been made between the different types of stents. Covered (total or partially) SEMS appears to be a better option for three reasons. First, upon full expansion SEMS effectively seal the puncture/dilation tract, which would in theory prevent leakage. Secondly, their larger diameter provides better long-term patency, which would decrease the need for stent revisions. Finally, if dysfunction by ingrowth or clogging occurs, management is somewhat less challenging than with plastic stents because a new stent (plastic or SEMS) can easily be inserted through the occluded SEMS in place. In contrast, exchanging a clogged plastic transmural stent usually requires over-the-wire replacement because free-hand removal involves the risk of track disruption with subsequent guidewire passage into the peritoneum. Uncovered SEMS could allow the leak of bile to peritoneum and possible biloma formation. These presumed advantages of covered SEMS must be balanced against the fact that transmural SEMS insertion and deployment are somewhat more demanding than they are at ERCP. In particular, the serious risk of foreshortening and bile peritonitis should be prevented with careful attention to detail.

What technique to use to drain the CBD in patient with a malignant stenosis of the lower part of the CBD? ERCP, or EUS-BD?

The question is posed today, and we have two recent randomized trials in the literature [11, 12] showing no difference between the two techniques. Bang et al. [12] randomized EUS-BD (n = 33) or ERCP (n = 34). The primary endpoint was the rate of adverse events. Secondary endpoints were technical success, treatment success (defined as decline in serum bilirubin by 50% at 2-week follow-up), reinterventions, and intraoperative technical outcome, when applicable. Follow-up was until death or minimum of 6 months. The rates of adverse events were 21.2% (6.1% moderate severity; others mild severity) in the EUS-BD group and 14.7% (5.9% moderate severity; others mild severity) in the ERCP group (risk ratio 0.69; 95% confidence interval, 0.24–1.97; p = 0.49). There were no procedure-related deaths. There was no significant difference in the rates of technical success (90.9% vs 94.1%, p = 0.67), treatment success (97 vs 91.2%, P = 0.61) or reinterventions (3.0 vs 2.9%, p = 0.99) between EUS-BD and ERCP cohorts, respectively. The endoscopic interventions did not impede subsequent pancreaticoduodenectomy that was performed in 5 of 33 (15.2%) patients in the EUS-BD and 5 of 34 patients (14.7%) in the ERCP group (p = 0.99). Given the similar rates of adverse events and treatment outcomes in this randomized trial, EUS-BD is a practical alternative to ERCP for primary biliary decompression in pancreatic cancer. Same conclusions were reported in the study of Paik et al. [11] (Table 4.1).

Table 4.1 Summary of the published literature on EUS-guided biliary drainage (HGE, CD, and rendezvous technique)

First author, year	*N*	Device for puncture	Technical success, *n*	Clinical success, *n*	Initial stent Fr (pl)	Initial stent SEMS (mm)	Early complications (*n*)
EUS-guided choledochoduodenostomy							
Giovannini, 2001 [13]	1	NK	1/1	1/1	10	–	None
Burmester, 2003 [6]	2	19G FT	1/2	1/1	8.5	–	Bile peritonitis (1)
Puspok, 2005 [14]	5	NK	4/5	4/4	7–10	–	None
Yamao, 2008 [15]	5	NK	5/5	5/5	7–8.5	–	Pneumo (1)
Ang, 2007 [16]	2	NK	2/2	2/2	7	–	Pneumo (1)
Fujita, 2008 [17]	1	19G FN	1/1	1/1	7	–	None
Tarantino, 2008 [18]	4	19G, 22G FN/NK	4/4	4/4	–[a]	–	None
Itoi, 2008 [19]	4	NK (2), 19G FN (2)	4/4	4/4	7, NBD	–	Bile peritonitis (1)
Horaguchi, 2009 [20]	8	19G	8/8	8/8	7	–	Peritonitis (1)
Hanada, 2009 [21]	4	19G FN	4/4	4/4	6–7	–	None
Park, 2009 [22]	4	19G FN/NK	4/4	4/4	–	10	None
Brauer, 2009 [17]	3	19G, 22G FN/NK	2/3	2/2	10	–	Pneumo cardiac failure
Maranki, 2009 [23]	4	19G 22G		[b]	10	10	[b]
Artifon, 2010 [24]	3	19G	3/3	3/3	–	10	None
Eum, 2010 [25]	2	19G	2/2	2/2	–	10	None
Hara, 2011 [26]	18	22G	17/18	17/17	7–8.5	–	Focal peritonitis (2) Hemobilia (1)
Ramírez-Luna, 2011 [27]	9	19G	9/9	8/9	7–10	–	Biloma (1)
Park, 2011 [28]	24	19G	22/24	20/22	7	10	Pneumo (7), bile peritonitis (2), Bleeding (2)[γ]
Artifon, 2012 [9]	13	19G	13/13	13/13		10	Bleed (1), bile leak (1)

(continued)

Table 4.1 (continued)

First author, year	N	Device for puncture	Technical success, n	Clinical success, n	Initial stent Fr (pl)	SEMS (mm)	Early complications (n)
Hara, 2011 [26]	18		17/18	16/17		10	Local peritonitis (2)
Attasaranya, 2012 [29]	9	19G	5/9	5/9	7		Perforation (1) Fever (2) Migration (1)
Kim, 2012 [30]	9	19G NK	9/9	9/9	8	–	Obstruction (1) Peritonitis (1) Migration (1)
Nicholson, 2012 [31]	5	19G	5/5	5/5	10	–	Migration (1)
Rebello, 2012 [32]	7	NK	7/7	6/7		10	None
Song, 2012 [33]	15	19G NK	13/15	13/15	10		Migration (4) Peritonitis (2) Cholangitis (1)
Hara, 2013 [34]	18	NK	17/18	16/18		10	Peritonitis (2)
Prachayakui, 2013 [35]	6	19G	6/6	5/6	10		Bile leakage (1)
Takada, 2013 [36]	17	19G NK	17/17	17/17	10		Migration (1)
Artifon, 2014 [37]	24	19G NK	22/24	17/24	10		Bile leak (1), perforation(n1), bleeding (1)
Dhir, 2015 [38]	68	19G	66/68	66/68	10		Bleeding (1)
Grupta, 2014 [39]	89	19G	75/89	75/89	–	–	Pneumoperitoneum (1) Bile leak (13) Bleeding (8) Pain (1) Cholangitis (4) Stent occlusion (2)
Hamada, 2014 [40]	3	NK	3/3	3/3		10	Cholangitis (1)
Kawakubo, 2014 [41]	44	19G NK	42/44	42/44	–	–	Bile leakage (3) migration (1) pneumoperitoneum (1) perforation (1)
Song, 2014 [42]	17	19G NK	17/17	16/17	10		Pneumoperitoneum (1) pain (1)
Bruckner, 2015 [43]	5	19G	5/5	5/5	8		None
Poincloux, 2015 [44]	30	19G NK	29/30	27/29	10		Death (1) Perforation (2)

Table 4.1 (continued)

First author, year	*N*	Device for puncture	Technical success, *n*	Clinical success, *n*	Initial stent Fr (pl)	SEMS (mm)	Early complications (*n*)
EUS-guided hepaticogastrostomy							
Burmester, 2003 [6]	1	19G FT	1/1	1/1	8.5		None
Artifon, 2007 [45]	1	19G FN	1/1	1/1	–	10	None
Bories, 2007 [46]	11	19G, 22G FN/CT	10/11	10/10	7	10	Cholangitis (2), ileus (1), biloma (1)
Will, 2007 [47]	4	19G FN	4/4	3/4	–	10	Cholangitis (1)
Chopin-Laly, 2009 [48]	1	–	1/1	1/1	–	–[a]	None
Park, 2009 [22]	9	19G FN/NK	9/9	9/9		10	None
Horaguchi, 2009 [20]	6	19G	6/6	5/6	7	–	None
Maranki, 2009 [23]	3	19G 22G	3	[b]	10	10	[b]
Park, 2010 [49]	5	19G	5/5	5/5	–	10	None
Martins, 2010 [50]	1	19G	1/1	0/1	–		Death (1)
Eum, 2010 [25]	1	19G	1/1	1/1	–	10	None
Artifon, 2011 [10]	1	19G	1/1	1/1	–	10	None
Ramírez-Luna, 2011 [27]	2	19G	2/2	2/2	7	–	Stent migration (1)
Park, 2011 [28]	17	19G	17/17	13/17	7	10	Pneumo (4), Bleeding (2)
Atassaranya, 2012 [29]	16	19G	13/16	13/16	7		Migration (2), peritonitis (1), abdominal pain (2), fever (1)
Kim, 2012 [30]	4	19G NK	3/4	2/4	8		Migration (2) Peritonitis (1)
Panpimanma, 2013 [51]	10	19G	8/10	7/10	10		Migration (2) Cholangitis (1)
Park, 2013 [52]	9	19G			10		
Park, 2013 [53]	6	19G NK	6/6	5/6	8		None
Prachayakui, 2013 [35]	15	19G	15/15	14/15	10		Pneumoperitoneum (1)

(continued)

Table 4.1 (continued)

First author, year	*N*	Device for puncture	Technical success, *n*	Clinical success, *n*	Initial stent		Early complications (*n*)
					Fr (pl)	SEMS (mm)	
Takada, 2013 [36]	6	19G NK	6/6	6/6	10		Bleeding (2) abdominal pain (1)
Artifon, 2014 [37]	25	19G NK	24/25	22/25	10		Bacteremia (1), biloma (2), and bleeding (3)
Gupta, 2014 [39]	145	19G	132/145	132/145	–	–	Pneumoperitoneum (11) Bile leak (14) Bleeding (18) Pain (4) Cholangitis (7)
Hamada, 2014 [40]	4	NK	4/4	5/4		10	Occlusion (1) Bleeding (1)
Kawakubo, 2014 [41]	20	19G NK	19/20	19/20	–	–	Bile leakage (2) migration (2) bleeding (1) cholangitis (1) biloma (1)
Ogura, 2014 [54]	20	19G	20/20	20/20	8		Migration (2), occlusion (1), peritonitis (1)
Paik, 2014 [55]	28	19G	27/28	24/28			Migration (1), bleeding (1)
Song, 2014 [42]	10	19G NK	10/10	10/10	10		Pneumoperitoneum (2) Bleeding (1)
Umeda, 2015 [56]	23	22G 19G	23/23	23/23	8		Bleeding (1), abdominal pain (3)
Poincloux, 2015 [44]	66	19G NK	65/66	61/66	10		Pneumoperitoneum (2) hematoma (1) Death (5) Bile leakage (5) Sepsis (2)
EUS-guided RendezVous							
Will, 2007 [47]	1	19G FN	–	–	–	–	–
Maranki, 2009 [23]	32	19G 22G	–	[b]	10	10	[b]
Poincloux, 2015 [44]	5	19G NK	5/5	5/5	10		None

HGE hepaticogastrostomy, *CD* choledoco-duodenostomy, *NK* needle knife, *FT* fistolotome, *FN* fine needle, *SEMS* self-expanding metal stent, *NBD* nasobiliary drainage, *CT* cystotome

[a]Unspecified

[b]Data are presented as an intrahepatic vs extrahepatic approach (these included HG, CD, and rendezvous technique). We could not obtain the raw data

4.7 Conclusion

EUS-BD is a useful tool in case of failure of ERCP with a high rate of technical success and clinical efficacy. Morbidity rate is high during biliary drainage requiring experienced team. Although data has demonstrated EUS-BD can be safe and effective, EUS-BD drainage remains one of the most technically challenging therapeutic EUS interventions.

At this time, we advocate that these procedures should only be performed in appropriately selected patients by experienced endoscopists trained in both, EUS and ERCP, with well-trained surgical back-up available.

References

1. Giovannini M, Pesenti C, Bories E, Caillol F. Interventional EUS: difficult pancreaticobiliary access. Endoscopy. 2006;38(Suppl 1):S93–5.
2. Kahaleh M. EUS-guided cholangio-drainage and rendezvous techniques. Tech Gastrointest Endosc. 2007;9:39–45.
3. Grimm H, Binmoeller KF, Soehendra N. Endosonography-guided drainage of a pancreatic pseudocyst. Gastrointest Endosc. 1992;38:170–1.
4. Giovannini M. EUS-guided pancreatic pseudocyst drainage. Tech Gastrointest Endosc. 2007;9:32–8.
5. Giovannini M. Ultrasound-guided endoscopic surgery. Best Pract Res Clin Gastroenterol. 2004;18:183–200.
6. Burmester E, Niehaus J, Leineweber T, Huetteroth T. EUS-cholangio-drainage of the bile duct: report of 4 cases. Gastrointest Endosc. 2003;57:246–51.
7. Giovannini M, Dotti M, Bories E, et al. Hepaticogastrostomy by echo-endoscopy as a palliative treatment in a patient with metastatic biliary obstruction. Endoscopy. 2003;35:1076–8.
8. Téllez-Ávila FI, Duarte-Medrano G, Gallardo-Cabrera V, Casasola-Sánchez L, Valdovinos-Andraca F. Endoscopic ultrasonography-guided transhepatic antegrade self-expandable metal stent placement in a patient with surgically altered anatomy. Endoscopy. 2015;47(Suppl 1):E643–4.
9. Artifon EL, Aparicio D, Paione JB, et al. Biliary drainage in patients with unresectable, malignant obstruction where ERCP fails: endoscopic ultrasonography-guided choledochoduodenostomy versus percutaneous drainage. J Clin Gastroenterol. 2012;46:768–74.
10. Artifon EL, Okawa L, Takada J, Gupta K, Moura EG, Sakai P. EUS-guided choledochoantrostomy: an alternative for biliary drainage in unresectable pancreatic cancer with duodenal invasion. Gastrointest Endosc. 2011;73:1317–20.
11. Paik WH, Lee TH, Park DH, Choi JH, Kim SO, Jang S, Kim DU, Shim JH, Song TJ, Lee SS, Seo DW, Lee SK, Kim MH. EUS-guided biliary drainage versus ERCP for the primary palliation of malignant biliary obstruction: a multicenter randomized clinical trial. Am J Gastroenterol. 2018;113(10):156.
12. Bang JY, Navaneethan U, Hasan M, Hawes R, Varadarajulu S. Stent placement by EUS or ERCP for primary biliary decompression in pancreatic cancer: arandomized trial (with videos). Gastrointest Endosc. 2018;88(1):9–17.
13. Giovannini M, Moutardier V, Pesenti C, Bories E, Lelong B, Delpero JR. Endoscopic ultrasound-guided bilioduodenal anastomosis: a new technique for biliary drainage. Endoscopy. 2001;33:898–900.
14. Puspok A, Lomoschitz F, Dejaco C, et al. Endoscopic ultrasound guided therapy of benign and malignant biliary obstruction: a case series. Am J Gastroenterol. 2005;100:1743–7.

15. Yamao K, Bhatia V, Mizuno N, et al. EUS-guided choledochoduodenostomy for palliative biliary drainage in patients with malignant biliary obstruction: results of long-term follow-up. Endoscopy. 2008;40:340–2.
16. Ang TL, Teo EK, Fock KM. EUS-guided transduodenal biliary drainage in unresectable pancreatic cancer with obstructive jaundice. JOP. 2007;8:438–43.
17. Fujita N, Noda Y, Kobayashi G, et al. Temporary endosonography-guided biliary drainage for transgastrointestinal deployment of a self-expandable metallic stent. J Gastroenterol. 2008;43:637–40.
18. Tarantino I, Barresi L, Repici A, Traina M. EUS-guided biliary drainage: a case series. Endoscopy. 2008;40:336–9.
19. Itoi T, Itokawa F, Sofuni A, et al. Endoscopic ultrasound-guided choledochoduodenostomy in patients with failed endoscopic retrograde cholangiopancreatography. World J Gastroenterol. 2008;14:6078–82.
20. Horaguchi J, Fujita N, Noda Y, et al. Endosonography-guided biliary drainage in cases with difficult transpapillary endoscopic biliary drainage. Dig Endosc. 2009;21:239–44.
21. Hanada K, Iiboshi T, Ishii Y. Endoscopic ultrasound-guided choledochoduodenostomy for palliative biliary drainage in cases with inoperable pancreas head carcinoma. Dig Endosc. 2009;21(Suppl 1):S75–8.
22. Park DH, Koo JE, Oh J, et al. EUS-guided biliary drainage with one-step placement of a fully covered metal stent for malignant biliary obstruction: a prospective feasibility study. Am J Gastroenterol. 2009;104:2168–74.
23. Maranki J, Hernandez AJ, Arslan B, et al. Interventional endoscopic ultrasound-guided cholangiography: long-term experience of an emerging alternative to percutaneous transhepatic cholangiography. Endoscopy. 2009;41:532–8.
24. Artifon EL, Takada J, Okawa L, Moura EG, Sakai P. EUS-guided choledochoduodenostomy for biliary drainage in unresectable pancreatic cancer: a case series. JOP. 2010;11:597–600.
25. Eum J, Park DH, Ryu CH, et al. EUS-guided biliary drainage with a fully covered metal stent as a novel route for natural orifice transluminal endoscopic biliary interventions: a pilot study (with videos). Gastrointest Endosc. 2010;72:1279–84.
26. Hara K, Yamao K, Niwa Y, et al. Prospective clinical study of EUS-guided choledochoduodenostomy for malignant lower biliary tract obstruction. Am J Gastroenterol. 2011;106:1239–45.
27. Ramírez-Luna MA, Téllez-Ávila FI, Giovannini M, et al. Endoscopic ultrasound- guided biliodigestive drainage is a good alternative in patients with unresectable cancer. Endoscopy. 2011;43:826–30.
28. Park DH, Jang JW, Lee SS, et al. EUS-guided biliary drainage with transluminal stenting after failed ERCP: predictors of adverse events and long-term results. Gastrointest Endosc. 2011;74:1276–84.
29. Attasaranya S, Netinasunton N, Jongboonyanuparp T, et al. The spectrum of endoscopic ultrasound intervention in biliary diseases: a single center's experience in 31 cases. Gastroenterol Res Pract. 2012;2012:680753.
30. Kim TH, Kim SH, Oh HJ, Sohn YW, Lee SO. Endoscopic ultrasound-guided biliary drainage with placement of a fully covered metal stent for malignant biliary obstruction. World J Gastroenterol. 2012;18:2526–32.
31. Nicholson JA, Johnstone M, Raraty MG, Evans JC. Endoscopic ultrasound-guided choledocoduodenostomy as an alternative to percutaneous trans-hepatic cholangiography. HPB (Oxford). 2012;14:483–6.
32. Rebello C, Bordini A, Yoshida A, et al. A one-step procedure by using linear echoendoscope to perform EUS-guided choledochoduodenostomy and duodenal stenting in patients with irresectable periampullary cancer. Endosc Ultrasound. 2012;1:156–61.
33. Song TJ, Hyun YS, Lee SS, et al. Endoscopic ultrasound-guided choledochoduodenostomies with fully covered self-expandable metallic stents. World J Gastroenterol. 2012;18:4435–40.

34. Hara K, Yamao K, Hijioka S, et al. Prospective clinical study of endoscopic ultrasound-guided choledochoduodenostomy with direct metallic stent placement using a forward-viewing echo-endoscope. Endoscopy. 2013;45:392–6.
35. Prachayakul V, Aswakul P. A novel technique for endoscopic ultrasound-guided biliary drainage. World J Gastroenterol. 2013;19:4758–63.
36. Takada JAM, Artifon LA. EUS-guided biliary drainage for malignant biliary obstruction in patients with failed ERCP. J Interv Gastroenterol. 2013;3:76–81.
37. Artifon EL, Marson FP, Gaidhane M, Kahaleh M, Otoch JP. Hepaticogastrostomy or choledochoduodenostomy for distal malignant biliary obstruction after failed ERCP: is there any difference? Gastrointest Endosc. 2015;81:950–9.
38. Dhir V, Itoi T, Khashab MA, et al. Multicenter comparative evaluation of endoscopic placement of expandable metal stents for malignant distal common bile duct obstruction by ERCP or EUS-guided approach. Gastrointest Endosc. 2015;81:913–23.
39. Gupta K, Perez-Miranda M, Kahaleh M, et al. Endoscopic ultrasound-assisted bile duct access and drainage: multicenter, long-term analysis of approach, outcomes, and complications of a technique in evolution. J Clin Gastroenterol. 2014;48:80–7.
40. Hamada T, Isayama H, Nakai Y, et al. Transmural biliary drainage can be an alternative to transpapillary drainage in patients with an indwelling duodenal stent. Dig Dis Sci. 2014;59:1931–8.
41. Kawakubo K, Isayama H, Kato H, et al. Multicenter retrospective study of endoscopic ultrasound-guided biliary drainage for malignant biliary obstruction in Japan. J Hepatobiliary Pancreat Sci. 2014;21:328–34.
42. Song TJ, Lee SS, Park DH, Seo DW, Lee SK, Kim MH. Preliminary report on a new hybrid metal stent for EUS-guided biliary drainage (with videos). Gastrointest Endosc. 2014;80:707–11.
43. Bruckner S, Arlt A, Hampe J. Endoscopic ultrasound-guided biliary drainage using a lumen-apposing self-expanding metal stent: a case series. Endoscopy. 2015;47:858–61.
44. Poincloux L, Rouquette O, Buc E, et al. Endoscopic ultrasound-guided biliary drainage after failed ERCP: cumulative experience of 101 procedures at a single center. Endoscopy. 2015;47:794–801.
45. Artifon EL, Chaves DM, Ishioka S, et al. Echoguided hepatico-gastrostomy: a case report. Clinics (Sao Paulo). 2007;62:799–802.
46. Bories E, Pesenti C, Caillol F, Lopes C, Giovannini M. Transgastric endoscopic ultrasonography-guided biliary drainage: results of a pilot study. Endoscopy. 2007;39:287–91.
47. Will U, Thieme A, Fueldner F, et al. Treatment of biliary obstruction in selected patients by endoscopic ultrasonography (EUS)-guided transluminal biliary drainage. Endoscopy. 2007;39:292–5.
48. Chopin-Laly X, Ponchon T, Guibal A, Adham M. Endoscopic biliogastric stenting: a salvage procedure. Surgery. 2009;145:123.
49. Park DH, Song TJ, Eum J, et al. EUS-guided hepaticogastrostomy with a fully covered metal stent as the biliary diversion technique for an occluded biliary metal stent after a failed ERCP (with videos). Gastrointest Endosc. 2010;71:413–9.
50. Martins FP, Rossini LG, Ferrari AP. Migration of a covered metallic stent following endoscopic ultrasound-guided hepaticogastrostomy: fatal complication. Endoscopy. 2010;42(Suppl 2):E126–7.
51. Panpimanmas S, Ratanachuek T. Endoscopic ultrasound-guided hepaticogastrostomy for advanced cholangiocarcinoma after failed stenting by endoscopic retrograde cholangiopancreatography. Asian J Surg. 2013;36:154–8.
52. Park DH, Jeong SU, Lee BU, et al. Prospective evaluation of a treatment algorithm with enhanced guidewire manipulation protocol for EUS-guided biliary drainage after failed ERCP (with video). Gastrointest Endosc. 2013;78:91–101.
53. Park SJ, Choi JH, Park DH, et al. Expanding indication: EUS-guided hepaticoduodenostomy for isolated right intrahepatic duct obstruction (with video). Gastrointest Endosc. 2013;78:374–80.

54. Ogura T, Kurisu Y, Masuda D, et al. Novel method of endoscopic ultrasound-guided hepatico-gastrostomy to prevent stent dysfunction. J Gastroenterol Hepatol. 2014;29:1815–21.
55. Paik WH, Park DH, Choi JH, et al. Simplified fistula dilation technique and modified stent deployment maneuver for EUS-guided hepaticogastrostomy. World J Gastroenterol. 2014;20:5051–9.
56. Umeda J, Itoi T, Tsuchiya T, et al. A newly designed plastic stent for EUS-guided hepatico-gastrostomy: a prospective preliminary feasibility study (with videos). Gastrointest Endosc. 2015;82:390–6.

EUS-Guided Gallbladder Drainage

5

Anthony Yuen Bun Teoh and Shayan Irani

5.1 Introduction

EUS-guided gallbladder drainage (EUS-GBD) is an established treatment for acute cholecystitis in patients that are a high-risk for cholecystectomy [1]. It provides an alternative to percutaneous drainage and laparoscopic cholecystectomy in these patients. With the development of lumen apposing metal stents, the procedure is associated with high rates of technical and clinical success with low rates of adverse events [2]. In this chapter, an overview of the techniques and outcomes of EUS-GBD will be provided. Furthermore, subsequent management of the gallbladder pathology using peroral cholecystoscopy will be discussed.

5.2 Development of EUS-GBD

Percutaneous gallbladder drainage/cholecystosotomy (PT-GBD) is associated with a significant risk of tube-related morbidity ranging from 58.8 to 75% [3]. Furthermore, recurrent acute cholecystitis can occur in up to 15.4% of the patients after percutaneous drainage [4]. The dyscosmesis and discomfort of a percutaneous drain led to the development of endoscopic drainage options for the gallbladder.

Endoscopic gallbladder drainage can be achieved by a transpapillary or transmural approach [2, 5]. Transpapillary drainage is performed at endoscopic retrograde cholangiopancreatography (ERCP). The gallbladder is cannulated through the cystic duct, allowing placement of usually a single double pigtail plastic stent. However,

A. Y. B. Teoh (✉)
Department of Surgery, Prince of Wales Hospital, The Chinese University of Hong Kong, Shatin, Hong Kong
e-mail: anthonyteoh@surgery.cuhk.edu.hk

S. Irani
Department of Gastroenterology, Virginia Mason Medical Center, Seattle, WA, USA

P. Sharma, N. Reddy (eds.), *Innovations in Gastrointestinal Endoscopy*,
https://doi.org/10.1007/978-981-15-9247-8_5

negotiating the tortuous cystic duct and its obstructing pathology (stone, stricture or mass) is not always feasible. Thus, the reported technical and clinical success rates of this approach are lower than EUS-GBD (83% vs 93% and 93% vs 97%, respectively). Furthermore, transpapillary placement of the stent does not allow treatment of the gallstones, and the patients may require periodic exchange of the stent.

The transmural approach involves placing a stent from the stomach or duodenum into the gallbladder under EUS guidance. The first reported case of transmural endoscopic ultrasound-guided gallbladder drainage was in 2007 in a patient with unresectable hilar cholangiocarcinoma with acute cholecystitis. This was successfully performed with only a 7 Fr double pigtail plastic stent [6]. Thereafter, increasing reports of endoscopic gallbladder drainage have been described.

In its infancy, EUS-guided gallbladder drainage was often performed by placing a naso-gallbladder drain (ENGBD) [7, 8]. In a randomized trial, ENGBD was compared to transpapillary drainage. The overall technical success rates, clinical success rates, and procedural times were comparable. While, the post-procedural pain score was significantly higher in the ENGBD group (1.3 ± 1.1 vs 0.4 ± 0.8, respectively; $P < 0.001$). In another randomized study comparing ENGBD to percutaneous drainage (PT-GBD), both procedures showed similar technical and clinical success rate, complications and conversions to open cholecystectomy [9]. However, the median post-procedure pain score was significantly lower after ENGBD than after PTGBD (1 vs 5; $P < 0.001$). These studies showed that ENGBD was feasible and useful for treatment of acute cholecystitis. But the presence of naso-gallbladder drain was still uncomfortable and cumbersome to manage.

Subsequently, EUS-GBD was performed using metal stents. Initially, tubular biliary metal stents were used for drainage [10]. Although an improvement over plastic stents, tubular metal stents are not ideal either for transmural gallbladder drainage. These stents do not impart luminal apposition, and their lack of flanges increased the risk of migration. Furthermore, they are often too long, with a risk of the ends causing contralateral wall injury or occlusion. The advent of lumen apposing stents (LAMS) provided an ideal stent for EUS-GBD [11]. These stents have several design characteristics. Besides being short and bi-flanged, they are available in large diameters allowing passage of even larger gallstones or the endoscope as needed for cholecystoscopy [12]. There are currently three different LAMS designs available in Asia and Europe, but only one type available in the United States. These stents have different appearances and also, based on some early data, have different lumen appositional forces. This was demonstrated in an ex vivo experiment using different LAMS to create gastrogastrostomies, gastrojejunostomies, cholecystoduodenostomies, and cholecystogastrostomies [11]. LAMS with high lumen appositional forces should be used in non-adherent organs like the gallbladder and the duodenum or jejunum for EUS-GBD and EUS-gastroenterostomies. Over the last few years, there have now been several case-series and comparative trials of EUS-GBD vs. PTGBD using LAMS [13–18]. These outcomes will be discussed later in the chapter.

5.3 Indications for EUS-GBD

The indications for EUS-GBD are as follows:

- For gallbladder drainage in high surgical-risk patients with acute cholecystitis [1]
- To enable removing a percutaneous cholecystostomy by allowing internal drainage [18]
- For drainage of malignant biliary obstruction in patients with failed ERCP and EUS-guided biliary drainage [19].

5.4 Technique of EUS-GBD

There are two described approaches of performing EUS-GBD which is mostly dependent on whether the LAMS has a cautery-enhanced tip or not (Fig. 5.1). The non-cautery enhanced method has to be performed over a guidewire. This involves puncturing the gallbladder with a 19-gauge needle, followed by guidewire insertion, track dilation, and stent placement. The second technique is the direct method that requires a cautery-enhanced LAMS. Using a pure cutting current, the stent is

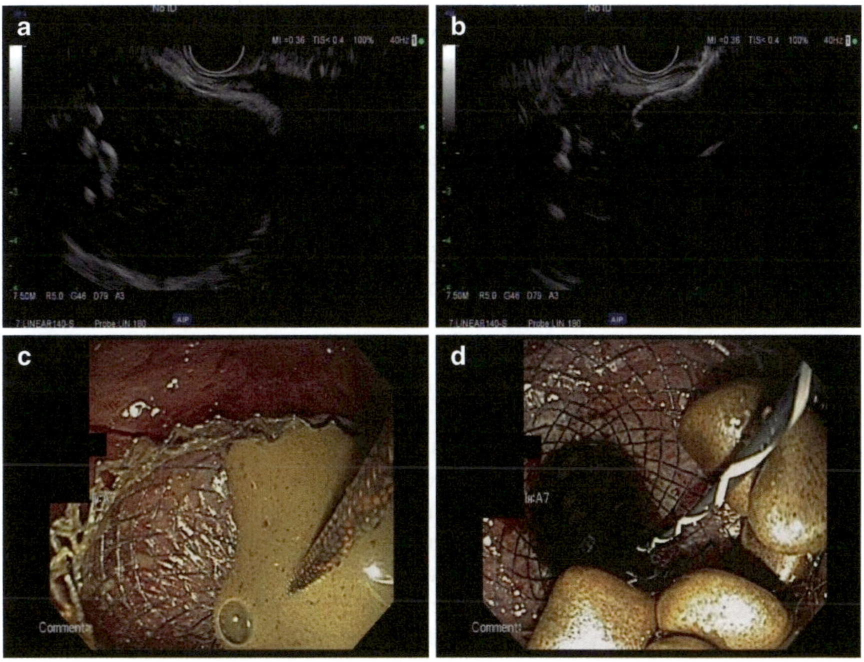

Fig. 5.1 Technical procedure of EUS-GBD. (**a**) EUS demonstrates gallbladder wall thickening with sludge and several shadowing calculi. (**b**) Gallbladder flange deployed under EUS guidance and pulled back snug. (**c**) Duodenal flange deployed revealing purulent bile. (**d**) Several cholesterol stones emerge through the stent and several more seen in the gallbladder

inserted through the duodenal/gastric wall into the gallbladder without the need for a guidewire. The gallbladder flange is then deployed, the stent pulled back snug followed by the deployment of the duodenal/gastric flange [20]. In patients with gallbladders that are contracted and fibrotic, with existing percutaneous drains, or in difficult scope positions or visualization, we tend to prefer an over-the-wire technique which provides some security of access in the rare case of stent misdeployment. The direct method is often employed in patients with acute cholecystitis, where the gallbladder is distended and easy to puncture. Although, in a comparative study, no significant differences in adverse events were observed whether drainage was from the stomach or duodenum [13], it is our preference to perform EUS-GBD when possible from the duodenum. This seems to reduce the risk of food causing stent occlusion, which is more commonly seen in the pre-pyloric antrum.

5.5 Outcomes of EUS-GBD

EUS-GBD boasts very high technical and clinical success rates ranging from 90 to 98.7% and 89 to 98.4%, respectively [16, 17, 21, 22]. EUS-GBD is currently most commonly performed as a definitive treatment for acute cholecystitis in high surgical-risk patients. Adverse events (AE) are infrequent and range from 4.8 to 22%. These include bleeding, recurrent cholecystitis, stent migration, and occlusion. Given the patient population tends to have multiple comorbidities (given non-surgical candidacy), care should be taken to minimize these as far as possible.

Four studies to date have compared EUS-GBD to PT-GBD [13–15, 23]. Three studies used LAMS and one study used biliary fully-covered self-expandable metal stents (FCSEMS). All studies reported comparable technical and clinical success rates between the two procedures. Teoh et al. reported significantly lower 1-year adverse events rates ($P < 0.001$) and readmission rates for re-intervention ($P < 0.001$) in the EUS-GBD group. The majority of adverse events in PT-GBD group were due to tube-related problems including leak, obstruction, or infection. This resulted in a significantly higher readmission and re-intervention rates in two studies. In the other two studies, similar 30-day adverse events rates were noted, but lower re-intervention rates were again noted in the EUS-GBD group. Irani et al. also reported lower post-procedural pain scores in the EUS-GBD group. In another study comparing EUS-GBD to PT-GBD in patients with acute cholecystitis secondary to malignant cystic duct obstruction, no difference in success rates and adverse events were observed. However, a shorter post-intervention hospital stay was noted in the EUS-GBD group [23]. Finally, a meta-analysis of comparative studies concluded that EUS-GBD is a promising alternative to PT-GBD in high-risk patients with acute cholecystitis, with equivalent success rates, improved pain scores, and lower re-intervention rates, with a lower morbidity than percutaneous drainage [3].

5.6 Follow-up After EUS-GBD

After successful resolution of cholecystitis with EUS-GBD, there are two options for stent management. One of the authors routinely performs follow-up peroral cholecystoscopy at 1 month after initial drainage [12]. The aim is to achieve stone clearance if they have not already passed spontaneously and to exchange the LAMS for double pigtail plastic stent to maintain the fistula (these being less traumatic than a LAMS long term). The technical success rate of cholecystoscopy has been 93.1%. Overall stone clearance rate was 88% after a mean (SD) number of 1.25 (0.46) sessions of cholecystoscopy. Fifty-six percent of patients had spontaneous stone passage and the remaining patients required stone removal. This can be done with stone-retrieval baskets and laser lithotripsy when needed.

The second option of leaving the LAMS in permanently is often employed in the very frail patients and in those who do not want to undergo a second procedure. In a study reporting the long-term outcomes of EUS-GBD [17], late adverse events were low at 7.1% and the 3-year stent patency was 86%, making this a reasonable approach as well.

5.7 Peroral Cholecystoscopy and Advanced Gallbladder Interventions

After EUS-GBD, the large diameter stents allow access for endoscopic assessment and interventions in the gallbladder [12, 24]. This has made cholecystoscopy an emerging option for patients. In the only study to date reporting this technique, magnifying endoscopy was performed in 10 patients (Fig. 5.2). In a patient with incidental gallbladder cancer, confocal endomicroscopy and EUS were performed. In vivo endocytoscopy was also possible and showed a layer of regular columnar cells with finger-like projections compatible with normal gallbladder mucosa. Laser

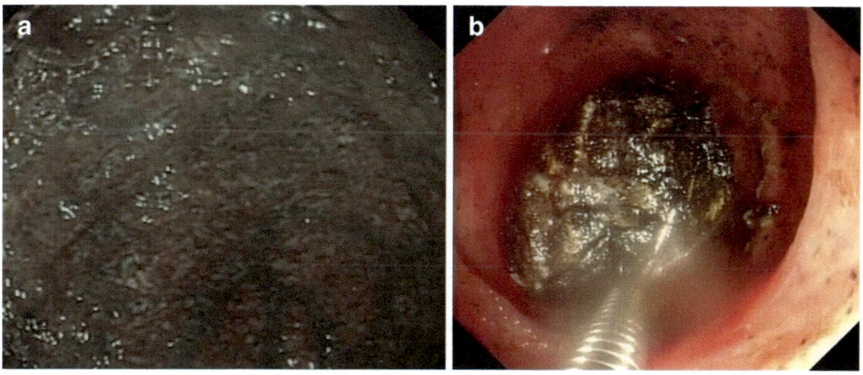

Fig. 5.2 Peroral cholecystoscopy after EUS-GBD. (**a**) Narrow band imaging of the gallbladder mucosa. (**b**) Basket mechanical lithotripsy of a gallstone during cholecystoscopy

lithotripsy was performed in a patient with very hard stones that failed to fragment with mechanical lithotripsy. One patient underwent polypectomy demonstrating a final pathology of inflammatory polyps.

5.8 Conclusion

In conclusion, EUS-GBD is an attractive option for the treatment of acute cholecystitis in the high surgical-risk patient. It has been shown to have similar technical and clinical success rates to PT-GBD but with benefits of fewer re-interventions and maybe fewer adverse events and lower post-procedure pain. It also allows for cholecystoscopy and advanced gallbladder interventions. A completed randomized study (Clinicaltrials.gov identifier: NCT02212717) is expected to provide further evidence for its established role in the management of cholecystitis.

References

1. Mori Y, Itoi T, Baron TH, et al. Tokyo guidelines 2018: management strategies for gallbladder drainage in patients with acute cholecystitis (with videos). J Hepatobiliary Pancreat Sci. 2018;25:87–95.
2. Anderloni A, Buda A, Vieceli F, et al. Endoscopic ultrasound-guided transmural stenting for gallbladder drainage in high-risk patients with acute cholecystitis: a systematic review and pooled analysis. Surg Endosc. 2016;30:5200–8.
3. Ahmed O, Rogers AC, Bolger JC, et al. Meta-analysis of outcomes of endoscopic ultrasound-guided gallbladder drainage versus percutaneous cholecystostomy for the management of acute cholecystitis. Surg Endosc. 2018;32:1627–35.
4. McKay A, Abulfaraj M, Lipschitz J. Short- and long-term outcomes following percutaneous cholecystostomy for acute cholecystitis in high-risk patients. Surg Endosc. 2012;26:1343–51.
5. Khan MA, Atiq O, Kubiliun N, et al. Efficacy and safety of endoscopic gallbladder drainage in acute cholecystitis: is it better than percutaneous gallbladder drainage? Gastrointest Endosc. 2017;85:76–87.e3.
6. Baron TH, Topazian MD. Endoscopic transduodenal drainage of the gallbladder: implications for endoluminal treatment of gallbladder disease. Gastrointest Endosc. 2007;65:735–7.
7. Kwan V, Eisendrath P, Antaki F, et al. EUS-guided cholecystenterostomy: a new technique (with videos). Gastrointest Endosc. 2007;66:582–6.
8. Lee SS, Park DH, Hwang CY, et al. EUS-guided transmural cholecystostomy as rescue management for acute cholecystitis in elderly or high-risk patients: a prospective feasibility study. Gastrointest Endosc. 2007;66:1008–12.
9. Jang JW, Lee SS, Song TJ, et al. Endoscopic ultrasound-guided transmural and percutaneous transhepatic gallbladder drainage are comparable for acute cholecystitis. Gastroenterology. 2012;142:805–11.
10. Widmer J, Singhal S, Gaidhane M, et al. Endoscopic ultrasound-guided endoluminal drainage of the gallbladder. Dig Endosc. 2014;26:525–31.
11. Teoh AY, Ng EK, Chan SM, et al. Ex vivo comparison of the lumen-apposing properties of EUS-specific stents (with video). Gastrointest Endosc. 2016;84:62–8.
12. Chan SM, Teoh AY, Yip HC, et al. Feasibility of per-oral cholecystoscopy and advanced gallbladder interventions after EUS-guided gallbladder stenting (with video). Gastrointest Endosc. 2017;85(6):1225–32.

13. Teoh AY, Serna C, Penas I, et al. Endoscopic ultrasound-guided gallbladder drainage reduces adverse events compared with percutaneous cholecystostomy in patients who are unfit for cholecystectomy. Endoscopy. 2017;49:130–8.
14. Irani S, Ngamruengphong S, Teoh A, et al. Similar efficacies of endoscopic ultrasound gallbladder drainage with a lumen-apposing metal stent versus percutaneous transhepatic gallbladder drainage for acute cholecystitis. Clin Gastroenterol Hepatol. 2017;15:738–45.
15. Tyberg A, Saumoy M, Sequeiros EV, et al. EUS-guided versus percutaneous gallbladder drainage: isn't it time to convert? J Clin Gastroenterol. 2018;52(1):79–84.
16. Dollhopf M, Larghi A, Will U, et al. EUS-guided gallbladder drainage in patients with acute cholecystitis and high surgical risk using an electrocautery-enhanced lumen-apposing metal stent device. Gastrointest Endosc. 2017;86(4):636–43.
17. Choi JH, Lee SS, Choi JH, et al. Long-term outcomes after endoscopic ultrasonography-guided gallbladder drainage for acute cholecystitis. Endoscopy. 2014;46:656–61.
18. Law R, Grimm IS, Stavas JM, et al. Conversion of percutaneous cholecystostomy to internal transmural gallbladder drainage using an endoscopic ultrasound-guided, lumen-apposing metal stent. Clin Gastroenterol Hepatol. 2016;14:476–80.
19. Imai H, Kitano M, Omoto S, et al. EUS-guided gallbladder drainage for rescue treatment of malignant distal biliary obstruction after unsuccessful ERCP. Gastrointest Endosc. 2016;84:147–51.
20. Teoh AY, Binmoeller KF, Lau JY. Single-step EUS-guided puncture and delivery of a lumen-apposing stent for gallbladder drainage using a novel cautery-tipped stent delivery system. Gastrointest Endosc. 2014;80:1171.
21. Walter D, Teoh AY, Itoi T, et al. EUS-guided gall bladder drainage with a lumen-apposing metal stent: a prospective long-term evaluation. Gut. 2016;65:6–8.
22. Kahaleh M, Perez-Miranda M, Artifon EL, et al. International collaborative study on EUS-guided gallbladder drainage: are we ready for prime time? Dig Liver Dis. 2016;48:1054–7.
23. Choi JH, Kim HW, Lee JC, et al. Percutaneous transhepatic versus EUS-guided gallbladder drainage for malignant cystic duct obstruction. Gastrointest Endosc. 2017;85:357–64.
24. Teoh AY, Chan AW, Chiu PW, et al. In vivo appearances of gallbladder carcinoma under magnifying endoscopy and probe-based confocal laser endomicroscopy after endosonographic gallbladder drainage. Endoscopy. 2014;46(Suppl 1 UCTN):E13–4.

Endoscopic Management of GERD

6

Pradev Inavolu, Nitin Jagtap, and Rakesh Kalapala

Gastroesophageal reflux disease (GERD) is a chronic condition associated with regurgitation of gastric contents, including gastric acid, pepsin, and pancreatobiliary secretions, into the esophagus causing symptoms [1]. It is a common clinical problem. In lifetime, 30–40% of the US population is affected by GERD. Worldwide, 5–25% of the population has symptoms of GERD in a 3-month period [2]. It can lead to negative impact on health-related quality of life [3–5]. GERD can lead to various complications which are erosive esophagitis, peptic strictures, Barrett's metaplasia, or subsequently adenocarcinoma [6].

6.1 Definition of Refractory GERD

Proton pump inhibitors (PPIs) are the most effective and safe therapeutic option for GERD. However, up to 15% of patients with erosive esophagitis (EE) are refractory for PPI. In subgroup of GERD patients with especially those with typical or extra-esophageal symptoms respond well to twice daily PPIs dosing. Esophageal acid exposure is a dose-dependent phenomenon, and increasing a PPI dose will normalize the pH parameters [7].

The American Gastroenterological Association (AGA) recommended twice-daily dosing for individuals with an inadequate response to once-daily dosing. AGA defines treatment failure as inadequate symptoms control to twice-daily PPI [8]. The concept of acid suppression in management of GERD has resulted from misconception that GERD is associated with increased esophageal exposure to only gastric acid, ignoring other components of refluxed gastric juice such as pepsin and pancreatobiliary secretion or the so-called non-acidic reflux [9]. Nonerosive reflux disease that is resistant to twice daily PPI might be attributed to the reflux of noxious substances other than hydrochloric acid such as bile acids [10]. A study has

P. Inavolu · N. Jagtap · R. Kalapala (✉)
AIG Hospitals, Hyderabad, India

P. Sharma, N. Reddy (eds.), *Innovations in Gastrointestinal Endoscopy*,
https://doi.org/10.1007/978-981-15-9247-8_6

Table 6.1 Reasons for poor response to PPI therapy

Reasons for treatment failure:
(a) Inadequate acid suppression: • Non-compliance to PPI • Genetic variation • *H. pylori* infection • Zollinger-Ellison syndrome
(b) Inadequate duration of treatment: • Nocturnal acid breakthrough • Non acid reflux • Esophageal hypersensitivity
(c) Other non-GERD-related conditions: • Functional dyspepsia • Rumination syndrome • Aerophagia • Achalasia cardia • Eosinophilic esophagitis

shown that 76% of patients with symptomatic reflux had abnormal esophageal exposure to both acid and bile reflux, and there was simultaneous acid and bile reflux in 70–91% of reflux episodes and in some severe forms had increasingly higher (89–100%) exposure [11]. Treatment failure might be explained by other pathological mechanism such as (Table 6.1) visceral hypersensitivity, bile reflux, delayed gastric emptying, eosinophilic esophagitis, and psychological comorbidity [12–15].

6.2 Approach to Refractory GERD

In patients with refractory GERD without alarm symptoms, first we need to consider appropriate dosing and compliance to PPI therapy. Further diagnostic testing is indicated if patients remain symptomatic on high-dose PPI (twice daily PPI). About 20–30% of erosive esophagitis (EE) and 10–40% of nonerosive reflux disease (NERD) patients do not respond to PPI therapy. EGD is important in patients with alarm symptoms despite therapy to rule out complications such as Barrett's esophagus [16].

The aim of EGD is to assess the presence or absence of erosive esophagitis and to exclude other non-GERD-related possibilities [17]. The erosive esophagitis on endoscopy is having high specificity for diagnosis of GERD. In nearly 90% of patient with refractory GERD, diagnostic endoscopy is normal [17], which makes its management challenging. NERD patients refractory to PPI need further evaluation (Fig. 6.1), which include prolonged pH monitoring with impedance testing, esophageal high-resolution manometry, and gastric function testing, and it is important to rule out non-acid GER, functional heartburn, or other non-GERD diseases such as achalasia or gastroparesis.

The ambulatory pH monitoring is commonly indicated for poor response to an empiric PPI trial (refractory symptoms) in patients with typical or atypical (extraesophageal) symptoms [18]. Esophageal pH monitoring can provide quantification

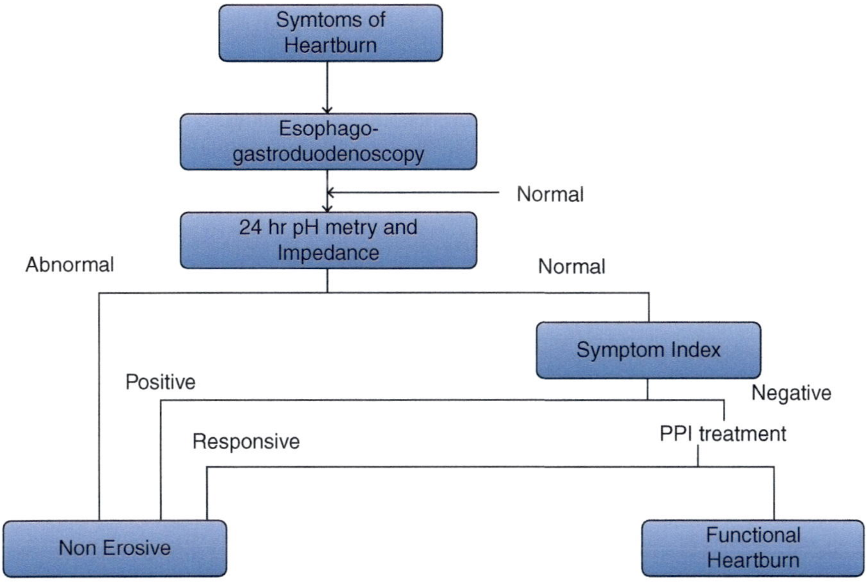

Fig. 6.1 Diagnostic approach of GERD

gastro-esophageal refluxate and evaluation of the relationship between symptoms and reflux events [19–24]. The *symptom index (SI)*, and *symptom association probability (SAP) are commonly used.* These symptom indices are important components for the assessment of the relationship between reflux episode and symptoms experienced by the patient. They are calculated using the data obtained by pH monitoring and using the patient's diary of symptoms recorded by the patient by pushing a button whenever he/she experiences any symptoms related to GERD. Though there are some conflicting evidences questioning the reproducibility and accuracy of SI and SAP in refractory GERD [25] (Fig. 6.2).

Daily use of PPIs is generally effective in the majority of patients with refractory GERD. However, up to 40% patients report persisting symptoms [26, 27]. Laparoscopic Anti-Reflux Surgery (LARS) is an effective alternative to chronic PPI use. Both surgeon and patients are reluctant for LARS because of invasive nature of therapy [28]. LARS might be associated with new onset short- and long-term dysphagia, gas-bloat syndrome, and bowel dysfunction [29]. To mitigate this problem, there is a strong desire to develop less invasive techniques which can solve the drawbacks of medical therapy and avoid the complications of LARS. Few endoscopic techniques/devices have been evaluated as alternative treatment options in the past; however, due to ineffective and safety concern, they were withdrawn from the market (Fig. 6.3).

The devices for endoscopic treatment of refractory GERD are as follows:

- Transoral incisionless fundoplication device (EsophyX®, Endo Gastric Solutions, Redmond, WA),

- Radiofrequency energy delivery system (Stretta®, Mederi Therapeutics, Inc., Greenwich, CT),
- Ultrasonic Surgical Endostapler device (MUSE™, Medigus, Omer, Israel),
- GERDx™ (G-SURG GmbH, Seeon-Seebruck, Germany), a recently launched endoscopic plication device. The interim report on short-term outcomes of GERDx™ showed improvement in objective reflux parameters and quality of life [30].

6.3 Endoscopic Anti-Reflux Therapies

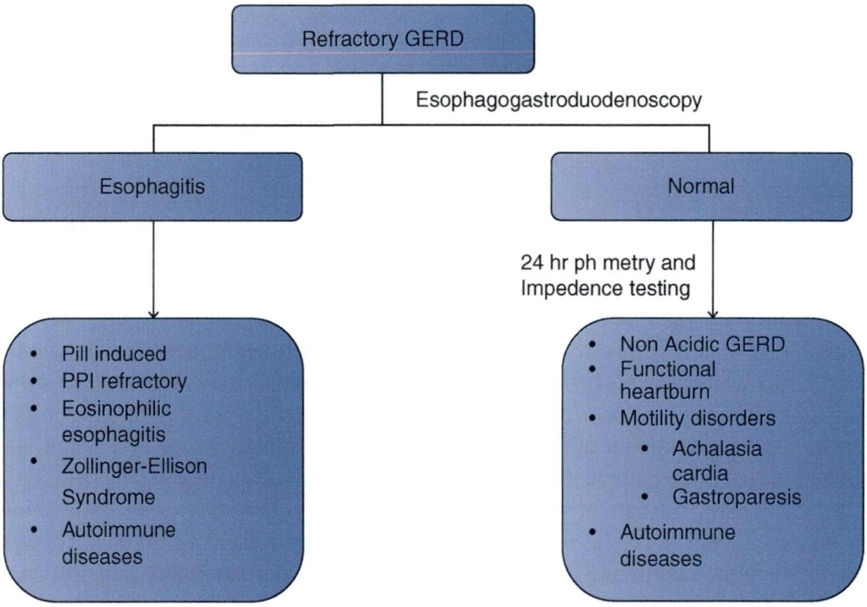

Fig. 6.2 Management algorithm for refractory GERD

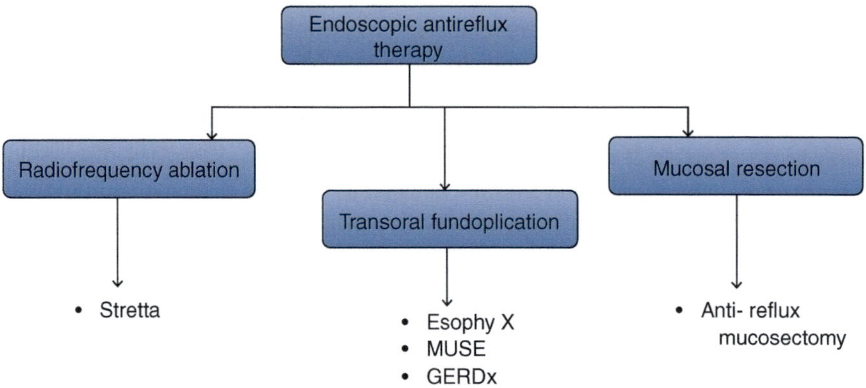

Fig. 6.3 Endoscopic anti-reflux therapies

6.4 Radiofrequency Ablation

The Stretta system (Mederi Therapeutics, Norwalk, CT, USA) apply the radiofrequency energy using a needle balloon catheter system to the LES muscle and gastric cardia. The catheter is rotated, and linear position of the balloon assembly system is changed (in relation to Z line) and multiple applications (up to 14) are delivered. The low power (5 W) energy with a thermocouple is delivered to avoid of high temperatures at muscularis (>85 °C) and mucosal (>50 °C). Regular irrigation is done to prevent injury to the mucosa (Fig. 6.4).

It is proposed that hypertrophy of the muscularis propria after RFA reduces transient LES relaxations [31, 32]. Fibrosis at the gastroesophageal junction (GEJ) was also seen after RFA. However, reduction GEJ compliance after RFA was noted, and it was normalized on administration of sildenafil, suggesting against fibrosis [33]. Multiple RCTs and a systemic review has established efficacy and durability of therapeutic response with RFA in patients with refractory GERD [34–39]. The 10-year follow-up data showed 72% normalization of GERD health-related quality of life (GERD-HRQL) and more than 50% reduction in PPI use in 64% of patients. Barrett's metaplasia regression was observed in 85% patients [38].

RFA showed significant improvement in heartburn scores and GERD-HRQL [39]. There was reduction in esophageal acid exposure time (EAET) and improvement De-Meester score of 44.4–28.5 ($p = 0.007$) [39]. The Society of American Gastrointestinal and Endoscopic Surgeons guidelines advocate the use of RFA in selected patients with GERD [40]. A recent meta-analysis of four RCTs showed no difference (in terms of EAET, LES pressure, ability to stop PPIs, or HRQL) in Stretta versus sham or PPIs in patients with GERD [41]. This may be due to very stringent criteria of pH normalization (pH <4 exposure time <4%) which is not an achievable goal even in successfully treated PPIs group [42]. Studies comparing RFA and ARS (laparoscopic Toupet fundoplication) showed varied results [43–46]. There are no RCTs comparing both.

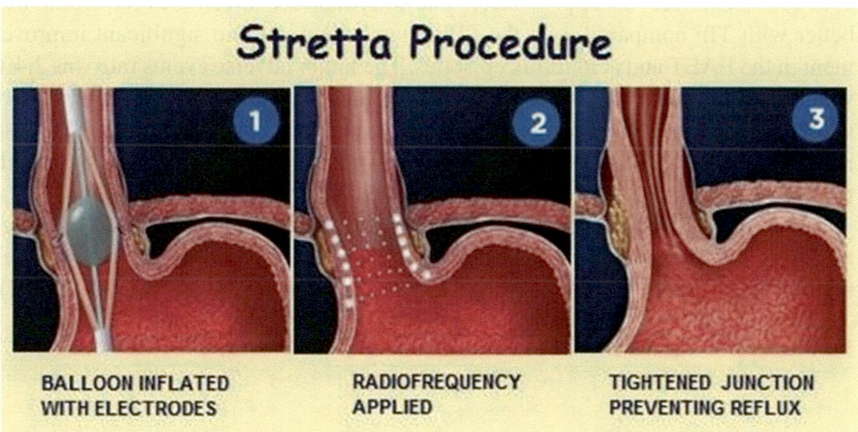

Fig. 6.4 Stretta procedure

Stretta (over other EARMs) can be performed under conscious sedation as a day care procedure, also it does not hamper subsequent therapy if indicated. More robust evidence for safety and efficacy is available compared to other endoscopic therapies. However, wide response rate (16–86%) and inadequate improvement in objective parameters like normalization of EAET are major drawbacks of Stretta [37]. On long-term follow-up, complete PPI cessation was achieved in 40% of patients [38]. RFA therapy is not suitable for patients with large hiatal hernia and severe esophagitis. Minor adverse event like chest pain in 50%, transient fever, and esophageal ulcerations are described. Inadvertent vagal nerve injury may be presumably the rarely reported adverse event of gastroparesis [47].

6.5 Transoral Incisionless Fundoplication

TIF is a minimally invasive procedure performed under general anesthesia which has undergone several modifications since its introduction, similar steps as ARS are performed. TIF procedure creates a valve of 2–4 cm in length and >270° circumferential wrap to reduce a hiatal hernia (≤2 cm). A fundoplication device (EsophyX; EndoGastric Solutions, Redmond, WA, USA) is gently introduced into the stomach under visualization of an endoscope. The device is retroflexed, and under the vision, a helical retractor is engaged into the tissue slightly distal to the Z line. The gastric fundus is folded up around the distal esophagus with the help of the tissue mold and chassis of the device. Later, an integrated suction apparatus is used to grasp the distal esophagus, to position it below the diaphragm. The apposed layers of esophageal and gastric fundus are anchored using H-shaped polypropylene fasteners. Further, these steps are repeated to obtain a full thickness, partial circumference, and gastroesophageal fundoplication (Fig. 6.5). Therefore about 20 fasteners are implanted during the procedure to obtain this valve.

The efficacy of TIF is reported in RCTs and systemic analysis [48–53]. In a systemic review, the pooled relative risk of response rate to TIF versus PPIs/sham was 2.44 (95% CI, 1.25–4.79; $p < 0.01$). The total number of refluxes reduction was better with TIF compared with the PPIs/sham group with no significant improvement in the EAET and acid reflux episodes. The major adverse events rate was 2.4% which include gastrointestinal perforation and bleeding [53]. The long-term follow-up study of 6 years showed cessation of PPIs or 50% or more reduction in dose noted in 87.8% and 84.4% at 2 and 3 years, respectively, with sustained response till the end of follow-up [54]. In same study, 33% were off PPI at 6 years [54].

TIF with ARS (Nissen and Toupet fundoplication) are equally effective in reduction in symptom frequency and severity with significantly shorter procedure times and hospital stay in TIF group [55]. GE junction morphology (Hill grade I to II),

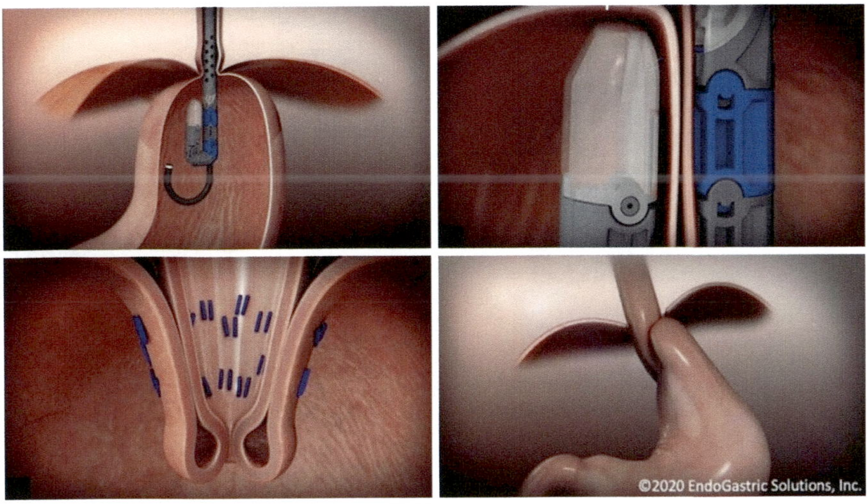

Fig. 6.5 Transoral incisionless fundoplication (TIF)

small (≤2 cm) or absent hiatal hernia, normal esophageal body motility, number of fasteners deployed during the procedure, persistence of typical symptoms on PPIs (GERD HRQL score ≥ 15), and an objectively confirmed diagnosis of GERD are predictors of better outcome [54, 56]. TIF is a less invasive outpatient procedure with fewer adverse events when compared to ARS, and revision ARS can be performed if needed [57]. Major adverse events with TIF are rare and include bleeding, perforation, and pneumothorax [58]. TIF showed encouraging results regarding symptom response and safety profile.

6.6 Medigus Ultrasonic Surgical Endostapler

The MUSE (Medigus Ltd., Omer, Israel) is a stapling device for transoral partial fundoplication [59, 60]. The device consists of a flexible endoscope, an endostapler, video camera, and an ultrasound transducer. The procedure is performed in retroflexion in the stomach; the device is withdrawn to the stapling level, which is usually 3 cm above the Z line. The stapler is then fired under the guidance of ultrasonic gap finder. The process is repeated until formation of a flap similar to laparoscopic fundoplication [59, 60] (Fig. 6.6).

In a multicenter study (n = 66 patients) with MUSE, there was a significant improvement in GERD-HRQL score in 73% of patients at 6 months. Approximately

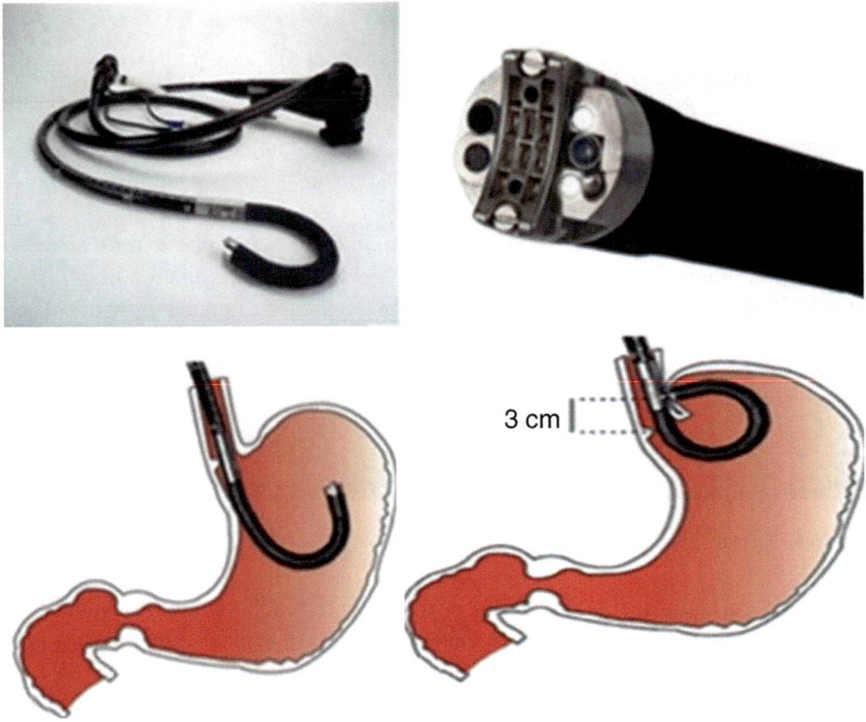

Fig. 6.6 Medigus ultrasonic surgical endostapler above the GE junction [61]

65% of patients could be completely off PPIs, and significant reduction in PPI dosage was observed in patients who continued PPIs after procedure. EAET showed a reduction at 6 months [59]. Two (of the initial 24 patients) serious adverse events were reported, including empyema/pneumothorax and upper gastrointestinal hemorrhage. No serious adverse events in the subsequent patient after modification of technique and stapling device. At 4-year follow-up, 69.4% were off PPIs after the TIF procedure. A significant reduction in GERD-HRQL scores and the daily dose PPI were observed [60]. In spite of encouraging emerging data with MUSE, long-term data is still limited. The ideal stapling site is not yet well established in vivo. In an ex vivo study the ideal stapling site was at 3 cm.

6.7 Endoscopic Full Thickness Plication (EFTP)

The procedure of EFTP has undergone several modifications since its introduction for treatment of GERD. Initially single suture was placed below gastro-esophageal junction, but, the results after single suture were not impressive as it might not have created an effective plication [62]. With modification multiple plications implants were deployed to achieve a robust and effective anti-reflux valve [63–65]. Initial

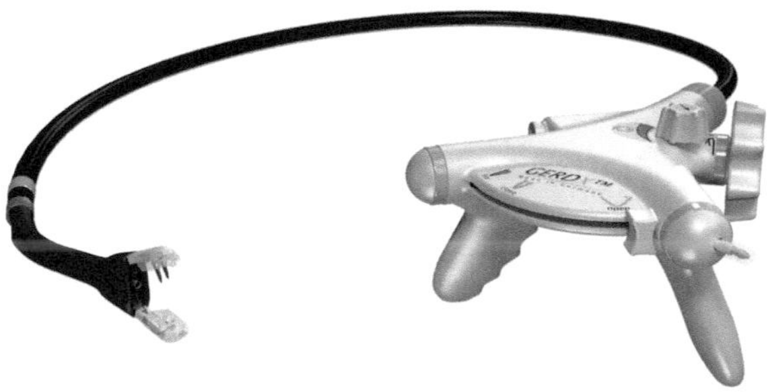

Fig. 6.7 GERDx

studies of EFTP were performed with the Plicator device (Ethicon Endo-surgery, Somerville, NJ, USA), which is not available commercially. A new device from a different manufacturer (GERDx System; G-SURG GmbH, Seeon-Seebruck, Germany) was introduced for full thickness plication (Fig. 6.7).

Prospective study of 36 patients with one or more plication implants showed symptoms improvement in 92%, and 89% of patients could be taken off PPIs at 1-year follow-up. It showed significant reduction in EAET [63]. A multicenter study showed more than 50% improvement in GERD-HRQL in 75% patients, and 70% of patients were taken off daily PPIs at 6 months. This improvement is maintained at 1-year follow-up [64, 65]. Post-procedure adverse events were minor that include abdominal pain, shoulder, and chest pain, with no long-term adverse events reported.

6.8 Anti-Reflux Mucosectomy

The ARMS procedure is based on the concept of natural healing after mucosal resection which will result in scar formation, sequentially leading to remodeling of gastric cardia flap valve; consequently, reducing reflux episodes. ARMS procedure was first performed almost 15 years ago; the data of the first series was published recently [66, 67].

Technically, ARMS involves gastric mucosal resection for about 2 cm and esophageal mucosa for about 1 cm in crescentic fashion [67]. After marking the field of resection with an electrocautery knife, submucosal injection by a solution of saline mixed with indigo-carmine dye is done. Then mucosal resection is performed along the lesser curvature; a gap equal to twice the scope diameter is left un-resected along the greater curvature side to avoid stricture formation. Hemostasis can be achieved by coagrasper (Fig. 6.8).

A pilot study ($n = 10$ patients) has shown reduction in EAET and improvement in flap valve grade, and PPI were discontinued in all patients after ARMS therapy [66]. ARMS procedure does not require any special devices or endoprostheses. There is need to establish amount of mucosal resection for adequate response in long term. Also, healing is natural and unpredictable event. Patients with hiatal hernia of more than 2 cm (large) are not ideal candidates for this procedure.

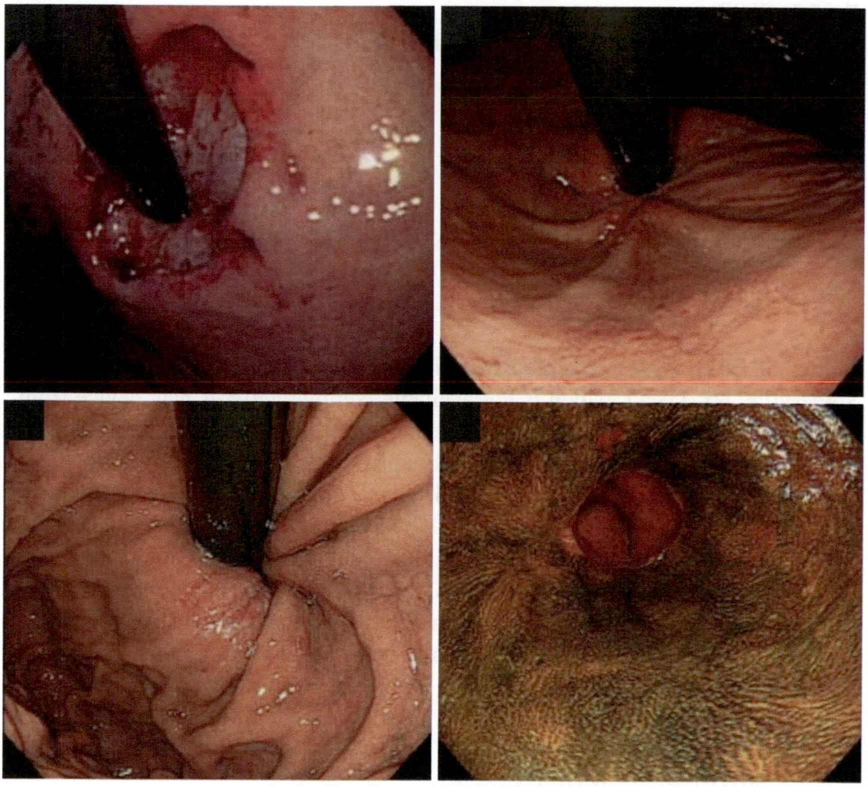

Fig. 6.8 ARMS - Anti Reflux Mucosectomy

6.9 EARMs: Strengths and Shortcomings

EARMs are emerging and a promising therapeutic option for refractory GERD which is minimally invasive. Compared to conventional surgery, endoscopic therapies have reduced hospital stay and fewer adverse events. Long term follow up data on Stretta (RFA) and emerging data on TIF, GERD-X and MUSE (Fundoplication techniques) show sustained treatment response.

Limitations

1. These devices have been tried in selected subgroup of patients with small hiatus hernia, minimal esophageal inflammation.
2. Although symptom response is reasonably good, objective improvement of impendence pH-metry parameters is less impressive. The available data suggests EARMs do reduce EAET, but often do not normalize. Normalization of EAET is an arduous goal to achieve, but cannot be disregarded due to potential risk of Barrett's esophagitis and esophageal adenocarcinoma. Similarly, there is

reduction in need for PPI but not its complete elimination in significant number of patients after endoscopic therapy.

3. Insufficient long-term data with some of the recently introduced EARMs and lack of comparative studies between different endoscopic modalities. Therefore, the better EARM procedure is not determined but with the long-term follow-up results of Randomized Control Trials from TIF and GERD-X devices will show the way forward for proper selection of the patients.

Procedure / Variable	Radiofrequency ablation (RFA-Stretta)	Transoral incisionless fundoplication (TIF)	Medigus ultrasonic surgical endostapler (MUSE)
Cessation (dose reduction) of PPI (treatment response)	16–80% [33, 34]	32–82% [53]	65% (83.8%—Dose reduction) [58, 59]
Sustained treatment response	41% at 10 years [37]	36% at 6 years [52]	69% at 4 years—Dose reduction [59]
Esophageal acid exposure—Normal	5–75% [33, 36]	37–89% [52]	37.1% [59]
Major adverse events	Aspiration pneumonia, gastroparesis [33, 35]	Bleeding, perforation, pneumothorax [53]	Bleeding, pneumothorax, pneumomediastinum [59]

References

1. Armstrong D. A critical assessment of the current status of non-erosive reflux disease. Digestion. 2008;78(Suppl. 1):46–54.
2. Katz PO. Lessons learned from intragastric pH monitoring. J Clin Gastroenterol. 2001;33(2):107–13.
3. Tack J, Becher A, Mulligan C, Johnson DA. Systematic review: the burden of disruptive gastro-oesophageal reflux disease on health-related quality of life. Aliment Pharmacol Ther. 2012;35(11):1257–66.
4. Toghanian S, Wahlqvist P, Johnson DA, Bolge SC, Liljas B. The burden of disrupting gastro-oesophageal reflux disease. Clin Drug Investig. 2010;30(3):167–78.
5. Williams JG, Roberts SE, Ali MF, Cheung WY, Cohen DR, Demery G, Edwards A, Greer M, Hellier MD, Hutchings HA, Ip B. Gastroenterology Services in the UK. The burden of disease, and the organisation and delivery of services for gastrointestinal and liver disorders: a review of the evidence. Gut. 2007;56(Suppl 1):1–13.
6. DiPalma JA. Management of severe gastroesophageal reflux disease. J Clin Gastroenterol. 2001;32(1):19–26.
7. Charbel S, Khandwala F, Vaezi MF. The role of esophageal pH monitoring in symptomatic patients on PPI therapy. Am J Gastroenterol. 2005;100(2):283–9.
8. Kahrilas PJ, Shaheen NJ, Vaezi MF. American Gastroenterological Association medical position statement on the management of gastroesophageal reflux disease. Gastroenterology. 2008;135(4):1383–91.

9. Oh DS, Hagen JA, Fein M, Bremner CG, Dunst CM, DeMeester SR, Lipham J, DeMeester TR. The impact of reflux composition on mucosal injury and esophageal function. J Gastrointest Surg. 2006;10(6):787–97.
10. McQuaid KR, Laine L, Fennerty MB, Souza R, Spechler SJ. Systematic review: the role of bile acids in the pathogenesis of gastro-oesophageal reflux disease and related neoplasia. Aliment Pharmacol Ther. 2011;34(2):146–65.
11. Vaezi MF, Richter JE. Role of acid and duodenogastroesophageal reflux in gastroesophageal reflux disease. Gastroenterology. 1996;111(5):1192–9.
12. Bredenoord AJ, Smout AJ. Refractory gastrooesophageal reflux disease. Eur J Gastroenterol Hepatol. 2008;20(3):217–23.
13. DeVault KR. The role of acid suppression in patients with non-erosive reflux disease or functional heartburn. Aliment Pharmacol Ther. 2006;23:33–9.
14. Iwakiri K, Kawami N, Sano H, Tanaka Y, Umezawa M, Kotoyori M, Hoshihara Y, Sakamoto C. Acid and non-acid reflux in Japanese patients with non-erosive reflux disease with persistent reflux symptoms, despite taking a double-dose of proton pump inhibitor: a study using combined pH-impedance monitoring. J Gastroenterol. 2009;44(7):708–12.
15. Fass R. Proton-pump inhibitor therapy in patients with gastro-oesophageal reflux disease. Drugs. 2007;67(11):1521–30.
16. Vaezi MF. Atypical manifestations of gastroesophageal reflux disease. Medscape Gen Med. 2005;7(4):25.
17. Richter JE. How to manage refractory GERD. Nat Clin Pract Gastroenterol Hepatol. 2007;4(12):658–64.
18. Hong SK, Vaezi MF. Gastroesophageal reflux monitoring: pH (catheter and capsule) and impedance. Gastrointest Endosc Clin N Am. 2009;19(1):1–22.
19. Pohl D, Tutuian R. Reflux monitoring: pH-metry, bilitec and oesophageal impedance measurements. Best Pract Res Clin Gastroenterol. 2009;23(3):299–311.
20. Johnson LF, DeMeester TR. Development of the 24-hour intraesophageal pH monitoring composite scoring system. J Clin Gastroenterol. 1986;8:52–8.
21. Johnson LF, Demeester TR. Twenty-four-hour pH monitoring of the distal esophagus. Am J Gastroenterol. 1974;62(4):325–32.
22. Richter JE, Bradley LA, DeMeester TR, Wu WC. Normal 24-hr ambulatory esophageal pH values. Dig Dis Sci. 1992;37(6):849–56.
23. Wiener GJ, Morgan TM, Copper JB, Castell DO, Sinclair JW, Richter JE. Ambulatory 24-hour esophageal pH monitoring. Dig Dis Sci. 1988;33(9):1127–33.
24. Wiener GJ, Richter JE, Copper JB, Wu WC, Castell DO. The symptom index: a clinically important parameter of ambulatory 24-hour esophageal pH monitoring. Am J Gastroenterol. 1988;83(4):358–61.
25. Slaughter JC, Goutte M, Rymer JA, Oranu AC, Schneider JA, Garrett CG, Hagaman D, Vaezi MF. Caution about overinterpretation of symptom indexes in reflux monitoring for refractory gastroesophageal reflux disease. Clin Gastroenterol Hepatol. 2011;9(10):868–74.
26. Dean BB, Gano AD Jr, Knight K, Ofman JJ, Fass R. Effectiveness of proton pump inhibitors in nonerosive reflux disease. Clin Gastroenterol Hepatol. 2004;2(8):656–64.
27. Sharma N, Agrawal A, Freeman J, Vela MF, Castell D. An analysis of persistent symptoms in acid-suppressed patients undergoing impedance-pH monitoring. Clin Gastroenterol Hepatol. 2008;6(5):521–4.
28. Finks JF, Wei Y, Birkmeyer JD. The rise and fall of antireflux surgery in the United States. Surg Endosc Other Interv Tech. 2006;20(11):1698–701.
29. Pointner R, Granderath FA. Laparoscopic fundoplication: when, how and what to do if it fails? Eur Surg. 2008;40(6):261–9.
30. Weitzendorfer M, Spaun GO, Antoniou SA, Tschoner A, Schredl P, Emmanuel K, Koch OO. Interim report of a prospective trial on the clinical efficiency of a new full-thickness endoscopic plication device for patients with GERD: impact of changed suture material. Surg Laparosc Endosc Percutan Tech. 2017;27(3):163–9.

31. Kim MS, Holloway RH, Dent J, Utley DS. Radiofrequency energy delivery to the gastric cardia inhibits triggering of transient lower esophageal sphincter relaxation and gastroesophageal reflux in dogs. Gastrointest Endosc. 2003;57(1):17–22.
32. Tam WC, Schoeman MN, Zhang Q, Dent J, Rigda R, Utley D, Holloway RH. Delivery of radiofrequency energy to the lower oesophageal sphincter and gastric cardia inhibits transient lower oesophageal sphincter relaxations and gastro-oesophageal reflux in patients with reflux disease. Gut. 2003;52(4):479–85.
33. Arts J, Bisschops R, Blondeau K, et al. A double-blind sham-controlled study of the effect of radiofrequency energy on symptoms and distensibility of the gastro-esophageal junction in GERD. Am J Gastroenterol. 2012;107:222–30.
34. Aziz AM, El-Khayat HR, Sadek A, Mattar SG, McNulty G, Kongkam P, Guda MF, Lehman GA. A prospective randomized trial of sham, single-dose Stretta, and double-dose Stretta for the treatment of gastroesophageal reflux disease. Surg Endosc. 2010;24(4):818–25.
35. Dughera L, Rotondano G, De Cento M, Cassolino P, Cisarò F. Durability of Stretta radiofrequency treatment for GERD: results of an 8-year follow-up. Gastroenterol Res Pract. 2014;2014:531907.
36. Corley DA, Katz P, Wo JM, Stefan A, Patti M, Rothstein R, Edmundowicz S, Kline M, Mason R, Wolfe MM. Improvement of gastroesophageal reflux symptoms after radiofrequency energy: a randomized, sham-controlled trial. Gastroenterology. 2003;125(3):668–76.
37. Coron E, Sebille V, Cadiot G, Zerbib F, Ducrotte P, Ducrot F, Pouderoux P, Arts J, Le Rhun M, Piche T, Bruley des Varannes S. Clinical trial: radiofrequency energy delivery in proton pump inhibitor-dependent gastro-oesophageal reflux disease patients. Aliment Pharmacol Ther. 2008;28(9):1147–58.
38. Noar M, Squires P, Noar E, Lee M. Long-term maintenance effect of radiofrequency energy delivery for refractory GERD: a decade later. Surg Endosc. 2014;28(8):2323–33.
39. Perry KA, Banerjee A, Melvin WS. Radiofrequency energy delivery to the lower esophageal sphincter reduces esophageal acid exposure and improves GERD symptoms: a systematic review and meta-analysis. Surg Laparosc Endosc Percutan Tech. 2012;22(4):2.
40. Auyang ED, Carter P, Rauth T, Fanelli RD, SAGES Guidelines Committee. SAGES clinical spotlight review: endoluminal treatments for gastroesophageal reflux disease (GERD). Surg Endosc. 2013;27(8):2658–72.
41. Lipka S, Kumar A, Richter JE. No evidence for efficacy of radiofrequency ablation for treatment of gastroesophageal reflux disease: a systematic review and meta-analysis. Clin Gastroenterol Hepatol. 2015;13(6):1058–67.
42. Richardson WS, Stefanidis D, Fanelli RD. Society of American Gastrointestinal and Endoscopic Surgeons response to "no evidence for efficacy of radiofrequency ablation for treatment of gastroesophageal reflux disease: a systematic review and meta-analysis". Clin Gastroenterol Hepatol. 2015;13(9):1700–1.
43. Liang WT, Yan C, Wang ZG, Wu JM, Hu ZW, Zhan XL, Wang F, Ma SS, Chen MP. Early and midterm outcome after laparoscopic fundoplication and a minimally invasive endoscopic procedure in patients with gastroesophageal reflux disease: a prospective observational study. J Laparoendosc Adv Surg Tech. 2015;25(8):657–61.
44. Yan C, Liang WT, Wang ZG, Hu ZW, Wu JM, Zhang C, Chen MP. Comparison of Stretta procedure and toupet fundoplication for gastroesophageal reflux disease-related extra-esophageal symptoms. World J Gastroenterol. 2015;21(45):12882.
45. Liang WT, Wu JM, Wang F, Hu ZW, Wang ZG. Stretta radiofrequency for gastroesophageal reflux disease-related respiratory symptoms: a prospective 5-year study. Minerva Chir. 2014;69(5):293–9.
46. Zhang C, Wu J, Hu Z, Yan C, Gao X, Liang W, Liu D, Li F, Wang Z. Diagnosis and antireflux therapy for GERD with respiratory symptoms: a study using multichannel intraluminal impedance-pH monitoring. PLoS One. 2016;11(8):e0160139.
47. Pandolfino JE, Krishnan K. Do endoscopic antireflux procedures fit in the current treatment paradigm of gastroesophageal reflux disease? Clin Gastroenterol Hepatol. 2014;12(4):544–54.

48. Hunter JG, Kahrilas PJ, Bell RC, Wilson EB, Trad KS, Dolan JP, Perry KA, Oelschlager BK, Soper NJ, Snyder BE, Burch MA. Efficacy of transoral fundoplication vs omeprazole for treatment of regurgitation in a randomized controlled trial. Gastroenterology. 2015;148(2):324–33.
49. Trad KS, Barnes WE, Simoni G, Shughoury AB, Mavrelis PG, Raza M, Heise JA, Turgeon DG, Fox MA. Transoral incisionless fundoplication effective in eliminating GERD symptoms in partial responders to proton pump inhibitor therapy at 6 months: the TEMPO randomized clinical trial. Surg Innov. 2015;22(1):26–40.
50. Trad KS, Simoni G, Barnes WE, Shughoury AB, Raza M, Heise JA, Turgeon DG, Fox MA, Mavrelis PG. Efficacy of transoral fundoplication for treatment of chronic gastroesophageal reflux disease incompletely controlled with high-dose proton-pump inhibitors therapy: a randomized, multicenter, open label, crossover study. BMC Gastroenterol. 2014;14(1):174.
51. Håkansson B, Montgomery M, Cadiere GB, Rajan A, Bruley des Varannes S, Lerhun M, Coron E, Tack J, Bischops R, Thorell A, Arnelo U. Randomised clinical trial: transoral incisionless fundoplication vs. sham intervention to control chronic GERD. Aliment Pharmacol Ther. 2015;42(11–12):1261–70.
52. Testoni PA, Mazzoleni G, Testoni SG. Transoral incisionless fundoplication for gastroesophageal reflux disease: techniques and outcomes. World J Gastrointest Pharmacol Ther. 2016;7(2):179.
53. Huang X, Chen S, Zhao H, Zeng X, Lian J, Tseng Y, Chen J. Efficacy of transoral incisionless fundoplication (TIF) for the treatment of GERD: a systematic review with meta-analysis. Surg Endosc. 2017;31(3):1032–44.
54. Testoni PA, Testoni S, Mazzoleni G, Vailati C, Passaretti S. Long-term efficacy of transoral incisionless fundoplication with Esophyx (Tif 2.0) and factors affecting outcomes in GERD patients followed for up to 6 years: a prospective single-center study. Surg Endosc. 2015;29(9):2770–80.
55. Toomey P, Teta A, Patel K, Ross S, Sukharamwala P, Rosemurgy AS. Transoral incisionless fundoplication: is it as safe and efficacious as a Nissen or Toupet fundoplication? Am Surg. 2014;80(9):860–7.
56. Bell RC, Fox MA, Barnes WE, Mavrelis PG, Sewell RW, Carter BJ, Ihde GM, Trad KS, Dargis D, Hoddinott KM, Freeman KD. Univariate and multivariate analyses of preoperative factors influencing symptomatic outcomes of transoral fundoplication. Surg Endosc. 2014;28(10):2949–58.
57. Witteman BP, Kessing BF, Snijders G, Koek GH, Conchillo JM, Bouvy ND. Revisional laparoscopic antireflux surgery after unsuccessful endoscopic fundoplication. Surg Endosc. 2013;27(6):2231–6.
58. Jain D, Singhal S. Transoral incisionless fundoplication for refractory gastroesophageal reflux disease: where do we stand? Clin Endosc. 2016;49(2):147.
59. Zacherl J, Roy-Shapira A, Bonavina L, Bapaye A, Kiesslich R, Schoppmann SF, Kessler WR, Selzer DJ, Broderick RC, Lehman GA, Horgan S. Endoscopic anterior fundoplication with the Medigus Ultrasonic Surgical Endostapler (MUSE™) for gastroesophageal reflux disease: 6-month results from a multi-center prospective trial. Surg Endosc. 2015;29(1):220–9.
60. Kim HJ, Kwon CI, Kessler WR, Selzer DJ, McNulty G, Bapaye A, Bonavina L, Lehman GA. Long-term follow-up results of endoscopic treatment of gastroesophageal reflux disease with the MUSE™ endoscopic stapling device. Surg Endosc. 2016;30(8):3402–8.
61. Gweon TG, Matthes K. Prospective, randomized ex vivo trial to assess the ideal stapling site for endoscopic fundoplication with medigus ultrasonic surgical endostapler. Gastroenterol Res Pract. 2016;31:2016.
62. Pace F, Costamagna G, Penagini R, Repici A, Annese V. Endoscopic antireflux procedures–an unfulfilled promise? Aliment Pharmacol Ther. 2008;27(5):375–84.
63. Koch OO, Kaindlstorfer A, Antoniou SA, Spaun G, Pointner R, Swanstrom LL. Subjective and objective data on esophageal manometry and impedance pH monitoring 1 year after endoscopic full-thickness plication for the treatment of GERD by using multiple plication implants. Gastrointest Endosc. 2013;77(1):7–14.

64. Von Renteln D, Schiefke I, Fuchs KH, Raczynski S, Philipper M, Breithaupt W, Caca K, Neuhaus H. Endoscopic full-thickness plication for the treatment of gastroesophageal reflux disease using multiple Plicator implants: 12-month multicenter study results. Surg Endosc. 2009;23(8):1866–75.
65. von Renteln D, Schiefke I, Fuchs KH, Raczynski S, Philipper M, Breithaupt W, Caca K, Neuhaus H. Endoscopic full-thickness plication for the treatment of GERD by application of multiple plicator implants: a multicenter study (with video). Gastrointest Endosc. 2008;68(5):833–44.
66. Satodate H, Inoue H, Fukami N, Shiokawa A, Kudo SE. Squamous reepithelialization after circumferential endoscopic mucosal resection of superficial carcinoma arising in Barrett's esophagus. Endoscopy. 2004;36(10):909–12.
67. Inoue H, Ito H, Ikeda H, Sato C, Sato H, Phalanusitthepha C, Hayee BH, Eleftheriadis N, Kudo SE. Anti-reflux mucosectomy for gastroesophageal reflux disease in the absence of hiatus hernia: a pilot study. Ann Gastroenterol. 2014;27(4):346.

Anti-reflux Mucosectomy and Anti-reflux Mucosal Ablation

7

Yuto Shimamura and Haruhiro Inoue

7.1 Introduction

Gastroesophageal reflux disease (GERD) is one of the most common gastrointestinal diseases, and its prevalence is increasing [1]. Although acid-suppressing drugs, such as proton pump inhibitors (PPI) and vonoprazan (P-CAB), are effective, some cases are refractory to or dependent on medical therapy [2–4]. GERD symptoms refractory to medication can significantly lower the quality of life and increase the risk of developing Barrett's esophagus-related diseases.

Surgical intervention is a mainstay of treatment in PPI-refractory cases. Nissen fundoplication, in which the fundus is wrapped around the lower esophagus to reinforce the lower esophageal sphincter, is the standard surgical approach, providing excellent short-term results with a low rate of adverse events. Although surgical fundoplication is effective, it may cause dysphagia and gas bloat syndrome, and some studies report high rates of relapse requiring repeat fundoplication [5]. To fill the gap between medical therapy and surgical intervention, various less-invasive endoscopic methods have been developed, mainly in Western countries, including transoral incisionless fundoplication (TIF) (EsophyX device; EndoGastricSolutions, Redmond, WA, USA) [6], Medigus Ultrasonic Surgical Endostapler (MUSE) (Medigus Ltd., Omer, Israel) [7], and Stretta (Mederi Therapeutics, Greenwich, CT, USA) [8], which are all currently available US Food and Drug Administration (FDA)-approved [9]. However, many studies of novel endoscopic anti-reflux procedures are limited to reports that demonstrate only good short-term symptomatic improvement but lack long-term efficacy data and that report a high cost for the procedure. Several previously developed endoscopic anti-reflux devices are no longer available due to safety issues. Therefore, minimally invasive procedures are currently not established as standard treatment.

Y. Shimamura · H. Inoue (✉)
Digestive Diseases Center, Showa University Koto Toyosu Hospital, Tokyo, Japan

P. Sharma, N. Reddy (eds.), *Innovations in Gastrointestinal Endoscopy*,
https://doi.org/10.1007/978-981-15-9247-8_7

In 2003, we reported that the scarring process around the cardia post-mucosal resection for high-grade dysplasia of Barrett's esophagus had an anti-reflux effect in a PPI-refractory GERD patient [10]. GERD was improved by the contraction and tightening of the cardiac opening during healing. No symptomatic recurrence has been seen, and the patient has remained off PPI for over 10 years. Based on this experience, ten patients with PPI-refractory GERD were treated with this method, which we reported as anti-reflux mucosectomy (ARMS) [11]. ARMS is considered a safe and effective endoscopic treatment that can be considered as a treatment of choice prior to surgical intervention. In addition, we have refined this technique, in which we perform mucosal ablation around the gastroesophageal junction to cause a healing process to re-form the cardiac opening. The technique is called anti-reflux mucosal ablation (ARMA). The concept of ARMA is similar to that of ARMS, aiming to contract and tighten the cardiac opening during healing to re-form the cardiac opening by ablating the mucosa. The scarring process narrows the hiatal opening by reconstructing the mucosal flap valve in order to suppress acid reflux. Our first clinical case was that of a patient who underwent ARMS, which was partially effective and then failed to enable discontinuation of PPI. Due to previous scarring, the performance of additional mucosectomy was considered too technically demanding and high risk. Ablation was performed with a Triangle-Tip Knife in spray coagulation mode to re-form the cardia. The GERD symptoms significantly resolved, and the patient was able to discontinue PPI postprocedure.

In this chapter, we provide an overview of current approaches, basic technical tips, and the outcomes of these procedures.

7.2 Anti-reflux Mucosectomy (ARMS) and Anti-reflux Ablation (ARMA)

7.2.1 Indications

Patients with typical GERD symptoms, such as heartburn or regurgitation, despite regular intake of acid-suppressing drugs, are considered for ARMS or ARMA. Patients with multiple comorbidities and those with postoperative states such as sleeve or distal gastrectomy may benefit from these procedures.

7.2.2 Exclusion Criteria

Patients with hiatal hernia over 3 cm or Hill's flap valve grade > III on gastroscopy and/or a primary esophageal motility disorder, such as achalasia or incomplete LES relaxation, should not be considered for these procedures.

7.2.3 Pre-assessment

Prior to ARMS or ARMA, pre-assessment EGD must be performed. This is to assess if there is any endoscopic evidence of esophagitis and to rule out large hiatal hernia. It is important to sufficiently insufflate the stomach to provide a good retroflex view to correctly assess herniation and to evaluate the gastroesophageal flap valve. Biopsy should be performed at the discretion of the endoscopist to exclude eosinophilic esophagitis. High-resolution manometry should be performed to rule out esophageal motility disorders, including achalasia, ineffective esophageal motility, and spastic esophageal disorders, among others. Ineffective esophageal motility associated with acid reflux is more resistant to endoscopic therapy, and the physician must be extracautious, as even mild stenosis can cause significant dysphagia. For patients with no erosive esophagitis, 24-h multichannel intraluminal impedance and pH monitoring (MII-pH) should be performed to accurately define the GERD phenotype.

7.2.4 Anti-reflux Mucosectomy (ARMS)

7.2.4.1 Technique

ARMS can be performed using the regular GIF-Q260J endoscope (Olympus Corp., Tokyo, Japan). Angulation of the scope should always be checked prior to the procedure. Insufficient retroflexion will result in poor-quality pre-assessment and will also cause difficulties in accessing the cardia, resulting in poor-quality procedure. ARMS can be performed in the endoscopy suite with intravenous sedation. However, general anesthesia is highly recommended because sufficient insufflation is needed for pre-assessment and for designing the area of resection. In addition, the procedure at the cardia is technically demanding in a patient under insufficient sedation. In our center, all cases are treated by the cap-EMR method (EMR-C). In this method, a large, hard cap with oblique cut (MAJ-296, Olympus) is used together with a thin-diameter crescent snare (SD-221L-25, Olympus). EMR with band ligation is an alternative EMR technique for ARMS [12]. ESD is an another option to resect the mucosa, but it can be highly technically demanding and time-consuming [13]. The EMR method is highly recommended for the ARMS procedure.

Step 1: *Designing*. Mucosectomy is planned around the gastric cardia, leaving parts of the mucosa intact at both the lesser and the greater curvatures. To prevent stricture, it is important not to include the esophageal side (squamous mucosa). The mucosal strips preserved along the lesser and greater curvatures should be approximately 1 cm long, mimicking the shape of a butterfly (Fig. 7.1). The width of the resection area should be around 2–3 cm.

Step 2: *Submucosal injection*. Saline with indigo carmine is injected into the submucosal layer to separate the mucosa from the muscularis propria layer using a 25-gauge needle with a 4-mm tip (Fig. 7.2a). Although other solutions are acceptable, saline is considered sufficient for the submucosal cushion. Injection is performed to ensure adequate lifting to avoid deep injury or perforation.

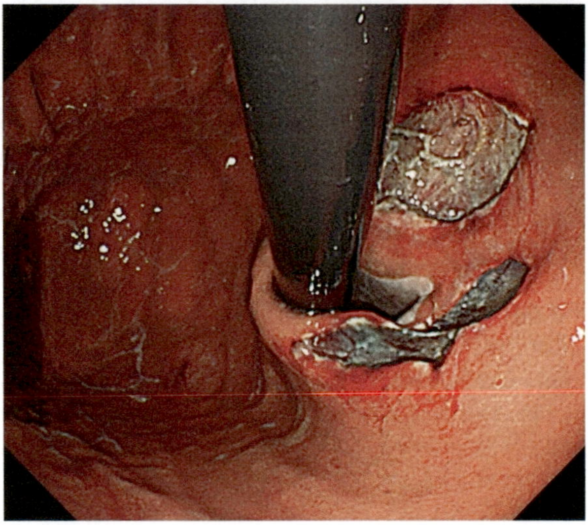

Fig. 7.1 Post-mucosal resection (post-ARMS). A butterfly shape can be seen, leaving the normal mucosa at the contralateral side of the cardia on the greater curvature and lesser curvature

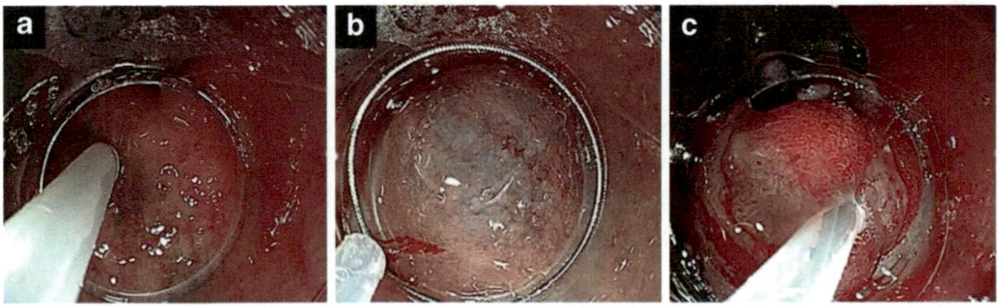

Fig. 7.2 (**a**) *Submucosal injection*: A normal saline solution with indigo carmine dye is injected into the submucosa. (**b**) *Prelooping*: A snare is fixed inside the rim of the cap. (**c**) *Mucosectomy*: The snare is closed and then resected with electrocautery

Step 3: *Mucosectomy*. Mucosectomy is performed by EMR or ESD. However, the EMR technique is highly recommended as it is safer with a shorter procedure time. The EMR-C method is the standard approach in our institution. A snare is prelooped on the internal circumferential ridge of the cap by lightly pressing against and suctioning the mucosa (Fig. 7.2b). After the ideal prelooping is done, sufficient suctioning of the targeted mucosal area is performed, and the targeted mucosal area is resected with an electrosurgical current (forced coagulation mode, 30 W, effect 3; VIO300D ERBE, Tübingen, Germany). EMR-C is performed in this manner until the marked mucosal area is completely resected (Fig. 7.2c). These resections should be performed in retroflex view. Approximately 2/3 to 4/5 of the circumference of the cardia should be resected, centering on the lesser curvature. Usually, mucosectomy is completed in about three to five times of EMR-C.

Step 4: *Hemostasis*. Hemostasis should always be performed with coagulation forceps (Coagrasper, FD-410LR, Olympus). All visible vessels should be identified and coagulated.

7.2.4.2 Management and Follow-up Post-ARMS

Management after ARMS is similar to that of EMR-C for esophageal or stomach tumor resection. The patient is allowed to have clear fluids 1 day after the procedure if there is no adverse event. Acid-suppressing drugs are prescribed for 4 weeks after ARMS and are then terminated if GERD symptom allows. Repeat endoscopy is usually performed 2–3 weeks after the procedure to assess the healing process and to look for signs of stenosis. If there is mild resistance to passing the endoscope, we perform endoscopic balloon dilatation as a preventive measure.

7.2.4.3 Outcome

Between April 2012 and May 2018, 109 patients with PPI-refractory GERD were treated with ARMS at our institution (Showa University Koto Toyosu Hospital, Tokyo, Japan). ARMS was performed in ESD for the initial nine patients and in EMR-C for the subsequent patients. The mean operation time was 54.7 min. There were two cases of postoperative bleeding, which were managed with endoscopic hemostasis not requiring blood transfusion. There was one case of minor perforation, which was treated with clipping. The clinical course of this patient was uneventful, without any prolonged hospitalization. These results show that ARMS can be performed without the risk of major adverse events. However, the rate of stenosis requiring more than three sessions of endoscopic balloon dilation was 14.4%. This rate improved significantly after we modified our resection design to the butterfly shape, as shown in Fig. 7.1. This shows the importance of leaving the mucosa unresected along both sides of the lesser and greater curvatures rather than performing circumferential resection. Only 1 patient of the 21 who underwent a butterfly resection required a single endoscopic balloon dilation.

With regard to efficacy, significant improvements in subjective and objective indicators of GERD were seen (Table 7.1). Two subjective scales, the Frequency Scale for the Symptoms of GERD (FSSG) and GerdQ, were used. The FSSG decreased from 25 to 12 ($p < 0.01$, $n = 88$) after 2–6 months and from 26 to 12 ($p < 0.01$, $n = 61$) after 1 year. The GerdQ decreased from 9 to 7 ($p < 0.01$, $n = 88$) after 2–6 months and from 10 to 7 ($p < 0.01$, $n = 61$) after 1 year. As for long-term outcome, 21 patients were followed for 3 years. The FSSG and GerdQ decreased from 28 to 10 and from 11 to 6, respectively. Although the MII-pH study was limited to 27 patients, both pre- and post-ARMS, significant improvements in acid

Table 7.1 Outcomes of ARMS ($n = 109$)

Outcome	Before ARMS	2–6 months after ARMS	*P* value
Symptom scores ($n = 88$)			
FSSG	25.1 ± 1.1	11.6 ± 0.8	<0.01
GerdQ	9.4 ± 0.3	6.6 ± 0.3	<0.01
MII-pH ($n = 27$)			
Acid exposure time (%)	20.8	6.9	<0.01
DeMeester composite score	64.4	24.9	<0.01

ARMS anti-reflux mucosectomy, *FSSG* Frequency Scale for the Symptoms of GERD, *MII-pH* multichannel intraluminal impedance and pH monitoring exposure time and DeMeester composite score were seen. The mean acid exposure time decreased from 20.8 to 6.9 ($p < 0.01$), and the mean DeMeester composite score decreased from 64.4 to 24.9 ($p < 0.01$). Forty-four percent (42/96) of the patients were able to discontinue PPI within 6 months. Of 59 patients who were followed for 1 year, 30 patients (51%) did not have any relapse of their symptoms, showing the sustainable effect of ARMS.

ARMS is being performed in other centers with promising results. Yoo et al. reported 33 cases of ARMS with EMR-C in patients with pathologic reflux disease and esophageal hypersensitivity [14]. Six months after ARMS, 63% of patients were able to discontinue PPIs, and 30% were able to reduce their PPI intake. The GERD questionnaire scores also improved significantly. Objective parameters, such as DeMeester score and acid exposure time on MII-pH, also improved. ARMS was reported to be safe, and there were only two patients with stenosis.

The first Indian study of ARMS, with 62 patients, was recently published, showing a similar profile to previously reported studies [15]. Five patients (8%) had stenosis requiring endoscopic balloon dilatation. Forty-five patients (72.5%) showed improvement in MII-pH, and 43 patients (69.4%) were able to discontinue PPIs. Thirty-eight patients (61.3%) showed sustained efficacy at 1-year follow-up.

These results showed promising safety and efficacy profiles. However, the sample sizes were small, and studies with larger sample sizes are warranted.

7.2.5 Anti-reflux Mucosal Ablation (ARMA)

7.2.5.1 Technique

ARMA can be performed using the regular GIF-Q260J endoscope (Olympus). Angulation of the scope should always be checked prior to the procedure. The procedure can be performed in the endoscopy suite with intravenous sedation or under general anesthesia. General anesthesia is preferred as sufficient insufflation is needed for good pre-assessment (designing) and for technical reasons.

Step 1: *Designing*. Ablation is planned mainly along the lesser curvature of the gastric cardia. As with ARMS, it is essential not to include the esophageal side (squamous mucosa) to prevent stricture. The circumferential gastric mucosa 1 cm distal to the squamocolumnar junction should be preserved as well. ARMA should be performed in retroflex view with sufficient insufflation, and ablation should be designed in the horseshoe shape (Fig. 7.3).

Step 2: *Ablation*. Mucosal ablation is performed with the Triangle-Tip KnifeJ (Olympus) in spray coagulation mode (50–120 W effect 2). The Triangle-Tip Knife without jet function can be used, as it has a wider triangle-tip to perform efficient ablation. The key technical point is to ablate deeply enough to reach the submucosal layer in semicircumferential shape with a width of approximately 2–3 cm. Submucosal injection is not necessary when performing ARMA.

Step 3: *Hemostasis*. Hemostasis should always be performed if and when visible vessels are identified.

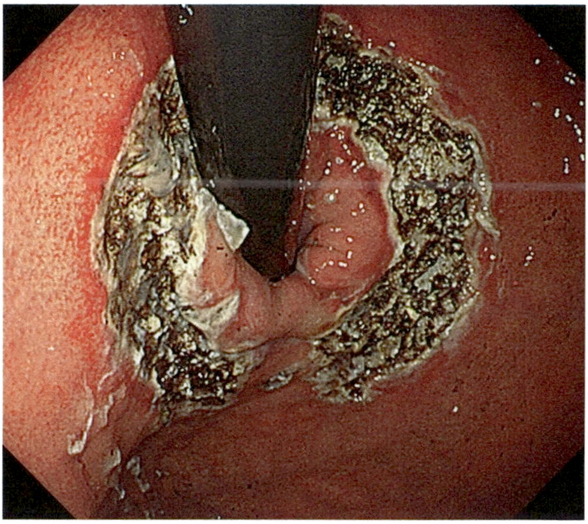

Fig. 7.3 Post-endoscopic ablation in horseshoe shape (1 SD wide normal mucosa preserved at the side of the greater curvature)

7.2.5.2 Postoperative Management

Management after ARMA is similar to that after ARMS. The patient is allowed to have clear fluids 1 day after the procedure if there is no adverse event. Acid-suppressing drugs are prescribed for 4 weeks after ARMS and are then terminated if GERD symptom allows. Repeat endoscopy is usually performed 2–3 weeks after the procedure to assess the healing process and to look for signs of stenosis. If there is mild resistance to passing the endoscope, we perform endoscopic balloon dilatation as a preventive measure.

7.2.5.3 Outcome

Twelve consecutive patients with PPI-refractory GERD underwent ARMA [16]. Two patients had a history of previous treatment with ARMS. There were no immediate adverse events such as bleeding or perforation. The mean operation time was 40.3 min. One patient developed dysphagia 2 weeks post-ARMA due to stricture, which was addressed with two sessions of endoscopic balloon dilatation.

Technical success was achieved in 100% of the patients. The clinical outcomes were as follows (Table 7.2). The median GERD-HRQL and FSSG scores significantly improved from 30.5 to 12 ($p = 0.002$) and from 25 to 10.5 ($p = 0.002$), respectively. The median DeMeester composite score also significantly improved from 33.5 to 2.8 ($p < 0.05$). Sixty-seven percent of patients (8/12) were able to discontinue PPI intake. The remaining three patients remained on PPI; however, their symptoms significantly improved.

Table 7.2 Outcomes of ARMA ($n = 12$)

Outcome	Before ARMA	2 months after ARMA	*P* value
Symptom scores (n = 12)			
FSSG	25	10.5	0.002
GERD-HRQL	30.5	12	0.002
MII-pH (n = 8)			
Acid exposure time (%)	9.0	0.5	0.068
DeMeester composite score	33.5	2.8	0.05

ARMA anti-reflux mucosal ablation, *FSSG* Frequency Scale for the Symptoms of GERD, *GERD-HRQL* GERD-Health Related Quality of Life Questionnaire, MII-pH, multichannel intraluminal impedance and pH monitoring

7.3 Conclusions

ARMS and ARMA are safe and feasible endoscopic treatments for PPI-refractory GERD.

There is no requirement for new, expensive, specialized equipment. These procedures can be performed with endoscopic techniques that are familiar to most therapeutic endoscopists. The greatest advancement in our endoscopic anti-reflux technique is that we have developed ARMA. We are currently investigating the optimal strategy to ablate the mucosa. Additional refinement of the technique and postoperative management may be able to fill in the gap between medical therapy and surgical intervention. Our experience has shown promising safety and efficacy profiles. However, the sample size was small, and studies with larger sample sizes and long-term follow-up are required. We have to keep appropriate selection of patients in mind. The short- and long-term outcomes of these procedures are favorable, but more studies are warranted.

References

1. Richter JE, Rubenstein JH. Presentation and epidemiology of gastroesophageal reflux disease. Gastroenterology. 2018;154:267–76.
2. Yadlapati R, DeLay K. Proton pump inhibitor-refractory gastroesophageal reflux disease. Med Clin North Am. 2019;103:15–27.
3. Delshad SD, Almario CV, Chey WD, Spiegel BMR. Prevalence of gastroesophageal reflux disease and proton pump inhibitor-refractory symptoms. Gastroenterology. 2020;158(5):1250–1261.e2.
4. Okuyama M, Nakahara K, Iwakura N, et al. Factors associated with potassium-competitive acid blocker non-response in patients with proton pump inhibitor-refractory gastroesophageal reflux disease. Digestion. 2017;95:281–7.
5. Hakanson BS, Lundell L, Bylund A, Thorell A. Comparison of laparoscopic 270 degrees posterior partial fundoplication vs total fundoplication for the treatment of gastroesophageal reflux disease: a randomized clinical trial. JAMA Surg. 2019;154:479–86.
6. Huang X, Chen S, Zhao H, et al. Efficacy of transoral incisionless fundoplication (TIF) for the treatment of GERD: a systematic review with meta-analysis. Surg Endosc. 2017;31:1032–44.

7. Kim HJ, Kwon CI, Kessler WR, et al. Long-term follow-up results of endoscopic treatment of gastroesophageal reflux disease with the MUSE endoscopic stapling device. Surg Endosc. 2016;30:3402–8.
8. Fass R, Cahn F, Scotti DJ, Gregory DA. Systematic review and meta-analysis of controlled and prospective cohort efficacy studies of endoscopic radiofrequency for treatment of gastroesophageal reflux disease. Surg Endosc. 2017;31:4865–82.
9. Committee AT, Thosani N, Goodman A, et al. Endoscopic anti-reflux devices (with videos). Gastrointest Endosc. 2017;86:931–48.
10. Satodate H, Inoue H, Yoshida T, et al. Circumferential EMR of carcinoma arising in Barrett's esophagus: case report. Gastrointest Endosc. 2003;58:288–92.
11. Inoue H, Ito H, Ikeda H, et al. Anti-reflux mucosectomy for gastroesophageal reflux disease in the absence of hiatus hernia: a pilot study. Ann Gastroenterol. 2014;27:346–51.
12. Monino L, Gonzalez JM, Vitton V, Barthet M. Anti-reflux mucosectomy with band ligation in the treatment of refractory gastroesophageal reflux disease. Endoscopy. 2019;51:E215–E6.
13. Ota K, Takeuchi T, Harada S, et al. A novel endoscopic submucosal dissection technique for proton pump inhibitor-refractory gastroesophageal reflux disease. Scand J Gastroenterol. 2014;49:1409–13.
14. Yoo IK, Ko WJ, Kim HS, et al. Anti-reflux mucosectomy using a cap-assisted endoscopic mucosal resection method for refractory gastroesophageal disease: a prospective feasibility study. Surg Endosc. 2020;34(3):1124–31.
15. Patil G, Dalal A, Maydeo A. Feasibility and outcomes of anti-reflux mucosectomy (ARMS) for proton pump inhibitor dependent Gastroesophageal reflux disease: first Indian study (with video). Digest Endosc. 2019.
16. Haruhiro Inoue, Mayo Tanabe, Enrique Rodríguez de Santiago, Mary Raina Angeli Abad, Yuto Shimamura, Yusuke Fujiyoshi, Akiko Ueno, Kazuya Sumi, Hideomi Tomida, Yugo Iwaya, Haruo Ikeda, Manabu Onimaru, (2020) Anti-reflux mucosal ablation (ARMA) as a new treatment for gastroesophageal reflux refractory to proton pump inhibitors: a pilot study. Endoscopy International Open 08 (02):E133-E138.

Biliary Radio Frequency Ablation (RFA)

8

Tae Jun Song and Dong Wan Seo

8.1 Introduction

Radiofrequency ablation (RFA) is a well-established locoregional thermal ablative treatment method that causes coagulative necrosis and eventually leads to local destruction of many malignancies [1]. RFA has been increasingly used for local control of premalignant and malignant tumors [2, 3].

During RFA, an active electrode at the tip of a specifically designed catheter creates a high-frequency alternating current. The subsequent thermal damage leads to coagulative necrosis and cellular death once the target temperature exceeds 48–50 °C [4]. Intracellular components such as heat shock proteins release after tumor necrosis and can cause immunologic reactions which activate antigen-presenting cells and enhance immunity directed against the tumor [5, 6].

Initially, RFA catheters were developed to perform through a surgical or a percutaneous route [7]. Recently, a biliary RFA catheter working over the guidewire has been developed and showed its safety and effectiveness in the animal study [8]. In subsequent studies, RFA has been used to increase stent patency in patients with malignant biliary strictures.

In this chapter, we performed a comprehensive review of the literature on the use of biliary RFA.

T. J. Song · D. W. Seo (✉)
Department of Internal Medicine, University of Ulsan College of Medicine, Asan Medical Center, Seoul, South Korea
e-mail: dwseoamc@amc.seoul.kr

P. Sharma, N. Reddy (eds.), *Innovations in Gastrointestinal Endoscopy*,
https://doi.org/10.1007/978-981-15-9247-8_8

8.2 Principles of RFA System

RFA is physically based on radiofrequency current and a high-frequency alternating current which produces ionic oscillation, thereby producing controlled frictional heat to destroy the tissue [1]. The thermal heat around the electrode induces coagulation necrosis. The term "coagulation necrosis" means irreversible thermal damage to cells whether or not cell death can be achieved according to the strict histologic criteria. The delivery of RF energy is directly proportional to the amplitude of oscillations, and the volume of coagulation necrosis can be expected according to the temperature and time. The main purpose of thermal tumor ablation therapy is to destroy the tumor using heat in a minimally invasive method.

When temperatures are increased to 42–45 °C in the body, cells become more susceptible to damage by other agents such as chemotherapy and radiation. However, these temperatures will not kill all cells. When temperatures are increased to 46 °C for 60 min, irreversible cellular damage can occur. The increase of the temperature to 50–52 °C markedly shortens the time necessary to induce cytotoxicity as 4–6 min. Between 60 and 100 °C, nearly instance protein coagulation which irreversibly damages the cells can occur. Temperatures greater than 105 °C induce tissue boiling, vaporization, and carbonization which usually retard optimal ablation due to a decrease in energy transmission. As a result, the ideal ablation temperature is between 60 and 100 °C [1].

The heat-sink effect of RFA should be considered during the RFA procedure. The heat-sink effect may occur when RFA was performed for lesions adjacent to large vessels. The inflow of cold blood at body temperature may impair the heating of the lesions closest to the blood vessels [9]. In hepatic hilum, bile duct and blood vessels including hepatic artery and portal vein are closely located. As a result, heat-sink effect and potential risk of vessel injury should be considered.

8.3 RFA Devices

For biliary RFA, there are two commercially available RFA catheters, the ELRA RF catheter (Taewoong Medical, Gyeonggi-Do, South Korea) and the Habib HPB-RF catheter (Boston Scientific Corp., Marlborough, MA, USA) [10, 11]. These RFA catheters are single-use and disposable devices that are designed for endoluminal delivery of RFA into the bile duct tumor over a guidewire.

The ELRA RF catheter has a 7Fr diameter and 175 cm length which can be inserted over a 0.025- or 0.035-inch guidewire. There are three types of the ELRA RF catheter, an 11 mm, 18 mm, and 22 mm, according to the probe lengths. RF power is supplied from the VIVA Combo generator (Taewoong Medical) which can control the power (range 0–200 W), temperature (range 5–95 °C) and time (range 10 s–10 min). Generally, recommended settings of biliary RFA are 80 °C of temperature, 10 W for 22 mm catheter, and 7 W for 11 or 18 mm catheter of power, and 1 or 2 min of time [4].

The HPB-RF catheter consists of an 8-Fr catheter with 180 cm in length, which can be used over a guidewire. The HPB-RF catheter has one size probe of 25 mm; the distance of two electrodes is 25 mm. This catheter allows connection to different RFA generators, such as RITA-1500X RF generator (Angiodynamics, Latham, NY, USA) and ERBE electrosurgical generator (Surgical Technology Group, Hampshire, UK). Most studies used settings of 7–10 W for up to 2 min so far [4].

8.4 Malignant Biliary Strictures

Malignant biliary strictures can occur due to hilar cholangiocarcinoma, pancreas head cancer, common bile duct (CBD) cancer, ampulla of Vater cancer or external compression secondary to lymph node (LN) metastasis. A large number of malignant biliary strictures are unresectable at presentation so that the palliation may be the aim of treatment in these patients. Adequate biliary drainage and resolution of obstructive jaundice are the most important palliation method for the patients' survival and quality of life with unresectable malignant biliary obstruction [12]. Self-expandable metal stents (SEMS) insertion is the standard palliative treatment for unresectable malignant biliary strictures with a life expectancy over 3 months [13, 14]. Although SEMS provide more favorable outcomes than that with a plastic stent, the patency of SEMS is still limited mainly due to tumor ingrowth or biliary sludge which cause stent occlusion [15]. Biliary RFA for unresectable malignant strictures before SEMS placement during ERCP procedure can be tried to prolong stent patency and increase overall survival (Fig. 8.1).

Until recently, several studies have evaluated the outcomes of biliary RFA in patients with unresectable malignant biliary strictures. The biliary RFA has been reported to be feasible and relatively safe. One study reported the significant increase of the bile duct diameter at the stricture site after biliary RFA [16]. Sharaiha et al. reported the results of a retrospective comparative study which evaluated the outcomes of SEMS insertion after biliary RFA ($n = 26$) versus SEMS insertion alone ($n = 40$) in patients with malignant biliary obstruction [17]. A total of 66 patients included 37 patients with cholangiocarcinoma and 29 patients with pancreatic cancer. This study showed no significant different differences between two groups. The same authors reported improved survival in patients treated by RFA before stent insertion compared with data from the Surveillance, Epidemiology, and End Results (SEER) database registry [18]. Patients with pancreatic cancer (14.6 vs. 5.9 months) and cholangiocarcinoma (17.7 vs. 6.2 months) showed significantly improved survival after biliary RFA. Another study by Kallis et al. also showed improvement of survival in patients with pancreatic cancer who had been treated with RFA plus SEMS placement compared with those who had SEMS placement alone (226 vs. 123.5 days) [19]. In a prospective study by Laleman et al., all 18 patients with malignant biliary strictures due to hilar cholangiocarcinoma ($n = 9$), pancreatic cancer ($n = 7$), and distal common bile duct (CBD) cancer ($n = 2$) could be undergone biliary RFA, and median stent patency was 110 days (16–374) with a median patient survival of 227 days (range 16–374) [20].

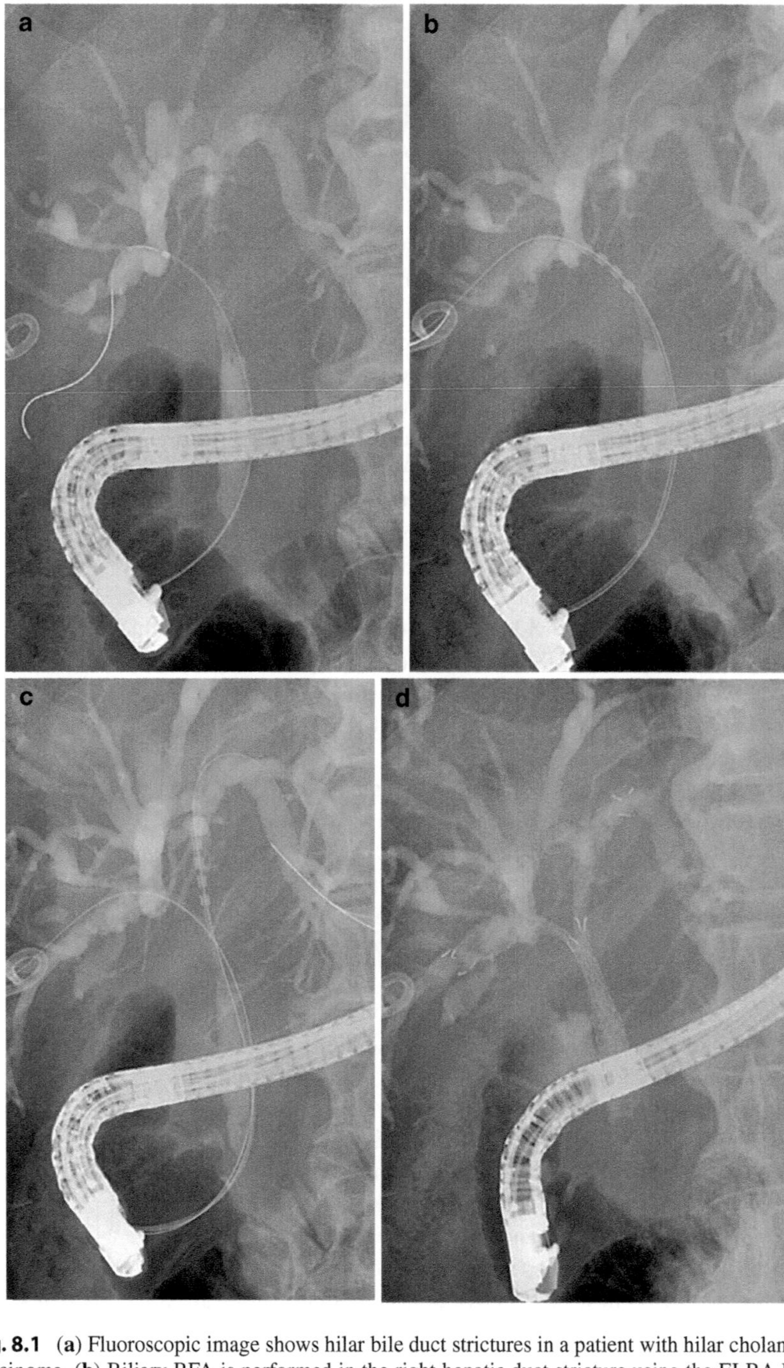

Fig. 8.1 (**a**) Fluoroscopic image shows hilar bile duct strictures in a patient with hilar cholangiocarcinoma. (**b**) Biliary RFA is performed in the right hepatic duct stricture using the ELRA RFA catheter (Taewoong Medical, Gyeonggi-Do, South Korea). (**c**) RFA is performed in the left intrahepatic duct. (**d**) After RFA, bilateral self-expandable metal stents are inserted in stent-in-stent manner

There have been studies that compared the outcomes of biliary RFA and photodynamic therapy (PDT). Although endoscopically delivered PDT has shown improved stent patency, biliary drainage, mortality, and quality of life, the associated phototoxicity requiring patients to avoid direct sunlight limits application of PDT [3]. In a retrospective, single-center study, survival after endobiliary RFA ($n = 16$) and PDT ($n = 32$) was not statistically different in patients with unresectable cholangiocarcinoma (a median survival of 9.6 versus 7.5 months). Cholangitis (0.13 vs. 0.05) and stent occlusion (0.06 vs. 0.02) occurred more frequently in RFA group [21]. In another study, 14 patients with malignant biliary strictures underwent biliary RFA, and 20 patients underwent PDT. RFA group showed a significantly lower rate of premature stent replacement (29% vs. 65%) and adverse events (AE) (21% vs. 40%) [22].

In a recent randomized trial, patients with Bisthmus type I or II hilar cholangiocarcinoma ($n = 19$) or distal CBD cancer ($n = 46$) underwent RFA with plastic stent placement or plastic stent placement alone. Patients in the RFA group showed significantly longer stent patency (6.8 vs. 3.4 months) and survival time (13.2 ± 0.6 vs. 8.3 ± 0.5 months). In this study, performing biliary RFA was the main prognostic factor for survival. AE rate was similar in both groups [23].

Recent systemic review and meta-analysis including a total of 505 patients also revealed that RFA was safe and was associated with improved stent patency in patients with malignant biliary strictures [24]. Patients in RFA group showed significantly longer stent patency (50 vs. 37 days) and survival time (285 vs. 248 days), although systemic chemotherapy was more frequently performed in the control group. Therefore, it may speculate that biliary RFA may trigger a systemic immunological response by thermal tumor necrosis in addition to cytoreduction. Abdominal pain was the most frequent AE related to biliary RFA.

In patients with altered anatomy due to previous surgery, biliary RFA followed by stenting also could be applied through percutaneous, endoscopic ultrasonography (EUS)-guided antegrade approach or using a single-balloon endoscope [25–27].

8.5 Biliary Involvement of Ampulla Adenoma

Biliary RFA can be applied for the management of biliary involvement of ampulla adenoma (Fig. 8.2). Remnant biliary adenoma after endoscopic snare papillectomy (ESP) can be treated with biliary RFA. Several case reports and small case series have reported that adenoma extended from ampulla to the CBD or pancreatic duct orifice can be successfully treated by biliary RFA with a good safety profile [28–30].

Recently, a prospective study on outcomes of biliary RFA for the treatment of adenomatous intraductal residual tumor after ESP in 20 patients, with low-grade dysplasia in 15 patients and high-grade dysplasia in 5 patients, showed a 70% of adenoma eradication at 1 year after single RFA session [31]. Biliary RFA was performed for 30 s with a power of 10 W at the distal CBD followed by SEMS or plastic stent placements. In this study, limited RF power and short duration were applied because of concern of pancreatitis. AE occurred in 40% of patients such as

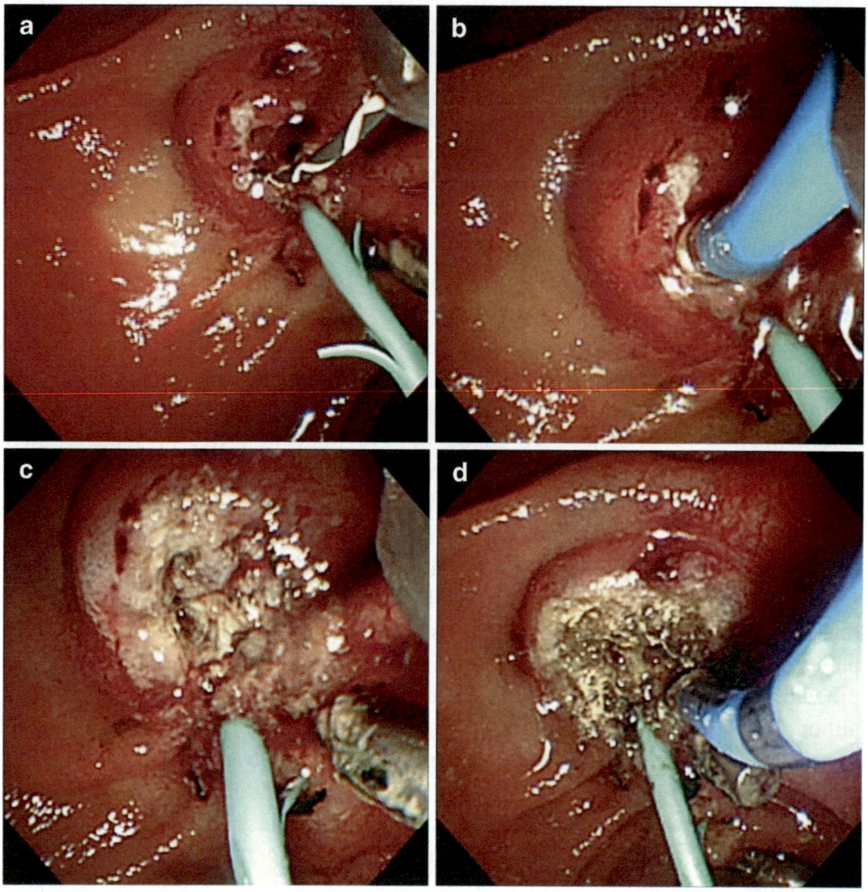

Fig. 8.2 (**a**) Endoscopic view of the papilla after endoscopic snare papillectomy. A 5Fr pancreatic stent is inserted. (**b**) The RFA catheter is placed at the distal common bile duct. (**c**) RFA is performed with 7 W power for 30 s. (**d**) After RFA, argon plasma coagulation is applied to ablate remnant adenoma

abdominal pain and cholangitis. The 15% of patients experienced mild pancreatitis. Biliary stricture after RFA occurred in 15% of patients during follow-up. When biliary RFA was performed to eradicate ampulla tumor, rectal nonsteroidal anti-inflammatory drugs or pancreatic stenting should be considered to prevent pancreatitis.

8.6 Treatment of Occluded SEMS

Biliary RFA may be used to ablate tumor ingrowth in occluded SEMS instead of additional stent insertion through occluded SEMS. The study by Nayar et al. evaluated biliary RFA treatment for occluded SEMS [32]. In this study, seven patients with occlusion of a previously inserted SEMS for malignant biliary stricture underwent biliary RFA. Among them, five patients (71%) needed additional stents placement for optimal drainage. During the mean follow-up period (range, 31–540 days), three patients (42.9%) died due to underlying malignancies at 31, 34, and 52 days after RFA. Therefore, based on the results so far, the role of RFA in patients with occluded SEMS remains uncertain and further studies are necessary.

In an animal study, biliary RFA was performed after uncovered SEMS placement, and histological examination after RFA treatment showed that ablation depth was decreased at the stented bile duct [33]. An in vitro study using a polyacrylamide-gel phantom model to simulate tumor ingrowth of uncovered SEMS also showed similar results. The placement of SEMS attenuated the effect of biliary RFA, and tumors outside the SEMS are unlikely to be affected by endoluminal RFA.

8.7 Safety of Biliary RFA

It is important for the endoscopist to know AEs of biliary RFA. AEs related to biliary RFA have been reported from 10 to 62% of patients including self-limited abdominal pain up to 50% of patients, cholangitis, acute cholecystitis, pancreatitis, liver abscess, and hemobilia from hepatic artery pseudoaneurysm [4, 24]. These wide variabilities in AEs may be due to differences in etiology, the location of stricture, bile duct wall thickness at the stricture site, the distance between bile duct and blood vessels, differences in RFA energy settings, type of biliary stents placed after RFA, and endoscopists' experiences. Serious AEs were rare.

8.8 Conclusions

Biliary RFA has been shown that it appears to be a promising adjuvant local treatment method. It can be applied for malignant biliary stricture, bile duct involvement of ampulla adenoma, or occluded SEMS by tumor ingrowth. The results of studies so far have suggested that biliary RFA can be technically feasible, can improve stent patency and patients' survival, and can be safely performed without serious AE. A prospective randomized trial compared biliary RFA with other treatment modalities such as PDT or radiation therapy is necessary. Biliary RFA can expand its indication to various biliary disease in the future.

References

1. Goldberg SN. Radiofrequency tumor ablation: principles and techniques. Eur J Ultrasound. 2001;13:129–47.
2. Song TJ, Seo DW, Lakhtakia S, et al. Initial experience of EUS-guided radiofrequency ablation of unresectable pancreatic cancer. Gastrointest Endosc. 2016;83:440–3.
3. McCarty TR, Rustagi T. New indications for endoscopic radiofrequency ablation. Clin Gastroenterol Hepatol. 2018;16:1007–17.

4. Larghi A, Rimbas M, Tringali A, et al. Endoscopic radiofrequency biliary ablation treatment: a comprehensive review. Dig Endosc. 2019;31(3):245–55. https://doi.org/10.1111/den.13298.
5. Schueller G, Kettenbach J, Sedivy R, et al. Heat shock protein expression induced by percutaneous radiofrequency ablation of hepatocellular carcinoma in vivo. Int J Oncol. 2004;24:609–13.
6. Haen SP, Pereira PL, Salih HR, et al. More than just tumor destruction: immunomodulation by thermal ablation of cancer. Clin Dev Immunol. 2011;2011:160250.
7. Mao EJ, Watson JB, Soares G, et al. Successful percutaneous endobiliary radiofrequency ablation for unresectable malignant biliary obstruction: a case report and review of the literature. J Gastrointest Cancer. 2014;45(Suppl 1):55–7.
8. Itoi T, Isayama H, Sofuni A, et al. Evaluation of effects of a novel endoscopically applied radiofrequency ablation biliary catheter using an ex-vivo pig liver. J Hepatobiliary Pancreat Sci. 2012;19:543–7.
9. Rhim H, Goldberg SN, Dodd GD 3rd, et al. Essential techniques for successful radio-frequency thermal ablation of malignant hepatic tumors. Radiographics. 2001;21 Spec No:S17–35; discussion S6–9.
10. Rustagi T, Jamidar PA. Intraductal radiofrequency ablation for management of malignant biliary obstruction. Dig Dis Sci. 2014;59:2635–41.
11. Cho JH, Lee KH, Kim JM, et al. Safety and effectiveness of endobiliary radiofrequency ablation according to the different power and target temperature in a swine model. J Gastroenterol Hepatol. 2017;32:521–6.
12. Loew BJ, Howell DA, Sanders MK, et al. Comparative performance of uncoated, self-expanding metal biliary stents of different designs in 2 diameters: final results of an international multicenter, randomized, controlled trial. Gastrointest Endosc. 2009;70:445–53.
13. Hong W, Sun X, Zhu Q. Endoscopic stenting for malignant hilar biliary obstruction: should it be metal or plastic and unilateral or bilateral? Eur J Gastroenterol Hepatol. 2013;25:1105–12.
14. Kaassis M, Boyer J, Dumas R, et al. Plastic or metal stents for malignant stricture of the common bile duct? Results of a randomized prospective study. Gastrointest Endosc. 2003;57:178–82.
15. Alis H, Sengoz C, Gonenc M, et al. Endobiliary radiofrequency ablation for malignant biliary obstruction. Hepatobiliary Pancreat Dis Int. 2013;12:423–7.
16. Figueroa-Barojas P, Bakhru MR, Habib NA, et al. Safety and efficacy of radiofrequency ablation in the management of unresectable bile duct and pancreatic cancer: a novel palliation technique. J Oncol. 2013;2013:910897.
17. Sharaiha RZ, Natov N, Glockenberg KS, et al. Comparison of metal stenting with radiofrequency ablation versus stenting alone for treating malignant biliary strictures: is there an added benefit? Dig Dis Sci. 2014;59:3099–102.
18. Sharaiha RZ, Sethi A, Weaver KR, et al. Impact of radiofrequency ablation on malignant biliary strictures: results of a collaborative registry. Dig Dis Sci. 2015;60:2164–9.
19. Kallis Y, Phillips N, Steel A, et al. Analysis of endoscopic radiofrequency ablation of biliary malignant strictures in pancreatic Cancer suggests potential survival benefit. Dig Dis Sci. 2015;60:3449–55.
20. Laleman W, van der Merwe S, Verbeke L, et al. A new intraductal radiofrequency ablation device for inoperable biliopancreatic tumors complicated by obstructive jaundice: the IGNITE-1 study. Endoscopy. 2017;49:977–82.
21. Strand DS, Cosgrove ND, Patrie JT, et al. ERCP-directed radiofrequency ablation and photodynamic therapy are associated with comparable survival in the treatment of unresectable cholangiocarcinoma. Gastrointest Endosc. 2014;80:794–804.
22. Schmidt A, Bloechinger M, Weber A, et al. Short-term effects and adverse events of endoscopically applied radiofrequency ablation appear to be comparable with photodynamic therapy in hilar cholangiocarcinoma. United European Gastroenterol J. 2016;4:570–9.
23. Yang J, Wang J, Zhou H, et al. Efficacy and safety of endoscopic radiofrequency ablation for unresectable extrahepatic cholangiocarcinoma: a randomized trial. Endoscopy. 2018;50:751–60.

24. Sofi AA, Khan MA, Das A, et al. Radiofrequency ablation combined with biliary stent placement versus stent placement alone for malignant biliary strictures: a systematic review and meta-analysis. Gastrointest Endosc. 2018;87:944–51.e1.
25. Acu B, Kurtulus OE. Feasibility and safety of percutaneous transhepatic endobiliary radiofrequency ablation as an adjunct to biliary stenting in malignant biliary obstruction. Diagn Interv Imaging. 2018;99:237–45.
26. Inoue T, Ito K, Yoneda M. Antegrade radiofrequency ablation and stenting for biliary stricture through endoscopic ultrasound-guided hepaticogastrostomy. Dig Endosc. 2018;30:793–4.
27. Inoue T, Ito K, Yoneda M. Radiofrequency ablation combined with multiple biliary metal stent placement using short-type single-balloon endoscope in patients with surgically altered anatomy. Dig Endosc. 2018;30:395–6.
28. Valente R, Urban O, Del Chiaro M, et al. ERCP-directed radiofrequency ablation of ampullary adenomas: a knife-sparing alternative in patients unfit for surgery. Endoscopy. 2015;47(Suppl 1 UCTN):E515–6.
29. Mehendiratta V, Desilets DJ. Use of radiofrequency ablation probe for eradication of residual adenoma after ampullectomy. Gastrointest Endosc. 2015;81:1055–6.
30. Rustagi T, Irani S, Reddy DN, et al. Radiofrequency ablation for intraductal extension of ampullary neoplasms. Gastrointest Endosc. 2017;86:170–6.
31. Camus M, Napoleon B, Vienne A, et al. Efficacy and safety of endobiliary radiofrequency ablation for the eradication of residual neoplasia after endoscopic papillectomy: a multicenter prospective study. Gastrointest Endosc. 2018;88:511–8.
32. Nayar MK, Oppong KW, Bekkali NLH, et al. Novel temperature-controlled RFA probe for treatment of blocked metal biliary stents in patients with pancreaticobiliary cancers: initial experience. Endosc Int Open. 2018;6:E513–E7.
33. Yoon WJ, Kim YT, Daglilar ES, et al. Evaluation of bipolar radiofrequency ablation for occluded self-expandable metal stents in the bile duct: in vivo and in vitro study. Endoscopy. 2015;47:1167–70.

Endoscopic Sleeve Gastroplasty

9

Daniel Maselli, Andrew C. Storm, and Barham Abu Dayyeh

9.1 Technical, Procedural, and Patient Considerations

ESG is performed under general anesthesia with the patient *nil* per os the night prior to the procedure. From its early implementation, the ESG has been performed using the FDA-cleared device for full-thickness endoscopic suturing system (Apollo Endosurgery, Austin, Texas, USA) [1–3]. Other endoscopic suturing devices are emerging but have yet to be extensively studied, including GERDX device (G-Surg GmbH, Seeon-Seebruck, Germany) and the Endomina device (Endo Tools Therapeutics, Gosselies, Belgium), among others [2, 3]. The Apollo device permits endoscopic suturing by utilizing a helix (corkscrew) tool to embed in the muscularis propria and retract the gastric wall between the suturing tower, thereby permitting full-thickness plications of gastric tissue [4]. The company recommends use of an esophageal overtube to prevent esophageal trauma during intubation with the suturing device, though the need for an overtube has been questioned [5]. Pre-marking of the intended suture line along the anterior and posterior walls of the stomach using argon plasma coagulation may be considered. To perform the ESG, the endoscopist places sutures in a retrograde fashion, which, when completed, will extend from the angle of the incisura to 1 cm below the gastroesophageal junction within the fundus. The procedure uses approximately 6–10 sutures, often in a triangular or "U-shaped" pattern, typically in the following order: starting from the anterior wall, down to the greater curvature, then to the posterior wall, and then brought back to the anterior wall about 1 cm proximally to the first suture bite (see Fig. 9.1) [6]. The stich is tightened to approximate the opposing gastric walls through serosal surface invagination, thus creating a tubular gastric sleeve with a lumen roughly 30% of the original stomach volume (see Fig. 9.2), with a small fundus cap (see Fig. 9.3c and d).

D. Maselli · A. C. Storm · B. A. Dayyeh (✉)
Division of Gastroenterology and Hepatology, Mayo Clinic, Rochester, MN, USA
e-mail: Maselli.Daniel@mayo.edu; AbuDayyeh.Barham@mayo.edu

P. Sharma, N. Reddy (eds.), *Innovations in Gastrointestinal Endoscopy*,
https://doi.org/10.1007/978-981-15-9247-8_9

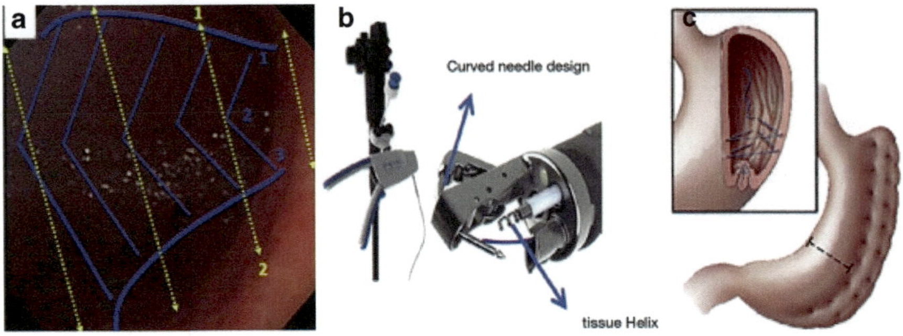

Fig. 9.1 (**a**) Suturing pattern used to create the ESG. (**b**) The full-thickness endoscopic suturing device used to create the ESG. (**c**) A longitudinal section depicting the invagination of the greater curvature of the stomach for creation of a narrow sleeve, reducing the functional capacity of the stomach by approximately 80%. (Reprinted with permission from Elsevier [Abu Dayyeh BK, Acosta A, Camilleri M, Mundi MS, Rajan E, Topazian MD, et al. Endoscopic sleeve gastroplasty alters gastric physiology and induces loss of body weight in obese individuals. Clin Gastroenterol Hepatology. 2017;15(1):37–43.e1])

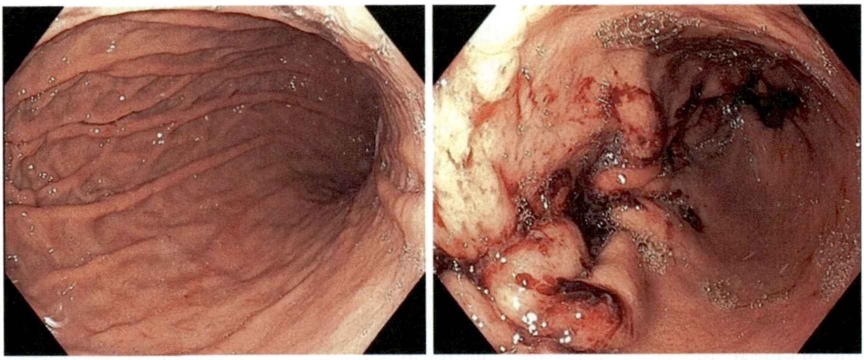

Fig. 9.2 Endoscopic sleeve gastroplasty prior to (left) and immediately upon completion of (right) the procedure. (Images courtesy of Andrew C. Storm, MD)

The suture is ultimately secured with a cinching device and held tightly in place by a needle and cinch T-tag at the respective ends. Procedural time varies by center and experience but is approximately 90 min.

Following the procedure, patients are either admitted to the hospital for a 24-h observation [4, 7] or discharged the same day [8]. A brief course of antibiotics, antiemetics, and analgesics is customary. Proton pump inhibitors (PPIs) have been continued anywhere from 3 days to 6 weeks [4, 6] and it is our practice to continue a PPI for at least 1 month post-procedure. Post-procedural dietary recommendations vary but generally follow a 1-month liquid diet, followed by pureed consistency for 2 weeks, and solids as tolerated thereafter [8, 9].

In the studies of ESG described here, patients were excluded if they had micro- or macroscopic abnormalities of gastric tissue that would compromise success of a

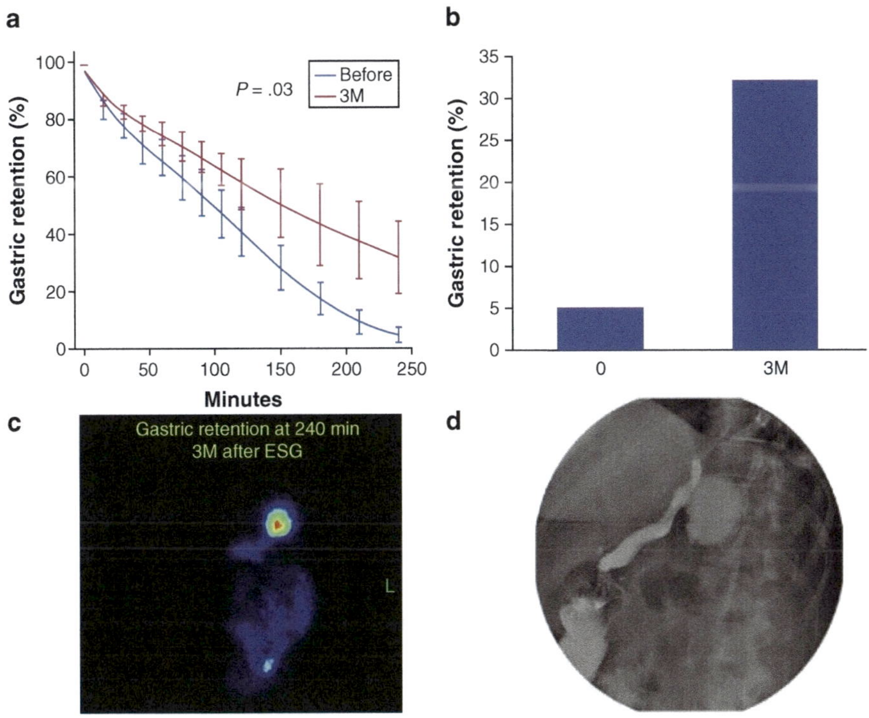

Fig. 9.3 (**a**) Changes in gastric emptying of solids at baseline and 3 months after ESG (means and standard error of the means presented). (**b**) Percent gastric retention of a solid meal at 240 min at baseline and 3 months after ESG. (**c**) Gastric scintigraphy at 240 min after solid meal ingestion, depicting retained solid mean in a small gastric fundus cap 3 months after ESG. (**d**) Upper gastrointestinal series with a radio-opaque contrast, demonstrating a sleeve effect with a small fundus cap. (Reprinted with permission from Elsevier [Abu Dayyeh BK, Acosta A, Camilleri M, Mundi MS, Rajan E, Topazian MD, et al. Endoscopic sleeve gastroplasty alters gastric physiology and induces loss of body weight in obese individuals. Clin Gastroenterol Hepatol. 2017;15(1):37–43.e1])

gastric plication procedure or prohibitively increase its risk, including a history of gastric cancer, family history of gastric cancer, active *Helicobacter pylori* infection, active gastritis or gastric ulcer, gastric intestinal metaplasia, vascular abnormalities, and prior foregut surgery. Patients were also routinely excluded if they had systemic conditions such as pregnancy/lactation, coagulation disorders, or decompensated organ failure [4, 6].

9.2 Operator Learning Curve

To evoke broad appeal, an endoscopic bariatric therapy must not only be an effective weight loss strategy but also imminently reproducible and implemented. While studies of ESG have invariably been carried out by endoscopists familiar with endoscopic suturing, it is nevertheless instructive to observe the performance characteristics with a novel technique. Hill et al defined the learning curve for ESG of a single endoscopist who performed 21 ESG procedures over a 9-month period after a 1 day training program [10]. Average procedural time and plication number decreased significantly over procedures and reached a plateau after 9 procedures, with 90% efficiency by 7 procedures. Abu Dayyeh et al. showed in a 25 subject case series of ESG that procedural time decreased from 217 ± 17 min in the average of the first 5 cases to 98 ± 4 min as the average of the last 5 cases ($P < 0.01$) [11]. Sharaiha et al observed that in a series of 91 ESG cases using B-spline regression that the number of procedures needed to achieve efficiency was 35 [4]. While precise numbers will vary, it is clear there is a trend toward greater efficiency within a manageable number of ESG procedures. These studies also highlight the growing importance and feasibility of incorporating dedicated bariatric therapy training within advanced endoscopic fellowship programs [12].

9.3 Physiologic Mechanisms

Gastric restriction is central tenant of most bariatric surgeries, and several studies have investigated the underlying physiologic mechanisms of various bariatric surgical procedures to induce weight loss [13–15]. While gastric pouch restriction is understood to be a fundamental principal of ESG, the physiologic underpinnings driving weight loss have not been fully elucidated. Abu Dayyeh et al. performed a physiologic appraisal in a subset of patients just prior to and 3 months after ESG [11]. ESG appeared to significantly alter satiation, rendering a 59% decrease in caloric consumption to reach maximum fullness ($P = 0.003$), as well as and satiety, prolonging time to half gastric emptying of solids by 90 min ($P = 0.03$) (see Fig. 9.3). Taken together, these findings suggest physiologic alterations in appetite, in the form of both satiation and satiety, play a role in a role in the mechanism of weight loss after ESG, though more work is required to define their relative contributions. In terms of hormonal alterations, despite significant weight loss, there were no observable statistical differences observed in levels of glucagon-like peptide-1, leptin, peptide YY, and fasting and post-prandial ghrelin by Abu Dayyeh and colleagues; however, Graus-Morales et al. did demonstrate a significant decrease in leptin 12 months following ESG [16]. There is still much to be learned about the neurohormonal and physiologic alterations that occur from ESG.

9.4 Patient Outcomes

9.4.1 Clinical Success in ESG: Percent Total Body Weight Loss

There are several studies that have retrospectively analyzed prospectively collected data from ESG subjects to approximate a customary primary end point of bariatric interventions: percent total body weight loss (%TBWL). Clinical success is defined as a %TBWL of at least 15% by the Preservation and Incorporation of Valuable Endoscopic Innovation Guidelines and has been associated with durable weight loss in endoscopic bariatric therapy [17, 18]. Subjects from earlier ESG studies have been in some cases incorporated into larger, multicenter retrospective studies [7, 11, 19]. The major studies and their implications will be described here.

In a single center study, Sharaiha et al. prospectively followed 91 consecutive patients (mean age 43.86 ± 11.26 years, 68% female, mean BMI 40.7 ± 7.0 kg/m^2) after ESG [4]. %TBWL was 14.4% at 6 months (80% follow-up rate), 17.6% at 12 months (76% follow-up rate), and 20.9% at 24 months (66% follow-up rate). Another single-center retrospective study in Spain of 148 patients (mean age 41.53 ± 10 years, 82% female, baseline BMI 35.11 ± 5.5 kg/m^2) found %TBWL at 17.5% at 12 months using a slightly modified stich pattern for the ESG [16]. Two robust assessments of ESG have come from two international, multicenter studies. Lopez-Nava et al. retrospectively analyzed 248 patients (mean age 44.5 ± 10 years, 73% female, baseline BMI 37.8 ± 5.6 kg/m^2) from three centers, two in the United States, and one in Spain [9]. At 6 months, %TBWL was 15.2%, and at 24 months it was 18.6%. Sartoretto et al. looked at 112 consecutive patients (mean age 45.1 ± 11.7 years, 69% female, baseline BMI 37.9 ± 6.7 kg/m^2) who underwent ESG in three centers, two in the United States and one in Australia [8]. %TBWL was 11.9% at 3 months and 14.9% at 6 months after ESG. A recent meta-analysis by Storm et al. of the 1607 ESGs performed to date showed a %TBWL of 15.784% at 6 months (95% CI 15.606–15.961), 17.107% at 12 months (95% CI 17.107–17.454), and 17.311% in the subgroup >18 months from ESG (95% CI 15.94–18.659) (see Fig. 9.4) [5]. Of note, there were no control or comparator arms in the aforementioned investigations. Nevertheless, these studies demonstrated that ESG facilitates clinically meaningful and durable weight loss.

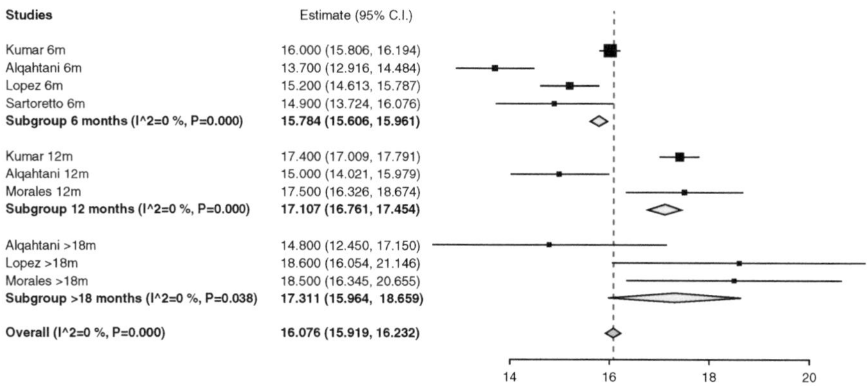

Fig. 9.4 Meta-analysis of percent total body weight loss after ESG in 1607 cases. (Reprinted with permission from Elsevier [Storm AC, Abu Dayyeh BK. Endoscopic sleeve gastroplasty for obesity: defining the risk and reward after more than 1600 procedures. Gastrointest Endosc. 2019;89(6):1139–40])

9.4.2 Comparison to Alternative Bariatric Procedures

While the studies reviewed in this chapter demonstrate a robust performance for long-term weight loss from ESG, without comparator arms, it is not clear how ESG fares compared to other endoscopic or surgical bariatric interventions. Two studies have endeavored to address this. Fayad et al. retrospectively reviewed consecutive patients at a single center who underwent ESG or an intragastric balloon (IGB) in the form of ReShape Integrated Dual Balloon System (ReShape Lifesciences, San Clemente, CA, USA) or the Orbera Intragastric Balloon System (Apollo Endosurgery, Austin, TX, USA), which were removed at 6 months. Both arms were subject to identical standards of post-procedural dietary, exercise, and medical follow-up. At 6 months, after controlling for sex, age, and baseline BMI, %TBWL was 19.5% for ESG (43.1% follow-up) and 15% for IGB (91.4% follow-up) ($P = 0.01$); by 12 months %TBWL was 21.3% for ESG (36.2% follow-up) and 13.9% for IGB (42.6% follow-up) ($P = 0.005$). While ESG subjects continued to lose weight between 6 and 12 months, those with IGB gained an average of 7.3 lbs. in weight after the IGB was removed at month 6. This study was limited by its inclusion of a greater proportion of men and higher baseline BMI in the ESG cohort, as well as by loss to follow up, but it does suggest that ESG brings about a statistically greater %TBWL compared to IGB, particularly in the longer term, as it is not subject to the same weight recidivism commonly observed after IGB removal.

Novikov et al. compared ESG to traditional bariatric surgeries—laparoscopic sleeve gastrectomy (LSG) and laparoscopic adjustable gastric banding (LAGB)—in a single-center retrospective cohort study of 278 obese patients [20]. While %TBWL was reported as greatest in LSG compared to LAGB and ESG (29.28% vs 13.30% vs 17.57%, respectively; $P < 0.001$), LSG had a statistically higher baseline BMI compared to ESG (47.22 ± 7.84 kg/m^2 vs 38.61 ± 6.98 kg/m^2, respectively); when BMI was stratified for BMI < 40 kg/m^2, there was no significant difference in %TBWL at 12 months when comparing the three techniques. ESG showed significantly lower rates of morbidity compared to surgical interventions and a reduced length-of-stay post-procedurally. The comparable effectiveness of ESG with standard bariatric surgery techniques, as well as the substantially reduced risk to the patient, provide compelling evidence for incorporating ESG into the armamentarium of bariatric intervention, particularly in those patients with BMI between 30 and 40 kg/m^2 or those with comorbidities that are prohibitive for surgery.

9.4.3 Outcomes in Obesity-Associated Conditions

While most of the investigations of ESG have used %TBWL as a marker of clinical success, Sharaiha et al. provided data to reinforce what was previously an assumption—namely that improvement in obesity-associated conditions would follow suit. 12 months after ESG, hemoglobin A1c (HA1c) decreased from $6.1 \pm 1.1\%$ to $5.5 \pm 0.48\%$ ($p = 0.05$), and in those with diabetes or pre-diabetes at baseline, HA1c improved from $6.6 \pm 1.2\%$ to $5.6 \pm 0.51\%$ ($P = 0.02$). In the same timeframe, serum triglycerides decreased from 131.84 ± 83.19 mmol/dL to 92.36 ± 39.43 mmol/dL

($P = 0.02$), and serum alanine aminotransferase decreased from 42.4 mg/dL to 22.0 mg/dL in men ($P = 0.05$), and 28.0 mg/dL to 20.0 mg/dL in women ($P = 0.01$). Despite improvement in the metabolic profile, there was no statistically significant difference in serum low-density lipoprotein levels after 12 months of ESG [4]. Alqahtani et al. showed that 13 of 17 patients with diabetes were in complete remission by month 3 after ESG, and the remaining four were on a decreased dose of diabetes medications [21].

9.4.4 Predictors of Clinical Success in ESG

Factors associated with increased likelihood of substantive %TBWL can be divided into patient and procedural factors. Patient characteristics that predicted more significant %TBWL include younger age [4] and greater adherence to nutritional and psychological follow-up [4, 6, 22]. Lopez-Nava et al observed that weight loss at 6 months was highly predictive of continued weight loss and maintenance at 24 months [9]. Lower baseline BMI was associated with greater percentage excess body weight loss but not total body weight loss, though percent excess body weight loss is not thought to be a reliable metric for clinical success in bariatric therapy because it is biased towards patients with BMI closer to non-obese ranges [8, 16]. Procedural characteristics associated with greater %TBWL likely include operator experience, as Sharaiha et al. demonstrated that the first 34 of 91 consecutive ESG cases had lower %TBWL compared to the remaining cases, even after adjusting for BMI and sex [4].

9.4.5 Adverse Events

Major intraprocedural complications have not been observed in ESG, though endoscopists continue to refine the technique outlined in the beginning of this chapter to improve safety. For instance, a report by Storm et al. demonstrated that the use of an esophageal overtube in more than 700 upper GI tract endoscopic suturing procedures was associated with an increased risk for minor esophageal mucosal trauma as compared to not using an esophageal overtube [23], and thus it is not our standard practice to employ an esophageal overtube in ESG. Immediate and mild post-procedural adverse events are so commonplace following ESG that they are often under-reported. These typically include the expected accommodative symptoms of nausea, cramping, and abdominal discomfort, which are observed in 38.4% to upwards of 92.4% of patients in the first 48 h following ESG and are almost universally successfully managed with pharmacologic therapy [4, 9, 11, 21].

Serious adverse events are rare and include bleeding, peri-gastric leak, and pulmonary complication. Upper gastrointestinal bleed (UGIB) was found in 2 of 112 patients in Sartoretto et al. and managed conservatively; 1 of 148 patients in Graus-Morales et al. and managed with sclerotherapy; and in 7 of 1000 patients in Alqahtani et al., 2 of whom received packed red blood cell transfusion and the remaining were managed with intravenous fluids [8, 16, 21]. Lopez-Nava et al reported one

Table 9.1 Serious adverse events in endoscopic sleeve gastroplasty across all major endoscopic sleeve gastroplasty reports totaling 1607 cases. (Recreated with permission from Elsevier [Storm AC, Abu Dayyeh BK. Endoscopic sleeve gastroplasty for obesity: defining the risk and reward after more than 1600 procedures. Gastrointest Endosc. 2019;89(6):1139–40])

Serious adverse events in ESG	Number of patients (frequency)
Intra-abdominal collection	7 (0.4%)
Hemorrhage requiring transfusion or endoscopic intervention	6 (0.4%)
Refractory symptoms requiring ESG reversal	3 (0.2%)
Pneumoperitoneum and pneumothorax	1 (0.1%)
Pulmonary embolism	1 (0.1%)
Perforation or death	0 (0%)

extra-gastric hemorrhage out of 248 patients, managed with blood tranfusion [9]. Peri-gastric leak with fluid collection was reported within the first 2 weeks in 2 of 248 (Lopez-Nava et al.), 1 of 91 (Sharaiha et al.), 1 of 91 (Novikov et al.), 1 of 112 (Sartoretto et al.), and 4 of 1000 (Alqahtani et al.) ESG cases [4, 8, 9, 20, 21]. At least 2 were explicitly due to dietary indiscretion with premature introduction of solid food [19, 20, 24]. All 9 were managed with antibiotics, 7 required percuteanous drainage, and all resolved without need for surgery. To reduce risk of peri-gastric leak, Abu Dayyeh et al. altered clinical protocol by avoiding reduction of the fundus, as the most posterior aspect of the fundus was considered the greatest risk for leak on account of its thin wall [11]. Other rare major adverse events of ESG include pneumothorax/pneumomediastinum in one patient, managed with a chest tube and antibiotics, and another patient with pulmonary embolism 72 hours after ESG [9].

A more recent meta-analysis by Storm et al. in 2019 of all major ESG reports (totalling 1607 ESGs) calculated the serious adverse event rates of intra-abdominal collection (0.4%), hemorrhage requiring transfusion or endoscopic intervention (0.4%), pneumoperitoneum or pneumomediastinum (0.1%), pulmonary embolism (0.1%), and perforation or death (0%) (see Table 9.1) [23].

9.5 Re-Do, Reversal, and Surgical Revision

Within the field of endoscopic bariatric therapies, the appeal of removable intragastric devices stems from their easy reversibility, should symptom intolerance or complications arise, and there is concern that endoscopic gastric plication would not afford ESG the same advantage; however, the available data show that ESG maintains plasticity and can still be manipulated or revised without considerable risk to the patient. There are only a few instances reported of need for re-do ESG available in the literature. Alqahtani et al. described 5 patients in their series of 1000 patients who underwent ESG who required re-do for weight regain during the trial [21]. In only one of these patients were the ESG sutures found to be intact. This experience parallels other reports that ESG can be easily "touched up" to achieve further weight reduction, an endeavor viewed as less challenging than the initial ESG procedure [25, 26].

Successful reversal of ESG with suture removal was reported only in Alqahtani et al., in which 3 of 1000 patients required reversal for intolerance of accommodative symptoms. Concerns over surgical revision of ESG arose from the theoretical challenges associated with increased gastric thickness from plication and the attendant focal devascularization [27]. Nevertheless, reported cases of clinically insignificant weight loss in two patients several months out from ESG showed that aside from adhesions found on nearby abdominal viscera, the stomachs otherwise appeared normal, and conversion to laparoscopic sleeve gastrectomy (LSG) was not technically distinguishable from patients without previous gastric manipulation [28]. This mirrors the experience of 8 of 1000 patients in Alqahtani et al. who were revised to LSG for insufficient weight loss, and none of these patients were found to have fully intact sutures [21]. The lack of technical challenge associated with surgical revision likely stems from the same etiology of insufficient weight loss—namely insufficiently imbricated gastric tissue during ESG—and should reassure surgical providers that those patients seeking surgical revision for inadequate %TBWL likely do not have dramatically or prohibitively altered anatomy from their prior ESG.

9.6 Areas for Future Research and Discussion

Given the increasingly recognized durability and minimal risk profile compared to similarly effective bariatric surgery, ESG has a promising role in managing obesity. Further work is needed to determine if weight loss is durable beyond 2 years, as well as to define the procedure's impact on physiologic underpinnings and obesity-associated cardiometabolic disease. Adding further complexity to the study of endoscopic bariatric therapies is the exploration of the potential synergism of combination therapies, such as the volume-restrictive effect of ESG and the neurohormonal and malabsorptive changes found in duodenal mucosal resurfacing or duodenal-jejunal bypass liner. In light of the growing abundance of endoscopic bariatric therapies that capitalize on unique anatomic and physiologic characteristics, identifying patient phenotypes in order to tailor endoscopic approaches to weight loss will likely improve the safety, tolerability, and sustained weight loss of these techniques. Further consideration is also required on how best to incorporate this growing field of endoscopic bariatric therapy into advanced endoscopy training.

References

1. Abu Dayyeh BK, Rajan E, Gostout CJ. Endoscopic sleeve gastroplasty: a potential endoscopic alternative to surgical sleeve gastrectomy for treatment of obesity. Gastrointest Endosc. 2013;78(3):530–5.
2. Wannhoff A, Hofmann C, Meier B, Birk D, Caca K. Endoscopic sleeve gastroplasty for severe obesity by full-thickness suturing using the GERDX device. Endoscopy. 2019;51(2):E34–5.

3. Wallstabe I, Oberaender N, Weimann A, Schiefke I. Endoscopic sleeve gastroplasty using the novel endomina device for morbidly obese patients. Endoscopy. 2018;50(11):E327–8.
4. Sharaiha RZ, Kumta NA, Saumoy M, Desai AP, Sarkisian AM, Benevenuto A, et al. Endoscopic sleeve gastroplasty significantly reduces body mass index and metabolic complications in obese patients. Clin Gastroenter Hepatol. 2017;15(4):504–10.
5. Storm AC, Abu Dayyeh BK. Endoscopic sleeve gastroplasty for obesity: defining the risk and reward after more than 1600 procedures. Gastrointest Endosc. 2019;89(6):1139–40.
6. Fayad L, Cheskin LJ, Adam A, Badurdeen DS, Hill C, Agnihotri A, et al. Endoscopic sleeve gastroplasty versus intragastric balloon insertion: efficacy, durability, and safety. Endoscopy. 2019;51(6):532–9.
7. Lopez-Nava G, Galvao MP, da Bautista-Castano I, Jimenez A, De Grado T, Fernandez-Corbelle JP. Endoscopic sleeve gastroplasty for the treatment of obesity. Endoscopy. 2015;47(5):449–52.
8. Sartoretto A, Sui Z, Hill C, Dunlap M, Rivera AR, Khashab MA, et al. Endoscopic sleeve gastroplasty (ESG) is a reproducible and effective endoscopic bariatric therapy suitable for widespread clinical adoption: a large, international multicenter study. Obes Surg. 2018;28(7):1812–21.
9. Lopez-Nava G, Sharaiha RZ, Vargas EJ, Bazerbachi F, Manoel GN, Bautista-Castano I, et al. Endoscopic sleeve gastroplasty for obesity: a multicenter study of 248 patients with 24 months follow-up. Obes Surg. 2017;27(10):2649–55.
10. Hill C, El Zein M, Agnihotri A, Dunlap M, Chang A, Agrawal A, et al. Endoscopic sleeve gastroplasty: the learning curve. Endosc Int Open. 2017;5(9):E900–e4.
11. Abu Dayyeh BK, Acosta A, Camilleri M, Mundi MS, Rajan E, Topazian MD, et al. Endoscopic sleeve gastroplasty alters gastric physiology and induces loss of body weight in obese individuals. Clin Gastroenterol Hepatol. 2017;15(1):37–43.e1.
12. Sullivan S, Kumar N, Edmundowicz SA, Abu Dayyeh BK, Jonnalagadda SS, Larsen M, et al. ASGE position statement on endoscopic bariatric therapies in clinical practice. Gastrointest Endosc. 2015;82(5):767–72.
13. Park CW, Torquati A. Physiology of weight loss surgery. Surg Clin North Am. 2011;91(6):1149–61, vii
14. Manning S, Pucci A, Batterham RL. Roux-en-Y gastric bypass: effects on feeding behavior and underlying mechanisms. J Clin Invest. 2015;125(3):939–48.
15. Chakravartty S, Tassinari D, Salerno A, Giorgakis E, Rubino F. What is the mechanism behind weight loss maintenance with gastric bypass? Curr Obes Rep. 2015;4(2):262–8.
16. Graus Morales J, Crespo Perez L, Marques A, Marin Arribas B, Bravo Arribas R, Ramo E, et al. Modified endoscopic gastroplasty for the treatment of obesity. Surg Endosc. 2018;32(9):3936–42.
17. Ginsberg GG, Chand B, Cote GA, Dallal RM, Edmundowicz SA, Nguyen NT, et al. A pathway to endoscopic bariatric therapies. Gastrointest Endosc. 2011;74(5):943–53.
18. Abu Dayyeh BK, Kumar N, Edmundowicz SA, Jonnalagadda S, Larsen M, Sullivan S, et al. ASGE Bariatric Endoscopy Task Force systematic review and meta-analysis assessing the ASGE PIVI thresholds for adopting endoscopic bariatric therapies. Gastrointest Endosc. 2015;82(3):425–438.e5.
19. Sharaiha RZ, Kedia P, Kumta N, DeFilippis EM, Gaidhane M, Shukla A, et al. Initial experience with endoscopic sleeve gastroplasty: technical success and reproducibility in the bariatric population. Endoscopy. 2015;47(2):164–6.
20. Novikov AA, Afaneh C, Saumoy M, Parra V, Shukla A, Dakin GF, et al. Endoscopic sleeve gastroplasty, laparoscopic sleeve gastrectomy, and laparoscopic band for weight loss: how do they compare? J Gastrointest Surg. 2018;22(2):267–73.
21. Alqahtani A, Al-Darwish A, Mahmoud AE, Alqahtani YA, Elahmedi M. Short-term outcomes of endoscopic sleeve gastroplasty in 1000 consecutive patients. Gastrointest Endosc. 2019;89(6):1132–8.
22. Lopez-Nava G, Galvao M, Bautista-Castano I, Fernandez-Corbelle JP, Trell M. Endoscopic sleeve gastroplasty with 1-year follow-up: factors predictive of success. Endosc Int Open. 2016;4(2):E222–7.

23. Storm AC, Vargas EJ, Matar R, Wong Kee Song LM, Sawas T, Bazerbachi F, et al. Esophageal overtubes provide no benefit to safety or technical success in upper gastrointestinal tract endoscopic suturing. Endosc Int Open. 2019;7(7):E919–21.
24. Barola S, Agnihotri A, Khashab MA, Kumbhari V. Perigastric fluid collection after endoscopic sleeve gastroplasty. Endoscopy. 2016;48(S1):E340–1.
25. Chang KJ. Endoscopic foregut surgery and interventions: the future is now. The state-of-the-art and my personal journey. World J Gastroenterol. 2019;25(1):1–41.
26. Kumta NA, Doshi R, Aronne LJ, Sharaiha RZ. Trimming the fat: endoscopic suturing for tightening of prior endoscopic sleeve gastroplasty. Gastrointest Endosc. 2017;85(1):253–4.
27. Movitz BR, Lutfi RE. Endoscopic sleeve gastroplasty: are we burning bridges? Surg Obes Relat Dis. 2017;13(12):2056–8.
28. Ferrer-Marquez M, Ferrer-Ayza M, Rubio-Gil F, Torrente-Sanchez MJ, Martinez Amo-Gamez A. [Revision bariatric surgery after endoscopic sleeve gastroplasty]. Cir Cir. 2017;85(5):428–431.

Full-Thickness Resection 10

Andreas Wannhoff, Horst Neuhaus, and Karel Caca

10.1 Introduction

Endoscopic full-thickness resection (EFTR) is a relatively new technique, which has greatly expanded the possibilities of endoscopic resection. It can be performed in upper and lower gastrointestinal tract. Typical indications include early mucosal neoplasms such as recurrent or residual adenomas in the colorectum, resection of subepithelial tumors (SET), and diagnostic EFTR. Different techniques can be used to perform EFTR. Exposed EFTR can be distinguished from non-exposed EFTR. In the latter case, the resection site is secured with a clip or suture prior to resection. The Full-Thickness Resection Device (FTRD) combines occlusion of resection site and resection itself in a single device. It is the best studied device for EFTR and mainly used for resection of difficult colonic adenomas. In the upper gastrointestinal tract, endoscopy and laparoscopy can be combined to achieve full-thickness resection. SETs are the major indication to perform full-thickness resection in the upper gastrointestinal tract.

A. Wannhoff · K. Caca (✉)
Department of Internal Medicine and Gastroenterology, Hospital Ludwigsburg, Ludwigsburg, Germany
e-mail: andreas.wannhoff@rkh-kliniken.de; karel.caca@rkh-kliniken.de

H. Neuhaus
Department of Internal Medicine, Evangelisches Krankenhaus Düsseldorf, Düsseldorf, Germany
e-mail: Horst.Neuhaus@evk-duesseldorf.de

P. Sharma, N. Reddy (eds.), *Innovations in Gastrointestinal Endoscopy*,
https://doi.org/10.1007/978-981-15-9247-8_10

10.2 Techniques and Devices for Endoscopic Full-Thickness Resection

10.2.1 Exposed Versus Non-exposed Full-Thickness Resection

To successfully perform EFTR, it is not only necessary to resect the target lesion but also to securely close the resulting transmural defect. Based upon the order of these two steps, exposed and non-exposed EFTR can be distinguished. In exposed EFTR full-thickness resection of the target lesion is performed first, followed by occlusion of the defect in the second step. This might result in a potential spoilage of neoplastic cells into the peritoneal cavity as well as an increased risk of bacterial contamination and peritonitis. Further, leakage of air and collapse of the lumen makes endoscopic closure of the resection defect more difficult and leads to development of pneumoperitoneum. In contrast, in non-exposed EFTR resection site is first secured with clips or other devices before the target lesion is resected [1, 2].

10.2.2 Full-Thickness Resection Device—FTRD

The FTRD system (Ovesco Endoscopy, Tuebingen, Germany) is the only currently commercially available device that combines resection and defect closure in one device (Fig. 10.1). It consists of a transparent cap, which is preloaded with a modified Over-The-Scope Clip (OTSC, Ovesco Endoscopy, Tuebingen, Germany) and a resection snare. The FTRD is mounted on the tip of a standard endoscope. The trigger for deployment of the clip runs through the endoscope's working channel, while the snare handle runs on the endoscope's outside underneath a flexible cover. To perform EFTR with the FTRD system the target lesion has to be incorporated into the transparent cap. This can be achieved by use of grasping forceps or a tissue anchor. It is advisable to mark the lesion's border prior to resection because the mounted FTRD significantly reduces visibility. After the lesion has been incorporated into the cap, the clip is deployed, and the snare is closed immediately thereafter. We use the following setting on the ERBE VIO (Erbe Elektromedizin GmbH, Tuebingen, Germany) high-frequency generator to finally resect the lesion: HIGH CUT, Effect 4, max. 180 W.

10.2.3 Clip-Assisted Full-Thickness Resection

Similar to resection with the FTRD, EFTR can be achieved by first applying an over-the-scope mounted clip (OTSC or Padlock Clip, Aponos Medical, Kingston, NH, USA) to secure the resection base with subsequent snare resection. In contrast to the FTRD system, which combines both steps in a single device, in our

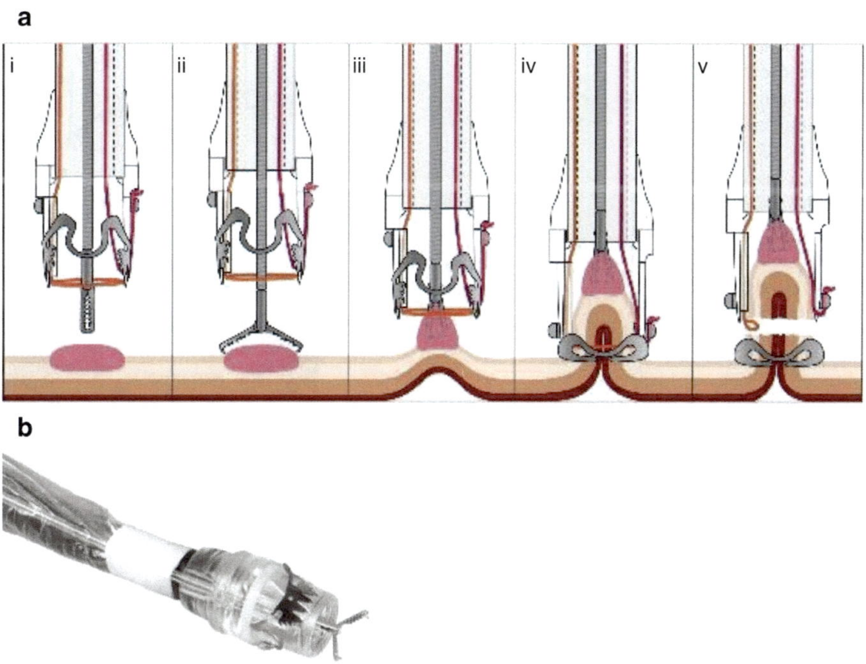

Fig. 10.1 The Full-Thickness Resection Device—FTRD. (**a**) The FTRD System is mounted on the tip of an endoscope. The snare handle runs under a transparent cover on the outside of the endoscope. (**b**) Utilization of the FTRD system consists of the following steps: (i + ii) Identification and grasping of the lesion, (iii) Pulling the lesion into the transparent cap, (iv) Releasing the over-the-scope clip, and (v) Snare resection of the lesion above the clip

experience, the risk of thermal injury is increased, and resected specimens are smaller.

10.2.4 Pure Endoscopic, Full-Thickness Resection Techniques in the Upper Gastrointestinal Tract

In the upper gastrointestinal tract, several different techniques have been described to perform pure endoscopic EFTR. While the resection is usually done either with a snare or ESD (endoscopic submucosal dissection) knife, the device for occlusion of the resulting wall defect differed between studies. Traditional through-the-scope clips as well as the OTSC have been used to close these wall defects. Further options for defect closure include the use of more specialized suturing devices such as the GERDX (G-Surg GmbH, Seeon, Germany), OverStitch (Apollo Endosurgery Inc., Austin, TX, USA), or Double-arm-bar Suturing System (Fig. 10.2). These devices can be used to close the resection site before resection and thus to perform non-exposed EFTR.

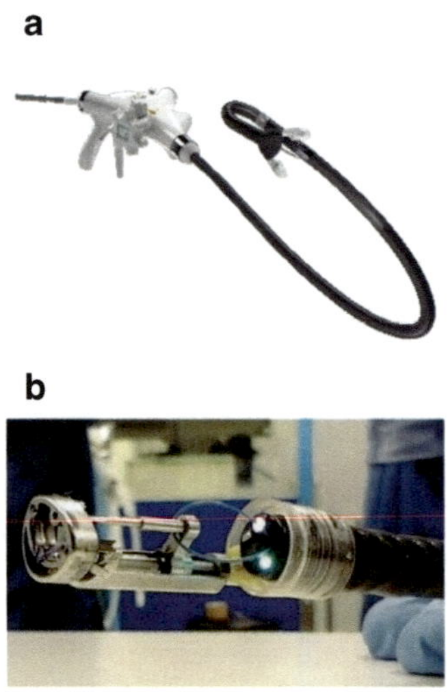

Fig. 10.2 Devices for pure endoscopic, non-exposed full-thickness resection in the upper gastrointestinal tract. (**a**) GERDX (G-Surg GmbH, Seeon, Germany) (Figure A with kind permission from the manufacture); (**b**) Double-arm-bar Suturing System (not yet commercially available, Figure from Mori et al. [3])

10.2.5 Combined Endoscopic and Laparoscopic Full-Thickness Resection

In contrast to pure endoscopic approaches, laparoscopic endoscopic cooperative surgery (LECS) combines endoscopy with laparoscopy to achieve full-thickness resection and close the resection defect. Classic LECS consists of the following steps: (1) endoscopic circumferential submucosal incision, (2) laparoscopic seromuscular incision over three-quarters of the circumference, (3) turning over the tumor into the abdominal cavity, and (4) closing the incision with a stapling device and retrieving the tumor laparoscopically. Several modifications of this technique have been developed. Inverted LECS was developed to reduce the risk of tumor cell dissemination into the peritoneal cavity. In contrast to the classic LECS procedure, the tumor is not turned into the abdominal cavity, and it is retrieved endoscopically. However, the gastric wall is opened and thus contamination of the abdominal cavity cannot be ruled out. In contrast, the CLEAN-NET procedure and Non-Exposed Endoscopic Wall-Inversion Surgery (NEWS) are forms of non-exposed full-thickness resection. For the CLEAN-NET procedure, seromuscular incision is done laparoscopically and the mucosa is preserved as a barrier (a "clean net"). The tumor is then pulled into the abdominal cavity, sutures are applied, and the tumor is resected. NEWS consists of the following steps: (1) marking around the tumor on the mucosal and serosal side, (2) submucosal injection, (3) laparoscopic seromuscular incision and suture, (4) endoscopic submucosal dissection, and (5) oral retrieval of the specimen (Fig. 10.3) [4].

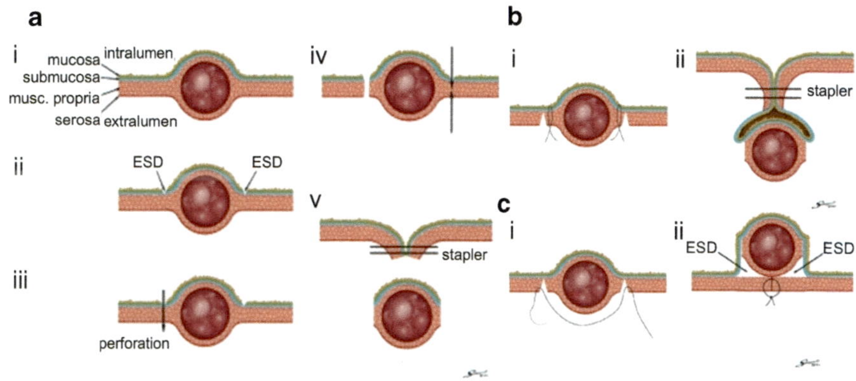

Fig. 10.3 Overview of different techniques of laparoscopic endoscopic cooperative surgery. Schematic overview of (**a**) Classic LECS procedure, (**b**) CLEAN-NET procedure, and (**c**) NEWS procedure (All figures from Hiki et al. [4]). For details on the procedures, see text

The major disadvantage of these combined procedures compared to pure endoscopic techniques is need for more resources (e.g., endoscopist, surgeon, anesthesiologist, operating room).

10.3 Gastric Full-Thickness Resection

Several studies have investigated variants of pure endoscopic full-thickness resection. In studies that utilized exposed EFTR, the subsequent closure of the resection site was done with through-the-scope clips, either alone or in combination with an endoloop, or with the OTSC. The OTSC was shown to be superior for closure of Natural Orifice Transluminal Endoscopic Surgery (NOTES) gastrostomies. The studies are summarized in Table 10.1.

Full-thickness suturing with the Double-arm bar Suturing System was compared to the OTSC and hand-sewn sutures in a porcine study and revealed similar strength to hand-sewn sutures [3]. EFTR with the device was shown feasible in a porcine model with five swines. Thus far, the OverStitch system has been evaluated in a porcine model only. It was used for successful defect closure after EFTR with an endoscopic robot device [12].

Non-exposed EFTR of gastric SET with the GERDX device (and its predecessor the Plicator, NDO Surgical Inc., Mansfield, NA, USA) and a resection snare was reported on 31 patients with a median tumor size of 20.5 mm. A R0 resection rate of 90% was achieved. Perforations occurred in three patients, all of which were

Table 10.1 Overview of selected studies on exposed, pure endoscopic full-thickness resection in the upper gastrointestinal tract. Summarized are the size, complete resection rate, the devices used for closure of the resection defect, and the complications that occurred in the different studies

Study	Patients, *n*	Mean size (range), cm	R0 resection rate, %	Device for closure	Compl.
Zhou 2011 [5]	26	2.8 (1.2–4.5)	100	TTS clips	None
Feng 2014 [6]	48	1.6 (0.5–4.8)	100	TTS clips	Five patients developed abdominal discomfort
Huang 2014 [7]	35	2.8 (2.0–4.9)	100	TTS clips	None
Shi 2013 [8]	20	1.5 (0.4–3.0)	100	TTS clips + Endoloop	Five patients with mild abdominal pain and increased body temperature and received antibiotics
Ye 2014 [9]	51	2.4 (1.3–3.5)	98	TTS clips + Endoloop	None
Schlag 2013 [10]	20	1.7 (0.7–3.0)	85	OTSC	In six patients, pure endoscopic resection was not possible and needed laparoscopic wedge resection, in one further patient the defect was closed with TTS clips
Guo 2015 [11]	23	1.2 (0.6–2.6)	100	OTSC	Localized peritonitis in two cases, no surgery needed

successfully treated by application of further sutures. The method was used for tumors of up to 48 mm in size (Fig. 10.4) [13].

Recently, first results of EFTR of small (up to 15 mm) gastric SETs with the FTRD in 29 patients were published. Resection was safe and feasible and allowed definite histological diagnosis in all cases. Complete resection was achieved in approximately two-thirds of the patients and thus might obviate the need for endoscopic follow-up in selected patients. From our own experience, EFTR with the FTRD might as well aid in the diagnosis of scirrhous gastric cancer, also known as linitis plastica.

Classic LECS as well as its variants have been evaluated for resection of SETs and early gastric cancer. Especially with regard to treatment of early gastric cancer there is only few data available and these techniques cannot yet be generally

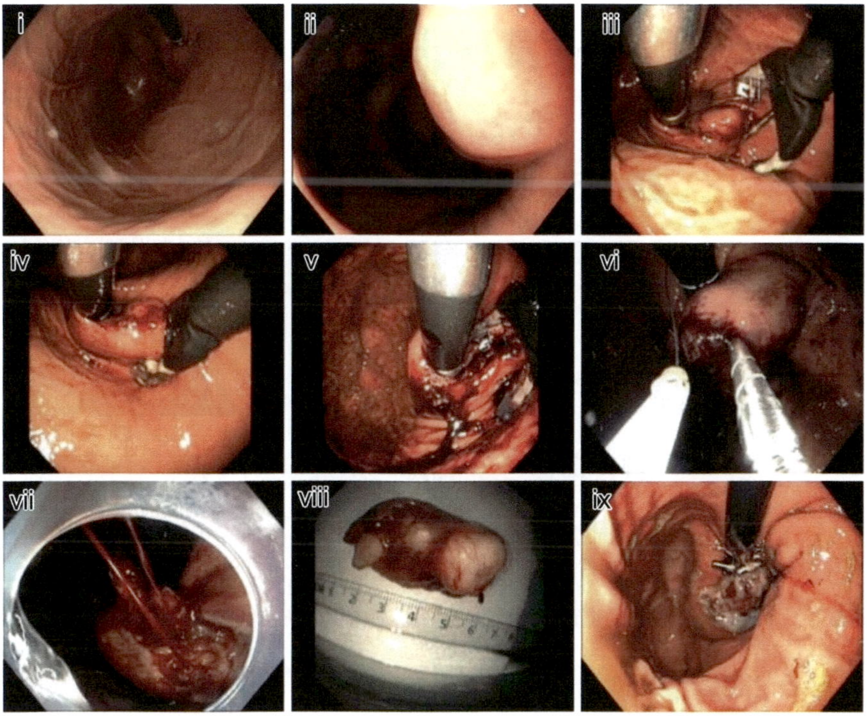

Fig. 10.4 Full-thickness resection of a gastric GIST with the GERDX device. Full-thickness resection with the GERDX device is performed as follows: (i + ii) Subepithelial tumor, (iii + iv) Application of the first suture underneath the tumor with the GERDX device, (v) Second suture, (vi) Snare resection using a double-channel endoscope with an anchoring device in the second working channel, (vii) Bleeding after resection that could be managed endoscopically with two TTS clips and one further full-thickness suture with the GERDX device, (viii) Resected specimen (Histology: GIST, R0 resection), and (ix) Resection site on the following day

recommended [4]. Classic LECS was reported for successful resection of a 6 cm, lateral-spreading early gastric cancer [14]. However, classic LECS is mostly considered for resection of SETs only because of the potential risk of tumor cell dissemination during exposed full-thickness resection. NEWS was combined with sentinel node dissection in a single patient with early gastric cancer [15]. In a further study, an approach that combined laparoscopic-assisted, endoscopic full-thickness resection and laparoscopic lymphadenectomy was reported in 14 patients. However, five of them had to be converted to surgical gastrectomy because of difficulties with wall closure, leakage, or ischemia [16].

10.4 Full-Thickness Resection in the Duodenum

EFTR has been described for resection of duodenal adenomas or subepithelial tumors in small and retrospective studies that either used the FTRD system or a clip-assisted technique (Fig. 10.5). Use of the FTRD in a retrospective study including

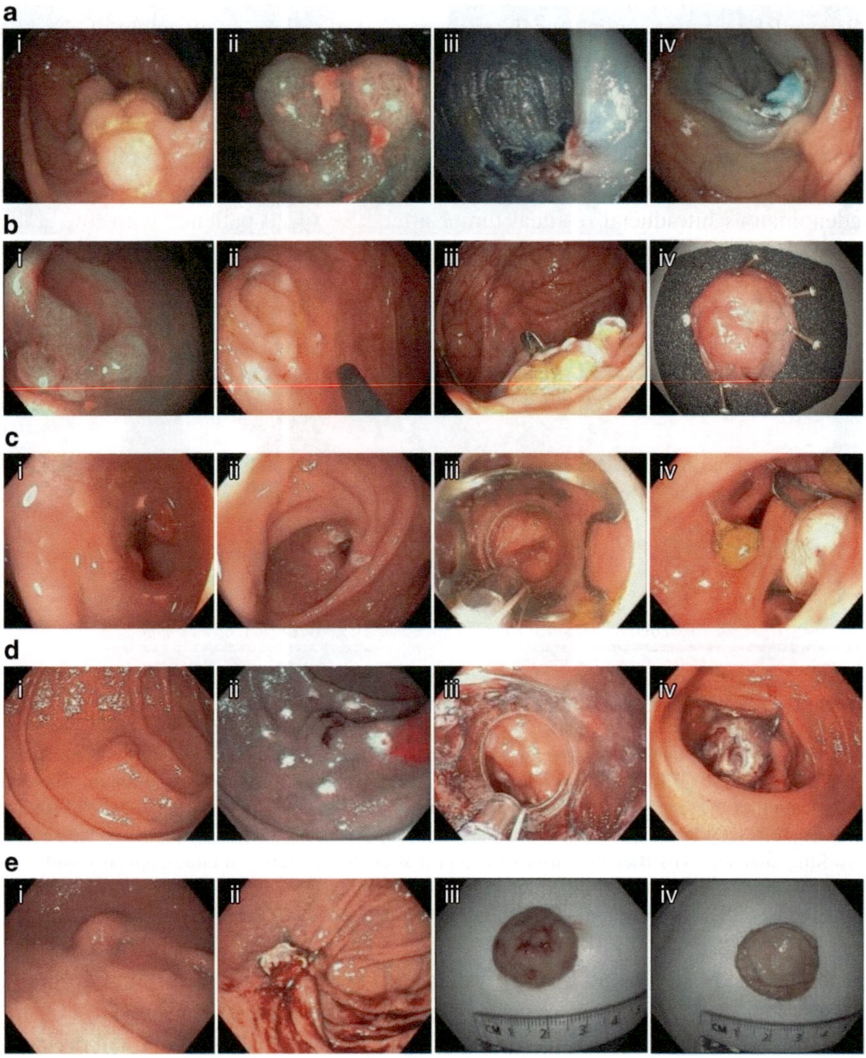

Fig. 10.5 Use of the FTRD for different indications in the upper and lower gastrointestinal tract. FTRD resection of different lesions is shown: (**a**) Hybrid EMR-FTRD resection for a recurrent adenoma with central on-lifting in the ascending colon, (**b**) Resection of a serrated adenoma at the orifice of the appendix, (**c**) Resection of two polyps at the orifice of a diverticulum, (**d**) Full-thickness resection of a duodenal adenoma, and (**e**) Resection of a gastrointestinal stroma tumor in the stomach

20 patients showed a successful resection in all cases and a R0 resection in 63.2%. Three events of minor bleeding were noted 1 day after the EFTR procedure, which all could be treated endoscopically [17]. The use of the Padlock Clip in combination with snare resection was described for treatment of supepithelial tumors in six patients [18].

10.5 Colorectal Full-Thickness Resection

10.5.1 Indications and Techniques

The major indication for EFTR in the colorectum is resection of "difficult adenomas." These include non-lifting lesions either due to scaring in residual or recurrent adenoma or due to submucosal tumor invasion. Further indications include the resection of adenomas at difficult anatomic locations (i.e., polyps at the orifice of the appendix or of a diverticulum). Besides this, resection of SETs in the rectum or diagnostic EFTR are further indications. The best studied and most-used device for colorectal EFTR is the FTRD system (Fig. 10.5a–d). In addition, clip-occlusion of the resection site and subsequent snare resection have been described.

10.5.2 Efficacy of Full-Thickness Resection in the Colorectum

The first retrospective study reporting on the use of the FTRD in the colorectum included 25 patients. The majority underwent FTRD resection because of a difficult adenoma, but the study also included patients with SET and one patient who underwent diagnostic EFTR. The target lesion could be reached with the FTRD mounted on top of the endoscope in 24 of 25 cases. The resection was technically successful in 83.3%, while histologically confirmed full-thickness resection was achieved in 87.5% and R0 resection in 75.0% of cases. The study reported no severe adverse events [19]. Since then, several further studies were published. Of these the most important ones are summarized in Table 10.2. A prospective multicenter study from Germany (WALL RESECT) is one of the few prospective studies and the largest study that investigated the FTRD system so far [23]. 181 patients were included and the main indication for FTRD was difficult adenoma again, which was the indication in 173 (79.0%) patients. This was followed by early cancer (stage T1) in 15 (8.3%), and SET in 23 (12.7%) of the patients. The target lesions were distributed throughout the colon and were reached with FTRD in 100% of the patients. The resection was technically successful in 89.5%, and R0 resection was achieved in 76.9%. In the subgroup of patients who underwent resection for difficult adenoma, the R0 resection rate was 77.7%.

A two-step method using an over-the-scope clip and a resection snare has been evaluated in the colon as well. There are two studies that either used the

OTSC or the Padlock Clip prior to resection [27, 28]. The studies reported the outcome in 17 and 26 patients, and the success rates in the two studies were 94% and 100%, respectively. However, one of the studies also included patients that underwent EFTR in the upper gastrointestinal tract. Due to the split approach, there is the need for withdrawal and reinsertion of the endoscope.

10.5.3 Complications of Colorectal Full-Thickness Resection

EFTR in the colon and rectum in general is safe and severe complications are rare. The overall rate of mostly minor adverse events can be approximated at 10% throughout the studies. These include bleeding, pain, postpolypectomy syndrome, or perforation (Table 10.3). Most of the complications can be treated conservative or endoscopically; surgery due to a complication was necessary in less than 2%. EFTR of lesions involving the orifice of the appendix might cause acute appendicitis and require subsequent surgery.

Table 10.2 Overview of studies on the FTRD in the colorectum. Summary of the major outcome parameters in studies on the FTRD system in the colon that included more than 10 patients

Study	Design	Patients, *n*	Lesion reached, %	Technical success, %	Full-thickness resection, %	R0 resection, %
Schmidt et al. 2015 [19]	Retrospective	25	96.0	83.3	87.5	75.0
Richter-Schrag et al. 2016 [20]	Retrospective	20	100.0	75.0	60.0	80.0
Valli et al. 2018 [21]	Combined retro- and prospective	60	96.7	96.7	85.0	76.7
Vitali et al. 2018 [22]	Prospective	12	100.0	100.0		83.3
Schmidt et al. 2018 [23]	Prospective	181	100.0	89.5	81.0	76.9
Aepli et al. 2018 [24]	Retrospective	33	97.0	87.9	80.6	87.9
Andrisani et al. 2018 [25]	Retrospective	114	96	94.3	91	90
van der Spek et al. 2018 [26]	Combined retro- and prospective	51	100.0	88.2	84.3	78.4

Table 10.3 Complications after FTRD resection in the colorectum. Overview of the complications reported in the 476 patients treated with FTRD in the studies summarized in Table 10.2

Adverse event	Number, *n* (% of 476)
Bleeding	18 (3.8)
Perforation	11 (2.3)
Postpolypectomy syndrome or pain	11 (2.3)
Appendicitis	5 (1.1)
Other	8 (1.7)
Emergency surgery	6 (1.3)

10.5.4 Special Situations

Early colorectal cancer seems an interesting target for EFTR. Results for FTRD resection of early colorectal cancer was reported in a subgroup analysis of the WALL RESECT study. This included 29 patients with early carcinoma as defined by histological examination. In 21 of these patients R0 resection was achieved. In addition to the eight patients with histologically incomplete resection, there were eight patients with a high-risk situation (depth of submucosal invasion >1000 μm) despite R0 resection. Thus, a total of 16 patients were evaluated for surgery. For 11 out of 13 patients with R0 resection and a low-risk situation, 3-month follow-up was available, which remained without signs of recurrent or residual disease in all cases [23]. Recently, a retrospective analysis of the national FTRD registry in Germany was published. In that study, 156 patients were included. Complete resection (R0) was reported for 71.8%, and 43.9% of the patients were classified as low risk based upon histological examination and underwent endoscopic follow-up. Discrimination between low-risk and high-risk status was possible after FTRD resection in almost all patients. Notably, patients that underwent FTRD resection after incomplete resection of a malign polyp showed low-risk situation in more than 80%, and surgery with oncological resection could be avoided in these cases [29].

Completed resection of colorectal lesions with the FTRD can be achieved for lesion up to 25 mm in size. For larger lesions, it is possible to combine EMR with FTRD. This hybrid EMR-FTRD technique allows endoscopic resection of large adenomas with a non-lifting part [30]. First, piece-meal EMR of the lifting area is performed and then FTRD resection of the non-lifting part is performed. A small retrospective study investigated this approach in 10 patients and no complications were reported.

EFTR of lesions involving the orifice of the appendix was shown to be possible in the abovementioned studies. However, a low rate of postinterventional appendicitis was noted. The WALL RESECT study included 34 patients who underwent FTRD resection at the orifice of the appendix and three of them developed acute appendicitis. Our own analysis (published as congress abstract only) of more than 40 patients revealed development of appendicitis in approximately one-fifth of the cases. It developed early after the resection as well as with latency of more than 1 month. A smaller study on seven patients showed a similar rate of appendicitis [31].

Rectal neuroendocrine tumors can as well securely and effectively be resected with the FTRD system.

Diagnostic full-thickness resection in the colorectum is possible in selected cases as well. These include the diagnosis of motility disorders as well as diagnosis of amyloidosis [32].

10.5.5 Follow-Up After FTRD Resection in the Colorectum

There is not yet a guideline recommendation on follow-up after EFTR of early mucosal neoplasms of the colorectum. Most centers perform first follow-up colonoscopy after 3 months. If the FTRD clip has not deployed spontaneously, which happens in approximately two-thirds of the patients, it should be removed with a special device to allow full inspection of the resection site [33].

10.6 Summary

Endoscopic full-thickness resection has greatly advanced the possibilities of endoscopic resection and allows endoscopic treatment of lesions that otherwise would have needed surgery. In the lower gastrointestinal tract, the main indication is resection of non-lifting adenomas. This can be done securely and efficiently with the FTRD system, which has been well evaluated in several studies. SETs are the main target of full-thickness resection in the upper gastrointestinal tract. Therefore, a variety of procedures are available, including pure endoscopic approaches as well as techniques combining endoscopy with laparoscopy. The preferred approach depends on the indication, location of the tumor as well as the local expertise. Sufficient personal skills and local resources to adequately manage potential complications are mandatorily needed before performing full-thickness resection in the upper or lower gastrointestinal tract.

References

1. Schmidt A, Meier B, Caca K. Endoscopic full-thickness resection: current status. World J Gastroenterol. 2015;21(31):9273–85. https://doi.org/10.3748/wjg.v21.i31.9273.
2. Mori H, Kobara H, Nishiyama N, Masaki T. Current status and future perspectives of endoscopic full-thickness resection. Dig Endosc. 2018;30(Suppl 1):25–31. https://doi.org/10.1111/den.13042.
3. Mori H, Kobara H, Fujihara S, Nishiyama N, Rafiq K, Oryu M, et al. Feasibility of pure EFTR using an innovative new endoscopic suturing device: the double-arm-bar suturing system (with video). Surg Endosc. 2014;28(2):683–90. https://doi.org/10.1007/s00464-013-3266-z.
4. Hiki N, Nunobe S, Matsuda T, Hirasawa T, Yamamoto Y, Yamaguchi T. Laparoscopic endoscopic cooperative surgery. Dig Endosc. 2015;27(2):197–204. https://doi.org/10.1111/den.12404.

5. Zhou PH, Yao LQ, Qin XY, Cai MY, Xu MD, Zhong YS, et al. Endoscopic full-thickness resection without laparoscopic assistance for gastric submucosal tumors originated from the muscularis propria. Surg Endosc. 2011;25(9):2926–31. https://doi.org/10.1007/s00464-011-1644-y.
6. Feng Y, Yu L, Yang S, Li X, Ding J, Chen L, et al. Endolumenal endoscopic full-thickness resection of muscularis propria-originating gastric submucosal tumors. J Laparoendosc Adv Surg Tech A. 2014;24(3):171–6. https://doi.org/10.1089/lap.2013.0370.
7. Huang LY, Cui J, Lin SJ, Zhang B, Wu CR. Endoscopic full-thickness resection for gastric submucosal tumors arising from the muscularis propria layer. World J Gastroenterol. 2014;20(38):13981–6. https://doi.org/10.3748/wjg.v20.i38.13981.
8. Shi Q, Chen T, Zhong YS, Zhou PH, Ren Z, Xu MD, et al. Complete closure of large gastric defects after endoscopic full-thickness resection, using endoloop and metallic clip interrupted suture. Endoscopy. 2013;45(5):329–34. https://doi.org/10.1055/s-0032-1326214.
9. Ye LP, Yu Z, Mao XL, Zhu LH, Zhou XB. Endoscopic full-thickness resection with defect closure using clips and an endoloop for gastric subepithelial tumors arising from the muscularis propria. Surg Endosc. 2014;28(6):1978–83. https://doi.org/10.1007/s00464-014-3421-1.
10. Schlag C, Wilhelm D, von Delius S, Feussner H, Meining A. EndoResect study: endoscopic full-thickness resection of gastric subepithelial tumors. Endoscopy. 2013;45(1):4–11. https://doi.org/10.1055/s-0032-1325760.
11. Guo J, Liu Z, Sun S, Liu X, Wang S, Ge N, et al. Endoscopic full-thickness resection with defect closure using an over-the-scope clip for gastric subepithelial tumors originating from the muscularis propria. Surg Endosc. 2015;29(11):3356–62. https://doi.org/10.1007/s00464-015-4076-2.
12. Chiu PW, Phee SJ, Wang Z, Sun Z, Poon CC, Yamamoto T, et al. Feasibility of full-thickness gastric resection using master and slave transluminal endoscopic robot and closure by overstitch: a preclinical study. Surg Endosc. 2014;28(1):319–24. https://doi.org/10.1007/s00464-013-3149-3.
13. Schmidt A, Bauder M, Riecken B, von Renteln D, Muehleisen H, Caca K. Endoscopic full-thickness resection of gastric subepithelial tumors: a single-center series. Endoscopy. 2015;47(2):154–8. https://doi.org/10.1055/s-0034-1390786.
14. Nunobe S, Hiki N, Gotoda T, Murao T, Haruma K, Matsumoto H, et al. Successful application of laparoscopic and endoscopic cooperative surgery (LECS) for a lateral-spreading mucosal gastric cancer. Gastric Cancer. 2012;15(3):338–42. https://doi.org/10.1007/s10120-012-0146-5.
15. Goto O, Takeuchi H, Kawakubo H, Sasaki M, Matsuda T, Matsuda S, et al. First case of non-exposed endoscopic wall-inversion surgery with sentinel node basin dissection for early gastric cancer. Gastric Cancer. 2015;18(2):434–9. https://doi.org/10.1007/s10120-014-0406-7.
16. Cho WY, Kim YJ, Cho JY, Bok GH, Jin SY, Lee TH, et al. Hybrid natural orifice transluminal endoscopic surgery: endoscopic full-thickness resection of early gastric cancer and laparoscopic regional lymph node dissection—14 human cases. Endoscopy. 2011;43(2):134–9. https://doi.org/10.1055/s-0030-1255955.
17. Bauder M, Schmidt A, Caca K. Endoscopic full-thickness resection of duodenal lesions-a retrospective analysis of 20 FTRD cases. United European Gastroenterol J. 2018;6(7):1015–21. https://doi.org/10.1177/2050640618773517.
18. Kappelle WFW, Backes Y, Valk GD, Moons LMG, Vleggaar FP. Endoscopic full-thickness resection of gastric and duodenal subepithelial lesions using a new, flat-based over-the-scope clip. Surg Endosc. 2018;32(6):2839–46. https://doi.org/10.1007/s00464-017-5989-8.
19. Schmidt A, Bauerfeind P, Gubler C, Damm M, Bauder M, Caca K. Endoscopic full-thickness resection in the colorectum with a novel over-the-scope device: first experience. Endoscopy. 2015;47(8):719–25. https://doi.org/10.1055/s-0034-1391781.
20. Richter-Schrag HJ, Walker C, Thimme R, Fischer A. [Full thickness resection device (FTRD). Experience and outcome for benign neoplasms of the rectum and colon]. Chirurg. 2016;87(4):316–25. https://doi.org/10.1007/s00104-015-0091-z.
21. Valli PV, Mertens J, Bauerfeind P. Safe and successful resection of difficult GI lesions using a novel single-step full-thickness resection device (FTRD((R))). Surg Endosc. 2018;32(1):289–99. https://doi.org/10.1007/s00464-017-5676-9.

22. Vitali F, Naegel A, Siebler J, Neurath MF, Rath T. Endoscopic full-thickness resection with an over-the-scope clip device (FTRD) in the colorectum: results from a university tertiary referral center. Endosc Int Open. 2018;6(1):E98–E103. https://doi.org/10.1055/s-0043-124079.
23. Schmidt A, Beyna T, Schumacher B, Meining A, Richter-Schrag HJ, Messmann H, et al. Colonoscopic full-thickness resection using an over-the-scope device: a prospective multicentre study in various indications. Gut. 2018;67(7):1280–9. https://doi.org/10.1136/gutjnl-2016-313677.
24. Aepli P, Criblez D, Baumeler S, Borovicka J, Frei R. Endoscopic full thickness resection (EFTR) of colorectal neoplasms with the full thickness resection device (FTRD): clinical experience from two tertiary referral centers in Switzerland. United European Gastroenterol J. 2018;6(3):463–70. https://doi.org/10.1177/2050640617728001.
25. Andrisani G, Soriani P, Manno M, Pizzicannella M, Pugliese F, Mutignani M, et al. Colo-rectal endoscopic full-thickness resection (EFTR) with the over-the-scope device (FTRD((R))): a multicenter Italian experience. Dig Liver Dis. 2019;51(3):375–81. https://doi.org/10.1016/j.dld.2018.09.030.
26. van der Spek B, Haasnoot K, Meischl C, Heine D. Endoscopic full-thickness resection in the colorectum: a single-center case series evaluating indication, efficacy and safety. Endosc Int Open. 2018;6(10):E1227–E34. https://doi.org/10.1055/a-0672-1138.
27. Fahndrich M, Sandmann M. Endoscopic full-thickness resection for gastrointestinal lesions using the over-the-scope clip system: a case series. Endoscopy. 2015;47(1):76–9. https://doi.org/10.1055/s-0034-1377975.
28. Backes Y, Kappelle WFW, Berk L, Koch AD, Groen JN, de Vos Tot Nederveen Cappel WH, et al. Colorectal endoscopic full-thickness resection using a novel, flat-base over-the-scope clip: a prospective study. Endoscopy. 2017;49(11):1092–7. https://doi.org/10.1055/s-0043-114730.
29. Kuellmer A, Mueller J, Caca K, Aepli P, Albers D, Schumacher B, et al. Endoscopic full-thickness resection for early colorectal cancer. Gastrointest Endosc. 2019;89(6):1180–1189.e1. https://doi.org/10.1016/j.gie.2018.12.025.
30. Meier B, Caca K, Schmidt A. Hybrid endoscopic mucosal resection and full-thickness resection: a new approach for resection of large non-lifting colorectal adenomas (with video). Surg Endosc. 2017;31(10):4268–74. https://doi.org/10.1007/s00464-017-5461-9.
31. Bronzwaer MES, Bastiaansen BAJ, Koens L, Dekker E, Fockens P. Endoscopic full-thickness resection of polyps involving the appendiceal orifice: a prospective observational case study. Endosc Int Open. 2018;6(9):E1112–E9. https://doi.org/10.1055/a-0635-0911.
32. Valli PV, Pohl D, Fried M, Caduff R, Bauerfeind P. Diagnostic use of endoscopic full-thickness wall resection (eFTR)—a novel minimally invasive technique for colonic tissue sampling in patients with severe gastrointestinal motility disorders. Neurogastroenterol Motil. 2018;30(1). https://doi.org/10.1111/nmo.13153.
33. Bauder M, Meier B, Caca K, Schmidt A. Endoscopic removal of over-the-scope clips: clinical experience with a bipolar cutting device. United European Gastroenterol J. 2017;5(4):479–84. https://doi.org/10.1177/2050640616671846.

Colonic Endoscopic Mucosal Resection 11

Michael X. Ma and Michael J. Bourke

Abbreviations

CSP	Cold snare polypectomy
CSPEB	Clinically significant post endoscopy bleeding
DMI	Deep mural injury
EEI	Enhanced endoscopic imaging
EMR	Endoscopic mucosal resection
GIT	Gastrointestinal tract
HGD	High-grade dysplasia
IMC	Intramucosal carcinoma
IPB	Intra-procedural bleeding
LGD	Low grade dysplasia
LMN	Lymph node metastases
LSL	Laterally spreading lesion
LVI	Lymphovascular invasion
MP	Muscularis propria
nCE	Chromoendoscopy
PPES	Post-polypectomy electrocoagulation syndrome
SMF	Submucosal fibrosis
SMI	Submucosal invasion
STSC	Snare tip soft coagulation

M. X. Ma
Department of Gastroenterology and Hepatology, Fiona Stanley Hospital, Perth, WA, Australia

M. J. Bourke (✉)
Department of Gastroenterology and Hepatology, Westmead Hospital, Sydney, NSW, Australia

University of Sydney, Sydney, NSW, Australia
e-mail: michael@citywestgastro.com.au

P. Sharma, N. Reddy (eds.), *Innovations in Gastrointestinal Endoscopy*,
https://doi.org/10.1007/978-981-15-9247-8_11

TSC	Topical submucosal chromoendoscopy
TTS	Through the scope
UEMR	Underwater endoscopic mucosal resection

11.1 Introduction

Endoscopic mucosal resection (EMR) is used to treat neoplastic lesions arising from the gastrointestinal tract (GIT) mucosa. EMR is the preferred therapy for colonic large laterally spreading lesions (LSLs) ≥20 mm in size, with >95% technical success and >90% avoiding surgery on long-term follow-up [1, 2]. EMR of colonic LSLs also holds significant morbidity and cost benefits when compared with surgery [1, 3]. This chapter discusses endoscopic assessment of large colonic polyps, technical aspects of EMR, and techniques to prevent and manage EMR-related complications.

11.2 Lesion Selection and Preparation

Careful endoscopic assessment of each lesion should be undertaken prior to EMR, particularly noting its size, anatomical location, and risk of submucosal invasion (SMI). Good quality bowel cleansing is essential to not only perform adequate lesion assessment but also to minimise contamination in case of perforation. Although larger LSLs may be more demanding to remove, lesion size itself does not preclude resectability. By combining a systematic approach with meticulous technique, even near circumferential and circumferential LSLs can be endoscopically resected [4, 5].

Only lesions with no or very low risk of lymph node metastases (LNM) are suitable for endoscopic resection. Given the absence of lymphovascular channels within the mucosa, LNM risk of lesions confined to the mucosa is negligible, and thus EMR is an appropriate treatment. This includes lesions with low-grade dysplasia (LGD) or high-grade dysplasia (HGD, sometimes also referred as intramucosal carcinoma [IMC]). For invasive lesions, depth of SMI determines the risk of LMN. For such lesions, endoscopic resection is generally not recommended. Lesions with very superficial SMI (sm1, superficial third of submucosa layer) may be an exception, where risk of LMN may be lower than risk of radical surgery, particularly in comorbid or elderly patients. For example colonic LSLs with sm1 have LNM risk as low at 3%, whereas sm3 lesions may have LNM risk may be as high as 25% [6]. Nonetheless, endoscopic submucosal dissection (ESD) is preferred for lesions with possible superficial SMI, as the en bloc specimen enables accurate histological assessment for local staging and curative resection.

Risk of SMI within a lesion can be determined by assessment of gross morphology and surface pit and vascular pattern.

11.2.1 Morphological Classification of Colonic LSLs

The Paris classification is a commonly used system to classify morphology of GIT lesions [7]. Three types of superficial lesions (type 0) are described: protruding (type 0-I), slightly elevated (type 0-II) and excavated (type 0-III) (Fig. 11.1). Further subclassifications of each subtype can be made, for example pedunculated (0-Ip), polypoid (0-Is), slightly elevated (0-IIa), flat (0-IIb) or slightly depressed (0-IIc). Slightly elevated (0-IIa) LSLs and polypoid lesions (0-Is) may also be categorised based on surface contour as granular ('bubbly' surface) or non-granular (a relatively smooth and firm surface). Lesions with mixed morphologies may be described using combinations of the Paris classification. For example a slightly elevated LSL with polypoid component is a Paris 0-IIa + Is lesion.

Certain morphologies are associated with a higher risk of SMI. Increasing lesion size is the main predictor of SMI for Paris 0-I lesions. For Paris 0-II lesions, type 0-IIb and type 0-IIc lesions harbour the greatest risk of SMI, whereas granular Paris 0-IIa LSLs harbour a very low risk of SMI (approximately 1%). Paris 0-III lesions have a high incidence of deep SMI and typically are not suitable for endoscopic resection [1, 8]. Table 11.1 describes SMI risk of colorectal LSLs based upon morphology and anatomical location [8].

11.2.2 Assessment of Surface Pit and Vascular Pattern

Chromoendoscopy (CE) and enhanced endoscopic imaging (EEI) are utilised to assess a lesion's surface pits and vascular pattern; areas of disruption may indicate underlying SMI. Both modalities are relatively easy to use and safe, with high sensitivity for detection of neoplasia throughout the GIT [9, 10]. CE involves the

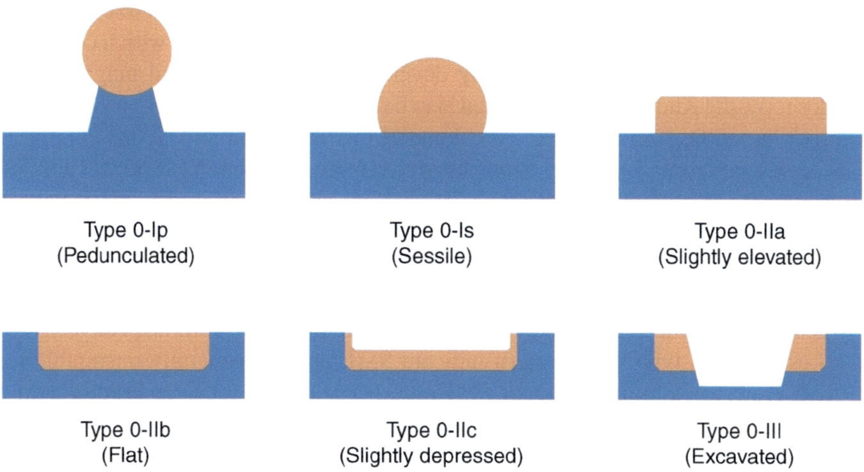

Fig. 11.1 Paris classification of gastrointestinal tract lesion morphology

Table 11.1 SMI risk in colorectal LSLs according to morphology and location

Morphology		Location in colon	Risk (%)
Paris 0-IIa granular	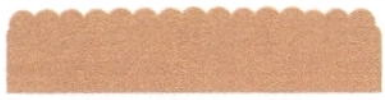	Proximal Distal	0.7 1.2
Paris 0-IIa non-granular		Proximal Distal	3.8 6.4
Paris 0-IIa + Is granular	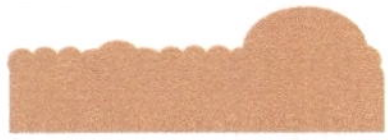	Proximal Distal	4.2 10.1
Paris 0-IIa + Is non-granular	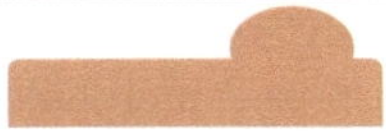	Proximal Distal	12.7 15.9
Paris 0-Is granular	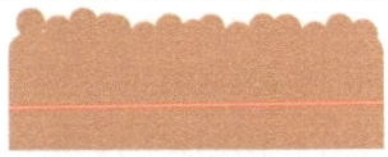	Proximal Distal	2.3 5.7
Paris 0-Is non-granular		Proximal Distal	12.3 21.4

Adapted from Burgess et al. 2017

topical application of absorptive (e.g. methylene blue) or contrast dyes (e.g. indigo carmine) to highlight abnormalities on the surface of lesions. Often, CE is combined with magnification endoscopy to better delineate fine surface microstructures.

Enhanced endoscopic imaging such as narrow band imaging (NBI, Olympus, Tokyo, Japan), i-Scan (Pentax, Tokyo, Japan) or Fujinon intelligent colour enhancement (FICE, Fujifilm, Tokyo, Japan) are also used to assess a lesion's fine surface structure. These modalities are now inbuilt functions of current-generation high-definition endoscopes and in contrast to CE, they do not require the preparation or physical application of dye mixtures during the procedure, saving time and costs. Studies comparing EEI with CE, mostly limited to diagnosis of colonic lesions, have found similar sensitivities and specificities [11].

The Kudo classification is a standardised and widely used system to classify the fine surface pit patten of LSLs. Five main categories are described which correlates with lesion histology [12]. Originally developed based on CE and magnification endoscopy, the Kudo classification can also be applied using high-definition colonoscopes, magnification and EEI. Type I and II pits are round and stellar in appearance, respectively. Both are considered to represent benign lesions (normal, hyperplastic or inflammatory). Type III pits are sub categorised to III-S (small, roundish, tubular pits) and III-L (larger, roundish, tubular pits), and represent tubular adenomas. Type IV pits are branch-like in appearance, representing lesions with villous histology. Type V pits are subcategories to Vi (irregular pits) and Vn (non-structural, amorphous pits), indicative of superficial or deep SMI, respectively.

Lesions with type V pit pattern indicate SMI, and are generally unsuitable for EMR. However, diminutive focal SMI may occasionally occur in lesions with a seemingly preserved pit pattern. Particular features that should alert endoscopists to an increased risk of covert SMI include recto-sigmoid located LSLs (odds ratio [OR] 1.91), lesions with Paris 0-IIc and 0-Is morphologies (OR 1.80 and OR 2.73, respectively), non-granular surface morphology (OR 2.80), increasing lesion size (OR 1.12 per 10 mm increase) and Kudo pit pattern V (OR 14.2) [8]. Other classification systems that assess surface vascular pattern (Sano and NBI International Colorectal Endoscopic [NICE] classification) [13, 14] are also validated to assess the histology of colorectal polyps.

11.3 Endoscopic Mucosal Resection Technique

Colonic EMR is performed using the 'inject and resect' method. With this technique, a submucosal injection is made below the target lesion to create a fluid cushion, separating it from the deeper muscularis propria (MP) layer, followed by snare resection (Fig. 11.2).

11.3.1 Patient Preparation

Patients should provide informed consent to the procedure, including awareness of EMR risks and treatment alternatives. Referrals should include a description of lesion size, location, Paris morphology and include colour images. The endoscopist should be aware of a patient's full medical history, particularly regular antithrombotic agents. Anti-platelet agents, with the exception of aspirin, are usually withheld for 7 days prior to the procedure. The duration of anticoagulant cessation depends on the medication, ranging between 5 and 7 days for warfarin and 2–3 days for the newer oral anticoagulants (NOACs). Temporary cessation of these medications may increase the risk of thrombosis, and some high-risk cases (e.g. recent coronary stent or significant thromboembolism) may require discussion with the patients' treating physician before proceeding.

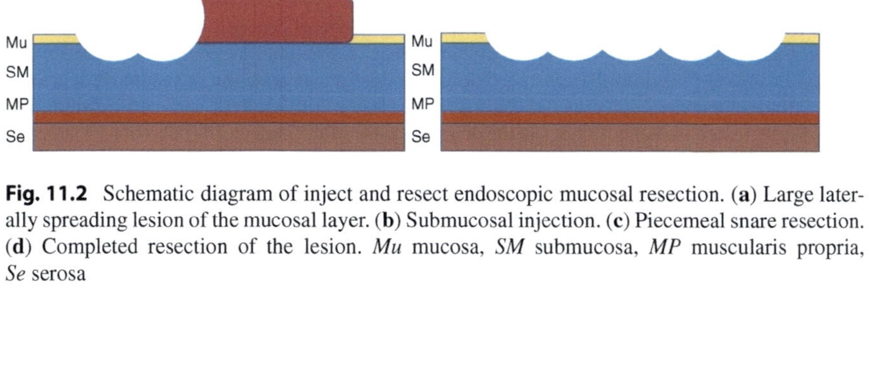

Fig. 11.2 Schematic diagram of inject and resect endoscopic mucosal resection. (**a**) Large laterally spreading lesion of the mucosal layer. (**b**) Submucosal injection. (**c**) Piecemeal snare resection. (**d**) Completed resection of the lesion. *Mu* mucosa, *SM* submucosa, *MP* muscularis propria, *Se* serosa

The lesion is optimally positioned at 6 o'clock, preferably on the non-dependant side (Fig. 11.3). This avoids obscuration of the working field by luminal contents and minimises extra-luminal contamination in the event of a perforation. Carbon dioxide insufflation significantly reduces post-procedural admissions for pain after EMR and should be routinely used instead of air [15]. For lesions in difficult positions such as those overlying the ileocaecal valve, extending over folds or flexures, access may be assisted by changing the position of the patient and/or use of a distal attachment cap. The adult colonoscope is generally preferred over the paediatric colonoscope as its larger working channel (3.7 mm compared with 3.2 mm, respectively) allows more specimens to be suctioned directly into a polyp trap instead of needing a retrieval net. However, for difficult to access positions, especially where retroflexion is required, the increased flexibility of the paediatric colonoscope may be advantageous.

11.3.2 Submucosal Injectate and Snares

The submucosal injectate includes a colloidal solution, epinephrine diluted to 1:100,000 and an inert dye (80 mg indigo carmine or 20 mg methylene blue per

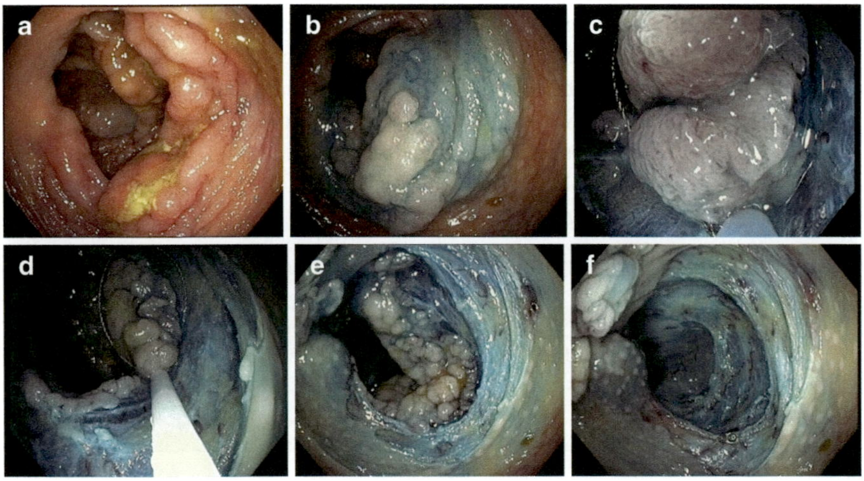

Fig. 11.3 EMR of a large 70 mm laterally spreading lesion of ascending colon. (**a**) The lesion involves approximately 60% of luminal circumference in proximal ascending colon, extending over 2–3 haustral folds into the caecum. The lesion does not involve the appendix or ileocaecal valve. Morphologically it is a granular, Paris 0-IIa + Is lesion with Kudo IV surface pit pattern. The lesion is positioned so that it is opposite the dependant side of the patient. (**b**) Submucosal injection with chromogelofusine + 1:100,000 adrenaline. (**c** and **d**) Snare resection. The edge of a previous resection is used as a guide for placement of the snare. When resecting over folds, the snare is placed parallel (rather than perpendicular) to the bowel wall to reduce the risk of entrapment of the muscularis propria. (**e** and **f**) Resection proceeds from distal to proximal to systematically resect all visible adenomatous tissue

500 mL solution). Fluid injection into the submucosa creates a cushion that reduces the risk of entrapment of the MP layer and deeper tissues by the snare, thereby avoiding deep mural injury (DMI) following resection. Colloid solutions such as succinylated gelatin (Gelofusin; Braun, Melsungen, Germany) are shown to reduce number of injections, resections and procedural duration compared with normal saline [16]. Diluted epinephrine reduces intra-procedural bleeding (IPB) and delays dispersion of the submucosal cushion, but does not affect the incidence of clinically significant post-procedural bleeding (CSPEB) [17]. The inert dye is avid for the submucosal connective tissue, but not the deeper MP layer, thus assisting identification of lesion margins and the submucosal resection plane.

Snares of different sizes, shape and wire type may be required to complete EMR. Specific snares are better suited to certain settings influenced by factors such as lesion size, location and morphology. Stiff spiral or braided snares (0.48 mm thickness wire of 15 mm, 20 and 25 mm diameter) are designed to increase tissue capture and are suited for piecemeal EMR. In most cases, the 15 mm snare provides adequate balance of efficacy and safety, but the choice of snare is a personal preference. Small, thin-wire snares (0.3 mm thickness wire of 10 mm diameter) are useful for difficult to remove tissue, such as peri-appendiceal lesions, areas of submucosal fibrosis, and small residual tissue at the EMR margin.

11.3.3 Resection Technique

11.3.3.1 Submucosal Injection

Prime the needle tip with submucosal injectate, place it tangentially to the lesion and be touching but not penetrating the mucosa. Next ask the assistant to commence injection whilst simultaneously penetrating the needle tip into the submucosa. Immediate elevation of the polyp indicates expansion of the submucosa and confirms the correct plane of injection. It is recommended to commence injection and resection in the most difficult to access area of the lesion, usually the caecal side that is behind or below a mucosal fold. Elevating this side moves the lesion towards the scope, aiding its access for resection. For lesions located partially or completely behind a fold, particularly in the right colon, retroflexion may be required to allow submucosal injection and elevation.

Submucosal injection is performed by simultaneously pulling back slightly on the injection catheter, gentle rotation of the colonoscope with slow upward tip deflection whilst keeping the needle tip within the submucosa. This method promotes distribution of the injectate into the submucosa, and allows the endoscopist to guide the direction of lift to move the LSL into a more accessible location. Finally, over-injection causes excessive tension, hinders visualisation and tissue capture, and should be avoided.

Poor lesion elevation can be caused by SMF or deep SMI. SMF may result from previous biopsy or ER attempts, reaction to submucosal injection of tattoo or prolapse over a fold by a bulky sessile lesion [18]. Endoscopic signs of SMF include the 'jet sign', where a fluid jet exits the lesion during injection, or 'canyoning effect', where the lesion peripheries elevate around a fixed central area [1, 18]. Inadequate elevation may also result from transmural injection; gentle withdrawal of the needle during injection assists location of the submucosal plane. Conversely, superficial mucosal injection results in immediate formation of a superficial blue bleb, but the lesion does not elevate. In the setting of deep SMI, tumour infiltration of the submucosa is another cause of non-elevation.

11.3.3.2 Snare Resection

Snare placement is essential for procedural efficacy and safety. Place the lesion in the 6 o'clock position, commence EMR on one side (usually the most difficult to access side) and continue resection systematically across the lesion, aiming to fully resect the lesion in as few pieces as possible. En bloc resection of LSLs ≤20 mm should be performed whenever possible as this assists histological assessment and is associated with less recurrence compared with piecemeal resection.

Open the snare fully over the lesion, and align it along the same plane as the tissue. Then angle down firmly with the up-down dial onto the fluid cushion while gently aspirating gas. The aspiration of gas reduces colonic wall tension and allows the tissue to 'fall' into the opened snare. When closing the snare over the edge of a lesion, aim to include a 2–3 mm rim of normal mucosa to ensure complete resection and avoid small residual islands of adenoma at the margins. Once adequately positioned, gradually close the snare whilst anchoring the catheter into the mucosa. Tight closure of the snare helps to exclude MP from the tissue within the snare. Premature resection with tight closure is unlikely, as generally it not possible to transect tissue of more than 10 mm with a braided or spiral snare without the use of diathermy.

We recommend the endoscopist controls the snare during closure and tissue transection as sensory feedback provides information regarding the safety and efficacy of excision. Safe tissue capture is confirmed by the following:

- Mobility: movement of the snare catheter quickly back and forth should result in independent movement of the tissue relative to the underlying colonic wall.
- Degree of closure: the snare should close to a distance of no more than 1 cm between thumb and fingers. If the endoscopist is unsure, the snare can be partially opened and tented into the lumen to allow any inadvertently captured MP to drop away, before repeating snare closure.
- Transection speed: transection should occur quickly. The snare is kept tightly closed while the foot pedal is depressed in short pulses. Usually, 1–3 pulses are sufficient to transect the polyp tissue. A longer transection raises concern of MP entrapment, SMF or SMI.

Microprocessor-controlled electrosurgery is essential for safe and effective EMR. The microprocessor senses tissue impedance and adjusts power output to avoid deep tissue injury. Fractionated current that alternates the cutting and coagulating cycles is preferred (e.g. Endo Cut mode Q, effect 3, cut duration 1, cut interval 6; ERBE, Türbingen, Germany). Low voltage coagulation (Soft Coag effect 4, maximum 80W; ERBE, Türbingen, Germany) can be used for haemostasis by gently placing the snare tip over any points of bleeding (STSC, snare tip soft coagulation). Following resection, irrigation of the submucosal defect aids assessment of residual adenoma, evidence of DMI and assists identification and control of IPB.

Use the edge of the EMR defect as a guide for the subsequent resection. The inside edge of the snare should be aligned along the defect margin, the snare placed over an area of adenoma, followed by the steps of tissue capture outlined above. This ensures a systematic approach to EMR and also reduces the risk of adenoma islands forming with the defect, which can be difficult to completely remove. Upon complete resection of all visible adenoma, STSC to the EMR margin is recommended to reduce recurrence at the EMR scar. Data from prospective randomised controlled trial showed that STSC to the EMR margin decreased adenomatous recurrence from 21 to 6% at first surveillance colonoscopy (RR 0.28, $P < 0.001$) without an increase in incidence of delayed bleeding or perforation [19].

Lesions containing a nodule (0-Is component) are best treated by first resecting the surrounding laterally spreading component, followed by resection of the nodule in one piece (Fig. 11.4). The nodule should be submitted separately for histological assessment as these are more likely to harbour SMI. All lesions suspected of harbouring SMI, other than those definitely located within the caecum, adjacent to the ileocaecal valve or in the low rectum, should have 2–3 tattoos placed at different points 2–3 cm distal to the resection site, to assist scar identification at surveillance, or localisation at surgery [18].

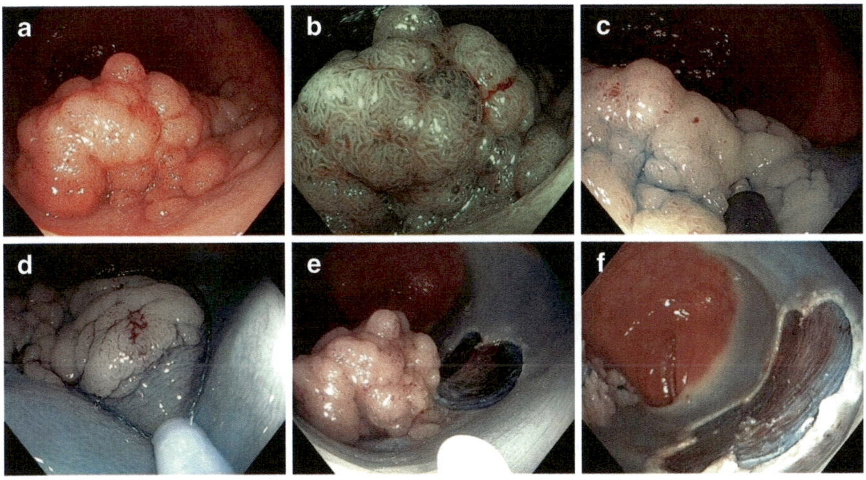

Fig. 11.4 EMR of 40 mm laterally spreading lesion from descending colon. (**a**) The lesion is morphologically a granular Paris 0-IIa + Is laterally spreading lesion. (**b**) On NBI the crypts are branched in keeping with a tubulovillous adenoma. (**c**) Submucosal injection with chromogelofusine solution + 1:100,000 adrenaline. (**d**) Snare resection commences at one lateral edge of the lesion, capturing a rim of normal mucosa to ensure complete resection. (**e**) The dominant large sessile component is removed last. (**f**) Snare tip soft coagulation applied to the resection margin to reduce likelihood of adenomatous recurrence

11.4 Variant Techniques

11.4.1 Piecemeal Cold Snare Polypectomy

EMR using electrosurgery is associated with a risk of delayed bleeding and perforation. Cold snare polypectomy (CSP) does not require thermal energy and is not associated with these risks, but it is limited to en bloc resection of small polyps (≤10 mm) only. For larger polyps, CSP performed in a piecemeal fashion with or without submucosal injection is reported to achieve complete excision whilst mitigating adverse events of EMR related to mural thermal injury. The data is so far limited, but recently published studies of piecemeal CSP for selected sessile adenomatous and large serrated polyps show good clinical efficacy with very few significant adverse events [20–23]. Larger, prospective and comparative studies are awaited.

11.4.2 Underwater EMR

Underwater EMR (UEMR) is performed in a decompressed colonic segment, in which water is infused to assist visualisation. Submucosal injection to lift polyps is not required in UEMR as the MP layer remains both circular and distant from the mucosal and submucosal layers, which 'float' within the lumen. As such, large pieces of mucosal tissue can be captured and removed by snare resection using electrosurgery. Since its first description in 2012, multiple studies have reported its efficacy and safety. A recently published systematic review of 10 studies including 508 non-polypoid colorectal lesions found a high complete resection rate (96.4%), low post-procedural bleeding of 2.85% and no cases of perforation [24]. Further prospective studies comparing UEMR with conventional inject and resect EMR are awaited.

11.5 Special Considerations

11.5.1 LSLs in the Anorectum

Lymphovascular drainage of the distal 5 cm of anorectum directly into the systemic circulation, bypassing the reticuloendothelial system of the portal system which drains the remaining colon. The reticuloendothelial system has a major role in sequestering enteric pathogens and prevention of bacteraemia during EMR. In contrast, resection of LSLs (≥30 mm) located in the distal anorectum is associated with significant bacteraemia, and prophylactic intravenous antibiotics are recommended larger LSLs. Somatic sensation supplies the dentate line, and addition of a long-acting local anaesthetic such as ropivacaine 0.5–0.75% to the submucosal injectate is effective for post-procedural analgesia. In this setting cardiac monitoring by electrocardiography is required. Lastly, haemorrhoidal vessels are thick walled, and are resistant to snare entrapment with adequate submucosal injection, and generally represents no additional bleeding risk from EMR [25].

11.5.2 Peri-Appendiceal and Ileocaecal Valve LSLs

EMR of LSLs involving the appendiceal orifice is challenging but can be successfully completed if <50% of the valve circumference is involved and deep margin within the appendix is adequately visualised. A small (10 mm), stiff thin-wire snare is useful for removing adenomatous tissue from within the orifice. ER around and within the orifice may precipitate appendicitis, and administration of a prophylactic intravenous antibiotic effective against enteric pathogens followed by a short 5- to 7-day oral course is recommended.

EMR of LSLs involving the ileocaecal valve (ICV) (Fig. 11.5) have higher risk of failure (OR 3.38) [1]. Access, particularly to the inferior lip, can be improved by use of a distal cap attached to a paediatric colonoscope. The cap helps to deflect mucosal folds and stabilise the scope. Extensive proximal extension of adenomatous tissue into the narrow terminal ileum and LSLs that involve both the superior and inferior lips prohibit complete EMR. A few adaptions are suggested for EMR of LSLs involving the ICV: (1) a small (10 mm), stiff thin-wire snare is preferred when working with the distal ileum due to space constraints, (2) submucosal injection should be conservative as excessive amounts can hamper endoscopic visualisation and lesion access, (3) careful attention should be paid to the anterior and posterior angles of the ICV, where residual tissue can be missed [26]. Lastly, the ICV submucosa is relatively adipose; underlying fat may be exposed following resection, but it is not necessarily a sign of deeper injury.

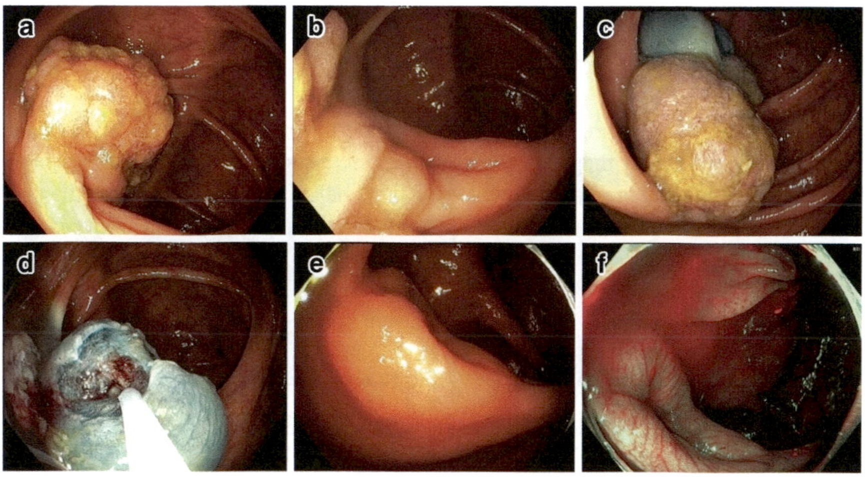

Fig. 11.5 EMR of large 35 mm sessile polyp from ileocaecal valve

11.5.3 Large Pedunculated Polyps

Pedunculated polyps represent about a third of all colonic polyps. Many are larger than 10 mm and contain a feeding arteriole within its stalk. Complete resection of a pedunculated polyp is achieved by transection of its pedicle. This minimises the risk of perforation, but risks bleeding from the feeding vessel, which can be severe. Increased risk of bleeding is associated with stalk thickness ≥5 mm, polyp head ≥20 mm in size, right colonic location, and presence of malignancy [27]. The risk of delayed bleeding following resection of pedunculated polyps can be reduced by mechanical prophylaxis with clips and/or nylon loops applied to the stalk, with or without pre-injection with diluted (1:10000) adrenaline [28, 29] (Fig. 11.6). Adequate ligation is confirmed by blanching of the polyp head. Following this, snare resection above the point of ligation with blended or coagulation current is performed. Pure cutting current is associated with an increased risk of immediate bleeding and should be avoided.

11.5.4 Lesions Previously Attempted for Resection

Previous attempts at resection or aggressive biopsies can cause significant SMF. Start submucosal injection and resection away from areas of obvious fibrosis to assist finding the submucosal plane. Small, stiff thin-wire snares are preferable. When fibrosis prevents snare capture of tissue, cold forceps avulsion followed by snare-tip soft coagulation (CAST) (Soft Coag effect 4, maximum 80W; ERBE, Türbingen, Germany) to the avulsed area is an effective technique to remove small residual islands [30]. A type 2 deep mural injury (DMI, see below section on 'perforation') may result and should be prophylactically closed by through the scope (TTS) clips to this area to prevent delayed perforation. A prospective multicentre study showed that two-stage EMR performed by tertiary centre endoscopists is a safe and effective salvage therapy after a failed single session, with 84% technical success and 82% of patients avoiding surgery on long-term follow-up [31].

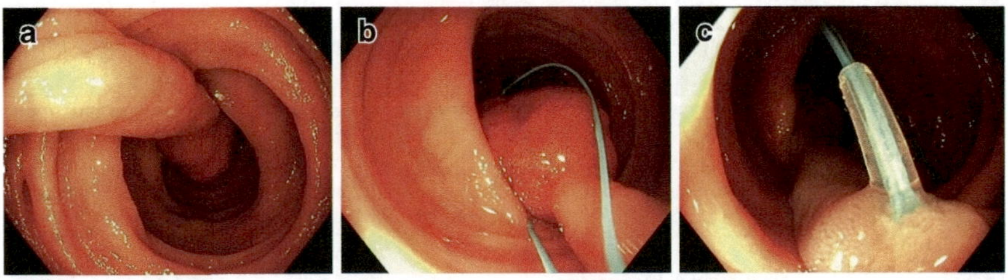

Fig. 11.6 Placement of nylon loop to stalk to large pedunculated polyp. (**a**) Large pedunculated polyp on long, thick stalk. (**b**) The nylon loop is opened above the polyp and gently manoeuvred over the head and down the stalk. (**c**) Once satisfactorily placed, the loop is tightened and deployed. Adequate placement is confirmed by ischaemic discolouration of the polyp ligated by the loop

11.6 Aftercare

Patients should be closely observed following colonic EMR. A two-stage management algorithm is suggested (see below). Patient discomfort and abnormalities in vital signs may herald perforation or significant bleeding, and should be promptly assessed. Most abdominal pain due to benign causes will resolve with simple analgesia such as intravenous acetaminophen. CT abdomen is indicated for persistent abdominal pain or clinical signs of peritonitis.

Patients who are asymptomatic and appear well with normal vital signs after a period of observation can be moved to second stage recovery. Following a successful trial of clear liquids and period of observation, patients may be discharged home on the same day with instructions to represent to hospital if they develop rectal bleeding, fevers or abdominal pain. Patients who become unwell during observation should be admitted for further investigation and management.

Repeat colonoscopy at 4–6 months is generally advised following the index procedure to assess for residual or recurrent adenoma. However, some factors may be predictive of a lower risk of recurrence. Recent evidence from a prospective multicentre study showed LSLs <40 mm, without IPB nor high-grade dysplasia had a 91% negative predictive value for residual or recurrent adenoma at first surveillance colonoscopy [32]. For lesions satisfying all these criteria, first surveillance colonoscopy could be delayed until 18 months after index EMR.

11.7 Managing Complications

The most frequent adverse events associated with colonic EMR are bleeding and perforation. Bleeding is the most common and can be intra-procedural or post-procedural, occurring up to 2 weeks after EMR. Severity ranges between self-limited oozing to brisk arterial bleeding; endoscopic haemostasis is achievable in most instances.

11.7.1 Intra-procedural Bleeding

Intra-procedural bleeding is defined as bleeding that persists for longer than 60 s or requiring endoscopic intervention. IPB occurs in up to 11% of cases, and is associated with increasing lesion size (OR 1.24/10 mm), Paris 0-IIa + Is lesion morphology (OR 2.12), lesions with villous histology (OR 1.84) and endoscopy centres that perform less than 75 EMRs per year (OR 3.78) [17]. Most cases of IPB are treatable endoscopically, although haemostasis methods require additional time and is associated with increased adenomatous recurrence (OR 1.68) [17].

IPB can be effectively treated by thermal modalities. Use of a voltage-limited microprocessor-controlled current helps to avoid deep thermal injury. STSC is an effective technique to control IPB arising from small arterioles or veins. It is performed by protruding the snare tip 2–3 mm beyond the catheter, gently touching the tip onto a bleeding point, followed by application of coagulating current (Soft Coag, effect 4, 80W; ERBE, Türbingen, Germany). Irrigation with the foot pump helps to localise the point of bleeding, and may also have a tamponade effect through expansion of fluid into the submucosa. For cases where STSC does not achieve haemostasis, additional treatment of the bleeding vessel with coagulating forceps (Soft Coag, effect 4, 80W; ERBE, Türbingen, Germany) or TTS clips may be used. Injection of dilute adrenaline should be used with another modality such as thermal ablation or mechanical haemostasis [18].

11.7.2 Delayed Bleeding

Delayed bleeding (clinically significant post endoscopic bleeding [CSPEB]) is defined as any bleeding occurring up to 30 days after EMR resulting in emergency room presentation, hospitalisation or requiring intervention. Based on data from a large multicentre study, the incidence of CSPEB is 6.2%, with increased risk associated with proximal colon location (OR 3.72), use of an electrosurgical current not controlled by a microprocessor (OR 2.03), and IPB (OR 2.16) [17]. Lesion size and patient comorbidities did not appear to predict CSPEB [17] (Fig. 11.7).

For most cases, CSPEB resolves spontaneously, although need for intervention is associated with hourly or more frequent haematochezia (OR 36.7), American Society of Anaesthesiologists grade ≥ 2 (OR 20.1) and need for transfusion (OR 18.7) [33]. These factors form the basis of an algorithm to manage post EMR CSPEB (Fig. 11.8). Prophylactic coagulation to non-bleeding vessels within the resection defect does not significantly decrease the incidence of CSPEB after EMR [34]. Closure of resection defects with clips may reduce the risk of CSPEB, particularly for proximal and larger LSLs [35].

11.7.3 Perforation

Perforation from colonic EMR occurs in 1–2% of cases [1]. Perforation is one of five categories of MP injury, collectively known as deep mural injury (DMI) (Table 11.2 and Fig. 11.9) [36]. Type 1 DMI is exposed but uninjured MP fibres and requires no treatment. In type 2 DMI, the distinction between submucosa and MP is unclear, usually due to SMF or CAST. As deep injury cannot be excluded, Type 2 DMI should be prophylactically clipped [37]. In type 3, 4 and 5 DMI, the injured MP is represented by concentric white rings within the MP, and should always be promptly closed by clips to avoid extension of injury or extraluminal contamination.

Endoscopically subtle MP injury is probably responsible for some cases of delayed perforations. In cases where there is poor staining of the EMR defect, topical irrigation using the injection solution (topical submucosal chromoendoscopy, TSC) can exclude uninjured submucosa or confirm MP injury [38]. Submucosal

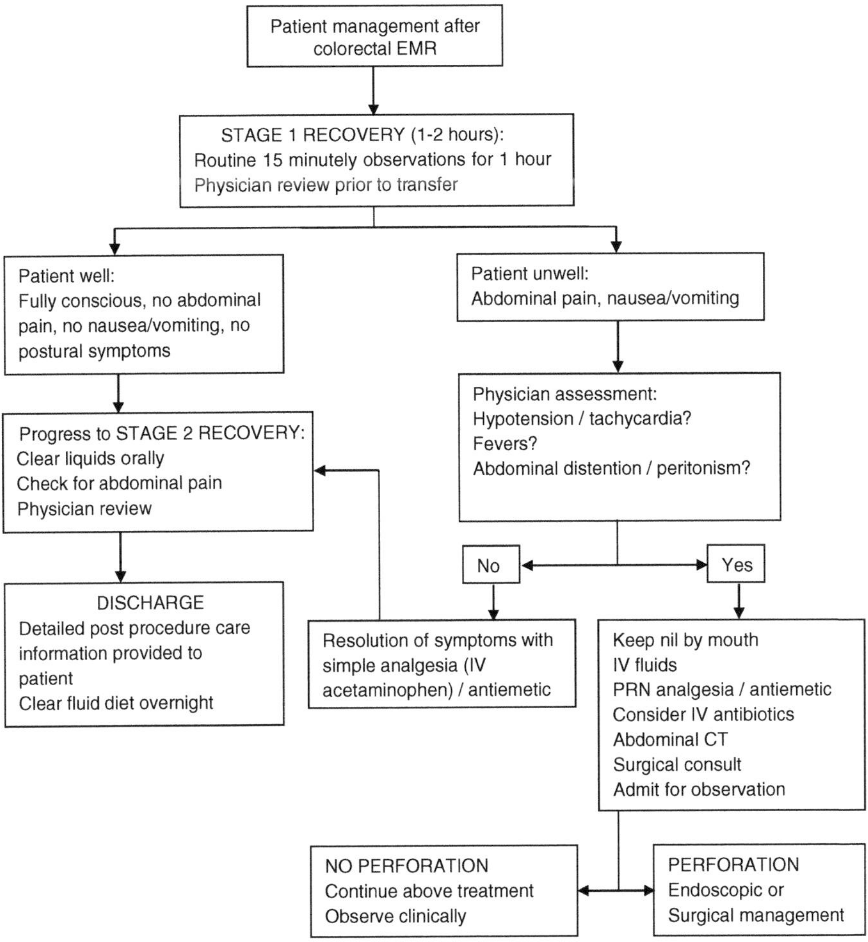

Fig. 11.7 Suggested management scheme following advanced resection of colorectal LSLs. (Adapted from Klein A & Bourke MJ Gastroenterology Clinics of North America 2015)

fibres avidly take up the dye, and a blue matt appearance reassures that no MP injury has occurred. Conversely, any exposed MP fibres will not take up the dye, and non-staining areas after TSC suggest deep injury and should be prophylactically treated by TTS clips.

TTS clips have similar tensile strength to surgical sutures, and are ideal for closure of ER-related perforations. Principles and technique perforation closure with clips include the following:

- Minimising gas insufflation to reduce tension on the defect. Administer anti-peristaltic agents to prevent peristalsis from contaminating the site.

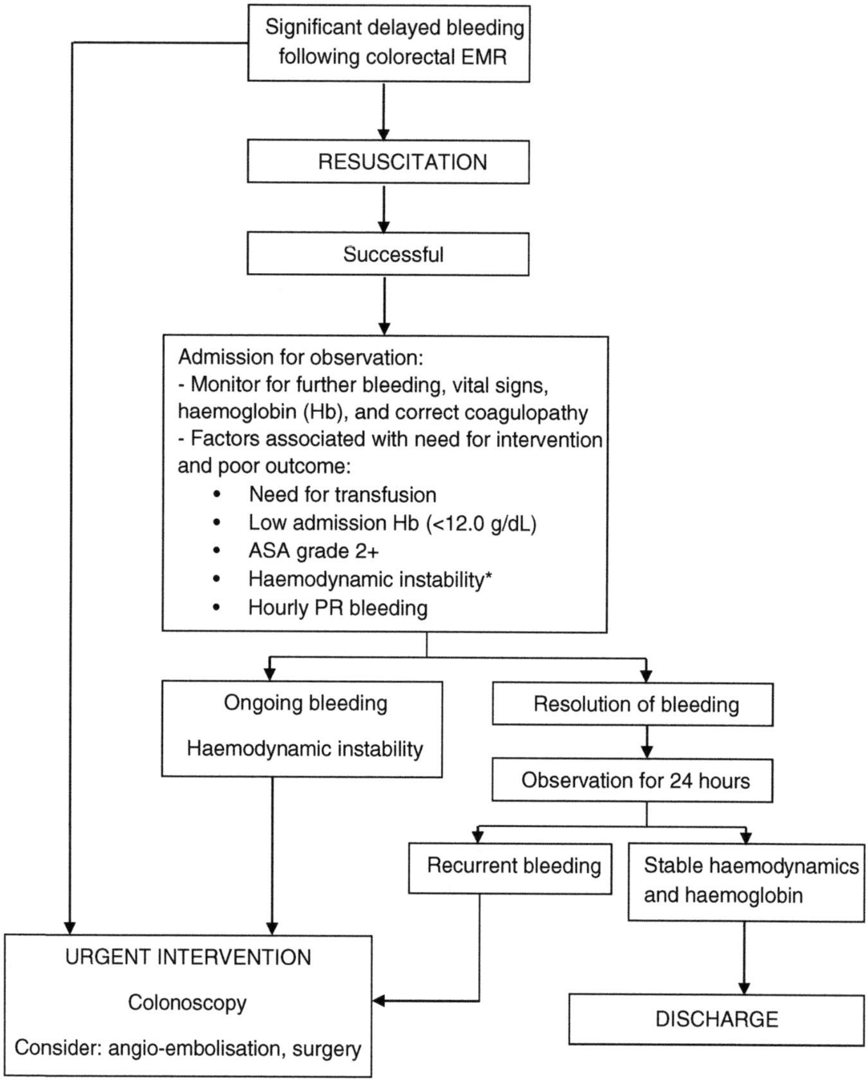

Fig. 11.8 Management algorithm for clinically significant post-EMR bleeding. *Haemodynamic instability defined as heart rate ≥100/min, systolic blood pressure ≤100 mmHg, or orthostatic decrease in SBP ≥20 mmHg. (Adapted from Burgess NB, Metz AJ, Williams SJ, et al. Clin Gastro Hep 2014)

Table 11.2 Sydney classification of deep mural injury (DMI) following EMR

Type 1	MP visible, but no mechanical injury. May have minimal thermal injury
Type 2	Focal or generalised loss of the submucosal plane raising concern for MP injury or rendering the MP defect uninterpretable
Type 3	MP injured, target or mirror target identified
Type 4	Hole within a white cautery ring, no observed contamination
Type 5	Hole within a white cautery ring, observed contamination

EMR endoscopic mucosal resection, *MP* muscularis propria

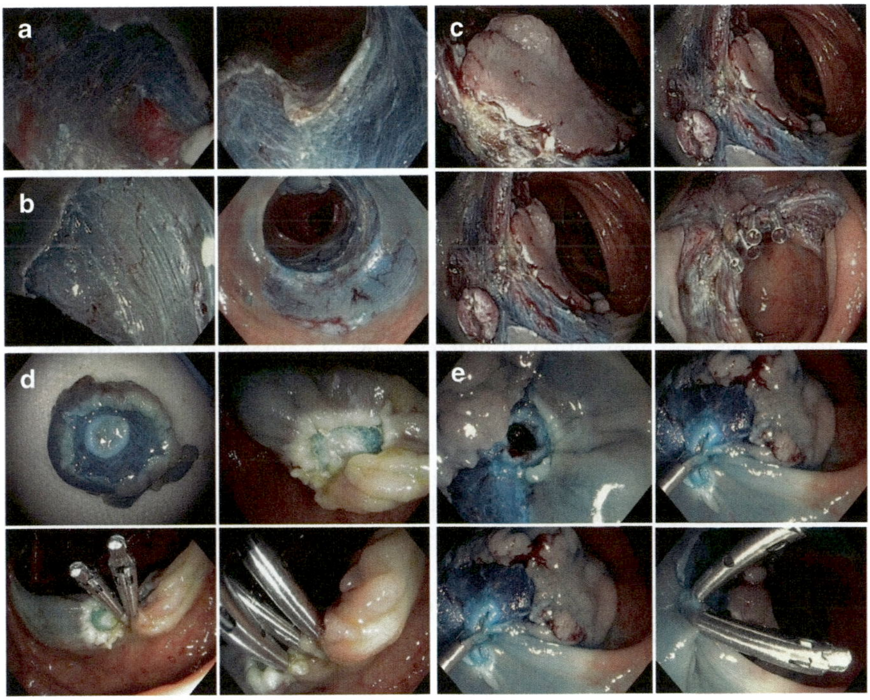

Fig. 11.9 Examples of deep mural injury and their management following EMR. (**a**) (Two images): Type 0. Normal finding. The submucosa is homogeneously stained with blue dye, without visible MP. Vessels may appear within or upon the blue layer. (**b**) (Two images): Type 1. Deeply resected submucosa, revealing the underlying parallel striations of the MP. Note the MP does not stain well and has a whiter appearance. There is no risk of delayed perforation. (**c**) (Four images): Type 2. Focal area of poor staining within the centre of the defect, usually due to submucosal fibrosis. However, this area cannot be adequately assessed for MP injury, and prophylactic closure with TTS clips is recommended. (**d**) (Four images): Type 3. The specimen TS (first image) is characterised by a whitish circle of resected MP on the transected surface of the specimen surrounded by blue stained submucosal tissue and encircled by white cauterised mucosa. This indicates partial or full thickness MP injury. TS should be promptly managed by TTS clips, and usually do not require operative management. (**e**) (Four images): Type 4. A perforation is demonstrated. Full thickness excision of MP has occurred without faecal contamination. These defects should be promptly closed to avoid peritoneal contamination. *EMR* endoscopic mucosal resection, *MP* muscularis propria, *TS* target sign, *TTS* through the scope. (Adapted from Ma MX, Bourke MJ, Best Prac Res Clin Gastroenterol 2016)

- Keep the working field clean by positioning the patient so fluid pools away from the defect.
- Remove adenomatous tissue adjacent to the defect if possible before placement of clips for DMI type 2 and 3. Prompt closure takes precedence in obvious perforations (DMI type 4 and 5).
- MP wounds are generally aligned perpendicular to the long axis of the colon. Clips are best placed from left to right to maintain access. Gravity should also be considered, and it is best to avoid placing a clip where it will fall across the working field.
- The initial clip can be placed just beyond the defect to elevate the bowel wall and facilitate subsequent clip placement. First suction the mucosa into the open clip, aiming to have the defect within the centre pivot of the clip. Gently press the clip against the mucosa, and with further suction, the lumen is deflated and the clip is closed. Confirm adequate convergence of the defect edges within the clip upon re-insufflation, and then deploy the clip.
- Endoscopic closure of perforations by suture devices is another option, although this requires endoscope exchange and reinsertion, risking extra-luminal contamination in the process and is probably best suited to large gaping perforations where clips are less likely to be effective.

Patients who are clinically well without signs of peritonitis after treatment for DMI type 2 and 3 may be safely discharged on the same day as their procedure. Extra-luminal gas seen on abdominal CT without intraperitoneal fluid after closure of a non-contaminated intra-procedural perforation in a patient who is well generally has a good prognosis. However, presence of extra-luminal fluid is a much more serious situation that requires careful clinical review and surgical consultation.

11.7.4 Post-polypectomy Electrocoagulation Syndrome and Delayed Perforation

Post-polypectomy electrocoagulation syndrome (PPES) results from transmural thermal injury to the bowel wall, with associated serosal inflammation and localised peritonitis. Patients may present hours to days after colonic EMR with fever, localised signs of peritonitis, raised inflammatory markers and absence of perforation on radiological imaging. The incidence of PPES is about 0.5% with risk factors including ER in the right colon, polyp size ≥20 mm, hypertension and lesions with a non-polypoidal morphology [27].

The risk of PPES is reduced by minimising transmission of electrocoagulation current to the submucosal layers of the bowel wall by adequate submucosal injection and tenting the snared lesion into the colonic lumen before resection by diathermy. Treatment is conservative with intravenous fluids, antibiotics and bowel rest.

Delayed perforation fortunately is rare, and, like PPES, may result from electrocoagulation-related thermal injury or subtle, unrecognised MP injury. Most patients present within 24 h of EMR, but delayed perforations may occur up to a week later. When suspected, urgent CT abdomen is required to establish the diagnosis. Delayed perforations are associated with a high rate of faecal peritonitis, and urgent surgery is usually required. Primary repair by laparoscopy may be possible if tissue appears healthy. Otherwise, faecal diversion by colostomy or ileostomy may be required.

11.8 Conclusion

Endoscopic mucosal resection is considered the first-line treatment for colonic large laterally spreading lesions. A strong evidence base exists supporting its efficacy, safety and cost-effectiveness compared with surgery. However, EMR is also a complex procedure, with potential serious risks. Keys to success include adequate training of endoscopist and support staff, careful lesion selection, attention to meticulous technique, management of complications and patient follow-up. Continuous evaluation of performance and review of contemporary literature are also crucial to maintaining optimal outcomes.

Conflict of Interest None.

Funding Sources and Sponsorship None.

References

1. Moss A, Bourke MJ, Williams SJ, Hourigan LF, Brown G, Tam W, et al. Endoscopic mucosal resection outcomes and prediction of submucosal cancer from advanced colonic mucosal neoplasia. Gastroenterology. 2011;140(7):1909–18.
2. Moss A, Williams SJ, Hourigan LF, Brown G, Tam W, Singh R, et al. Long-term adenoma recurrence following wide-field endoscopic mucosal resection (WF-EMR) for advanced colonic mucosal neoplasia is infrequent: results and risk factors in 1000 cases from the Australian colonic EMR (ACE) study. Gut. 2015;64(1):57–65.
3. Jayanna M, Burgess NG, Singh R, Hourigan LF, Brown GJ, Zanati SA, et al. Cost analysis of endoscopic mucosal resection vs surgery for large laterally spreading colorectal lesions. Clin Gastroenterol Hepatol. 2016;14(2):271–8, e1–2.
4. Tutticci N, Klein A, Sonson R, Bourke MJ. Endoscopic resection of subtotal or completely circumferential laterally spreading colonic adenomas: technique, caveats, and outcomes. Endoscopy. 2016;48(5):465–71.
5. Tutticci N, Sonson R, Bourke MJ. Endoscopic resection of subtotal and complete circumferential colonic advanced mucosal neoplasia. Gastrointest Endosc. 2014;80(2):340.
6. Nascimbeni R, Burgart LJ, Nivatvongs S, Larson DR. Risk of lymph node metastasis in T1 carcinoma of the colon and rectum. Dis Colon Rectum. 2002;45(2):200–6.

7. Participants in the Paris W. The Paris endoscopic classification of superficial neoplastic lesions: esophagus, stomach, and colon. Gastrointest Endosc. 2003;58(6):S3–S43.
8. Burgess NG, Hourigan LF, Zanati SA, Brown GJ, Singh R, Williams SJ, et al. Risk stratification for covert invasive cancer among patients referred for colonic endoscopic mucosal resection: a large multicenter cohort. Gastroenterology. 2017;153(3):732–42.e1.
9. Coletta M, Sami SS, Nachiappan A, Fraquelli M, Casazza G, Ragunath K. Acetic acid chromoendoscopy for the diagnosis of early neoplasia and specialized intestinal metaplasia in Barrett's esophagus: a meta-analysis. Gastrointest Endosc. 2016;83(1):57–67.e1.
10. Brown SR, Baraza W, Din S, Riley S. Chromoscopy versus conventional endoscopy for the detection of polyps in the colon and rectum. Cochrane Database Syst Rev. 2016;4:CD006439.
11. dos Santos CE, Lima JC, Lopes CV, Malaman D, Salomao AD, Garcia AC, et al. Computerized virtual chromoendoscopy versus indigo carmine chromoendoscopy combined with magnification for diagnosis of small colorectal lesions: a randomized and prospective study. Eur J Gastroenterol Hepatol. 2010;22(11):1364–71.
12. Kudo S, Rubio CA, Teixeira CR, Kashida H, Kogure E. Pit pattern in colorectal neoplasia: endoscopic magnifying view. Endoscopy. 2001;33(4):367–73.
13. Ikematsu H, Matsuda T, Emura F, Saito Y, Uraoka T, Fu KI, et al. Efficacy of capillary pattern type IIIA/IIIB by magnifying narrow band imaging for estimating depth of invasion of early colorectal neoplasms. BMC Gastroenterol. 2010;10:33.
14. Hewett DG, Kaltenbach T, Sano Y, Tanaka S, Saunders BP, Ponchon T, et al. Validation of a simple classification system for endoscopic diagnosis of small colorectal polyps using narrow-band imaging. Gastroenterology. 2012;143(3):599–607.e1.
15. Dellon ES, Hawk JS, Grimm IS, Shaheen NJ. The use of carbon dioxide for insufflation during GI endoscopy: a systematic review. Gastrointest Endosc. 2009;69(4):843–9.
16. Moss A, Bourke MJ, Metz AJ. A randomized, double-blind trial of succinylated gelatin submucosal injection for endoscopic resection of large sessile polyps of the colon. Am J Gastroenterol. 2010;105(11):2375–82.
17. Burgess NG, Metz AJ, Williams SJ, Singh R, Tam W, Hourigan LF, et al. Risk factors for intraprocedural and clinically significant delayed bleeding after wide-field endoscopic mucosal resection of large colonic lesions. Clin Gastroenterol Hepatol. 2014;12(4):651–61, e1–3.
18. Ferlitsch M, Moss A, Hassan C, Bhandari P, Dumonceau JM, Paspatis G, et al. Colorectal polypectomy and endoscopic mucosal resection (EMR): European Society of Gastrointestinal Endoscopy (ESGE) clinical guideline. Endoscopy. 2017;49(3):270–97.
19. Klein A, Tate DJ, Jayasekeran V, Hourigan L, Singh R, Brown G, et al. Thermal ablation of mucosal defect margins reduces adenoma recurrence after colonic endoscopic mucosal resection. Gastroenterology. 2019;156(3):604–13.e3.
20. Piraka C, Saeed A, Waljee AK, Pillai A, Stidham R, Elmunzer BJ. Cold snare polypectomy for non-pedunculated colon polyps greater than 1 cm. Endosc Int Open. 2017;5(3):E184–e9.
21. Choksi N, Elmunzer BJ, Stidham RW, Shuster D, Piraka C. Cold snare piecemeal resection of colonic and duodenal polyps >/=1 cm. Endosc Int Open. 2015;3(5):E508–13.
22. Tate DJ, Awadie H, Bahin FF, Desomer L, Lee R, Heitman SJ, et al. Wide-field piecemeal cold snare polypectomy of large sessile serrated polyps without a submucosal injection is safe. Endoscopy. 2018;50(3):248–52.
23. Tutticci NJ, Hewett DG. Cold EMR of large sessile serrated polyps at colonoscopy (with video). Gastrointest Endosc. 2018;87(3):837–42.
24. Spadaccini M, Fuccio L, Lamonaca L, Frazzoni L, Maselli R, Di Leo M, et al. Underwater EMR for colorectal lesions: a systematic review with meta-analysis (with video). Gastrointest Endosc. 2019;89(6):1109–1116.e4.
25. Holt BA, Bassan MS, Sexton A, Williams SJ, Bourke MJ. Advanced mucosal neoplasia of the anorectal junction: endoscopic resection technique and outcomes (with videos). Gastrointest Endosc. 2014;79(1):119–26.
26. Nanda KS, Tutticci N, Burgess NG, Sonson R, Williams SJ, Bourke MJ. Endoscopic mucosal resection of laterally spreading lesions involving the ileocecal valve: technique, risk factors for failure, and outcomes. Endoscopy. 2015;47(8):710–8.

27. Ma MX, Bourke MJ. Complications of endoscopic polypectomy, endoscopic mucosal resection and endoscopic submucosal dissection in the colon. Best Pract Res Clin Gastroenterol. 2016;30(5):749–67.
28. Paspatis GA, Paraskeva K, Theodoropoulou A, Mathou N, Vardas E, Oustamanolakis P, et al. A prospective, randomized comparison of adrenaline injection in combination with detachable snare versus adrenaline injection alone in the prevention of postpolypectomy bleeding in large colonic polyps. Am J Gastroenterol. 2006;101(12):2805; quiz 913
29. Kouklakis G, Mpoumponaris A, Gatopoulou A, Efraimidou E, Manolas K, Lirantzopoulos N. Endoscopic resection of large pedunculated colonic polyps and risk of postpolypectomy bleeding with adrenaline injection versus endoloop and hemoclip: a prospective, randomized study. Surg Endosc. 2009;23(12):2732–7.
30. Tate DJ, Bahin FF, Desomer L, Sidhu M, Gupta V, Bourke MJ. Cold-forceps avulsion with adjuvant snare-tip soft coagulation (CAST) is an effective and safe strategy for the management of non-lifting large laterally spreading colonic lesions. Endoscopy. 2018;50(1):52–62.
31. Tate DJ, Desomer L, Hourigan LF, Moss A, Singh R, Bourke MJ. Two-stage endoscopic mucosal resection is a safe and effective salvage therapy after a failed single-session approach. Endoscopy. 2017;49(9):888–98.
32. Tate DJ, Desomer L, Klein A, Brown G, Hourigan LF, Lee EY, et al. Adenoma recurrence after piecemeal colonic EMR is predictable: the Sydney EMR recurrence tool. Gastrointest Endosc. 2017;85(3):647–56.e6.
33. Burgess NG, Williams SJ, Hourigan LF, Brown GJ, Zanati SA, Singh R, et al. A management algorithm based on delayed bleeding after wide-field endoscopic mucosal resection of large colonic lesions. Clin Gastroenterol Hepatol. 2014;12(9):1525–33.
34. Bahin FF, Naidoo M, Williams SJ, Hourigan LF, Ormonde DG, Raftopoulos SC, et al. Prophylactic endoscopic coagulation to prevent bleeding after wide-field endoscopic mucosal resection of large sessile colon polyps. Clin Gastroenterol Hepatol. 2015;13(4):724–30, e1–2
35. Pohl H, Grimm IS, Moyer MT, Hasan MK, Pleskow D, Elmunzer BJ, et al. Clip closure prevents bleeding after endoscopic resection of large colon polyps in a randomized trial. Gastroenterology. 2019;89(6):1109–1116.e4.
36. Burgess NG, Bassan MS, McLeod D, Williams SJ, Byth K, Bourke MJ. Deep mural injury and perforation after colonic endoscopic mucosal resection: a new classification and analysis of risk factors. Gut. 2017;66(10):1779–89.
37. Swan MP, Bourke MJ, Moss A, Williams SJ, Hopper A, Metz A. The target sign: an endoscopic marker for the resection of the muscularis propria and potential perforation during colonic endoscopic mucosal resection. Gastrointest Endosc. 2011;73(1):79–85.
38. Holt BA, Jayasekeran V, Sonson R, Bourke MJ. Topical submucosal chromoendoscopy defines the level of resection in colonic EMR and may improve procedural safety (with video). Gastrointest Endosc. 2013;77(6):949–53.

12 Endoscopic Mucosal Resection for Early Esophageal and Gastric Cancers

Suneha Sundaram, Prateek Sharma, and Madhav Desai

12.1 Introduction

Esophageal and gastric cancer are two of the top 10 most common cancers and the third and sixth leading causes of cancer death worldwide, respectively [1, 2]. The lifetime risk of developing gastric cancer is 0.84% with a 0.36% overall lifetime risk of death [3]. Esophageal cancer carries a 0.5% lifetime risk of diagnosis for all races and sexes, with a higher predominance in white males, and a 0.45% lifetime risk of death overall [3]. The treatment of early esophageal and gastric cancer has changed drastically with the advancement of endoscopic technologies and techniques. Endoscopic mucosal resection (EMR) has emerged ahead of surgical treatment for early stage esophageal and gastric cancers because of its combined diagnostic and therapeutic value, safety, and improvement in overall mortality.

The gastrointestinal tract wall consists of four layers: mucosa (made up of the epithelium, lamina propria, and muscularis mucosa), submucosa, muscularis propria, and the adventitia. One of the most important prognostic factors for both cancer types is the depth of invasion. Based on TNM staging, T1a cancer is limited to the mucosa and has considerably better prognosis than T1b cancers that extend just into the submucosa [4–8]. Unfortunately, most cases of these gastrointestinal cancers are advanced at the time of diagnosis when patients present after symptoms develop [2, 9]. Latest data from 2010 to 2016 shows that less than 20% of esophageal cancers are localized at the time of diagnosis, and the 5-year survival rate with nodal involvement or further metastasis is dismal (~25% and 5%, respectively) [3]. For advanced gastric cancer, surgery is considered the only curative treatment and

S. Sundaram · M. Desai (✉)
Department of Gastroenterology, Kansas City VA Medical Center, Kansas City, MO, USA

P. Sharma
Department of Gastroenterology, Kansas City VA Medical Center, Kansas City, MO, USA

Division of Gastroenterology, Hepatology and Motility, Department of Internal Medicine, University of Kansas School of Medicine, Kansas City, MO, USA

P. Sharma, N. Reddy (eds.), *Innovations in Gastrointestinal Endoscopy*,
https://doi.org/10.1007/978-981-15-9247-8_12

carries significant risk [9]. Hence, it is vital to establish biopsy-proven diagnosis and staging early on for both conditions to determine the most appropriate treatment options.

There are multiple imaging modalities to aid with staging; however, each has its limitations. Endoscopic ultrasound (EUS) can be used to determine local lymph node invasion and has been shown to be more sensitive in detection of T1b lesions but less sensitive for distant metastasis. Computed tomography (CT) imaging is used to determine distant metastasis, but patient will still require biopsy for histopathological diagnosis [6]. Alternatively, electronic chromoendoscopy and advanced imaging is used as an adjunct in endoscopic evaluation to identify mucosal and surface vascular abnormalities that suggest mucosal invasion and guides endoscopic therapy including EMR. A major advantage of EMR is the combined ability to directly visualize anatomy, remove lesions that can be analyzed for histopathology and provide information for staging and lymphovascular involvement. Additionally, lesions <20 mm could be removed en bloc with EMR and may be curative if lateral and deep margins are clean. The diagnostic and therapeutic effect of EMR makes it a promising treatment option. Appropriate patients with T1b or more advanced cancer should be referred for esophagectomy or gastrectomy with or without adjuvant radiation and chemotherapy.

12.2 Endoscopic Mucosal Resection

EMR involves separating the mucosa from the submucosal layer and removing the mucosal lesion, potentially en bloc. Strip biopsy is the conventional EMR method before the development of newer tools and techniques. In strip biopsy, a submucosal bleb is created, but the target lesion is removed by simple polypectomy snare without the use of a cap. The two commonly used methods today, specifically in early esophageal and gastric cancers, are the later developed cap and multiband ligation-assisted method. These are also referred to as the "lift and cut" and "suck and snare" techniques, respectively. First, we will discuss the general concept and technique of EMR and then discuss the specifics of these methods.

12.2.1 EMR Technique

First, the entire length of the esophagus is examined by high-definition white-light imaging (WLI) endoscopy before any intervention is attempted. Dye-based (e.g., Lugol's iodine, indigo carmine, or acetic acid) or electronic chromoendoscopy [e.g., narrow band imaging (NBI), i-scan, BLI] with or without optical magnification has an adjunctive role in characterizing the lesion's cellular and vascular pattern to determine if there is concern for submucosal invasion. Lugol's iodine stains the glycogen present in normal epithelium thereby differentiating it from the contrastingly unstained dysplastic epithelium with its lack of glycogen. Some concerns with Lugol's iodine are the additional procedure time, clinical side effects including substernal pain and irritation, but mostly it has low specificity for esophageal neoplasia. NBI and BLI use short wavelength light that is particularly absorbed by hemoglobin, illustrating highly vascular patterns in mucosa with a brown discoloration. Supplemental magnification with near focus option further enhances these details. Subtle epithelial abnormalities can identify cancer not visible on WLI. Certain vascular and mucosal changes have been identified to predict depth of invasion [10–12]. When compared to WLI alone, NBI has been shown to be clinically useful for the detection of early esophageal and gastric cancer lesions and should be considered in surveillance of high-risk patients [4, 7, 10, 13, 14]. In cases where submucosal invasion is suspected, EUS has been used to assess depth of invasion; however, accuracy is not high [7, 15].

Once identified, the target lesion can be demarcated by applying electrocautery circumferentially in a staccato-like pattern at least 2 mm away from suspected lateral margins. This helps to achieve complete inclusion of the lesion in the cap and snare, or if a piecemeal resection is necessary, it helps to re-identify the lesion in the setting of any distortion caused from cautery or obscured view from bleeding. It is paramount that the location of all biopsies taken is precisely mapped. If submucosal invasion is identified on histology of any lesion, the exact location should be known for any subsequent treatment. Prague classification of the circumferential and maximum extent of Barrett's esophagus, if present, is also important to report for eradication therapy and subsequent surveillance [2, 6, 8, 10, 13, 16].

Next, if submucosal injection is required, a needle is inserted tangentially through the mucosa of the identified lesion. To separate the mucosa from the muscle layer, fluid is injected in the submucosal layer with the goal of creating a visible "saline cushion." The amount of fluid needed can vary and is determined by the endoscopist based on visualization of a mucosal bleb. Commonly used fluids include hypertonic saline, diluted epinephrine, fibrinogen, sodium hyaluronate, and hydroxypropyl methyl cellulose. These solutions increase safety by decreasing bleeding post-resection and by creating longer lasting "cushions" before resorption compared to normal saline alone. There are several benefits specifically related to this part of the procedure. Separating these two tissue layers reduces the likelihood of perforation by preventing damage to the muscle layer during electrocautery and biopsy removal. Also, absence of a saline bleb may indicate submucosal invasion and can be a sign of more advanced cancer, requiring alternate treatment [6, 13, 14, 17].

For the final steps, a transparent cap that is affixed to the tip of the endoscope is positioned over the demarcated lesion. Together with a specialized snare, the lesion is captured, cut, and removed. Both the cap and multiband methods utilize a cap and snare to resect the lesion; but, as the name suggests, the "suck and cut" band technique additionally uses suction to create a pseudopolyp with the band before cutting. This method does not require submucosal fluid injection. Each technique will be discussed in further detail next.

The submucosal side of the resected specimen is affixed to a slide with formalin. The specimen is serially sectioned and stained with H&E. Frozen-section analysis correlates well with permanent section analysis and can be used for real-time decision-making and may prevent the need for multiple invasive procedures [5, 13].

If pathology suggests the cancer is invasive, the patient should be referred for other treatment options and is protected from unnecessary additional resections.

12.2.2 Cap-Assisted Method

The cap method was first described in the early 1990s for esophageal, stomach, and colonic mucosal lesions [18]. It is also referred to as the “lift and cut” technique based on the lifting of the mucosa by the saline cushion and grasping forceps before cutting the defined lesion.

This method always utilizes submucosal fluid injection to form a visible bleb. The transparent cap is placed at the distal end of the endoscope. These caps have a unique groove where a customized crescent-shaped snare will be “pre-looped.” To do this, the cap is placed over the lesion and slight suction is applied to seal the cap. The snare is inserted into the endoscope channel and opened so that the outer sheath is fixed to the rim of the cap. The cap and snare are both positioned to encompass the entire target lesion. Suction or grasping forceps is used to pull the mucosa into the cap and the snare is closed around the lesion. The specimen is removed by use of electrocautery with selection of settings for optimal blending of cut and coagulation. Caps can range in shape, flexibility, and size. Oblique (oval) caps are usually used for larger or more tangential esophageal lesions. Straight (flat and circular) caps are medium capacity and could be used for smaller lesions (<1 cm). Caps can be hard or soft with an outer diameter ranging from 12.9 to 18 mm. The crescent-shaped snare is highly pliable and more flexible for use with the cap than a conventional snare. There are now specialized single-use mucosectomy kits with the specific size, shape, material cap desired, and the crescent-shaped snare included.

Concerns about this method include risk of perforation; however, this risk is present in most procedures involving removal of esophageal tissue. Snares can also lose shape with multiple uses, so a new kit is required for each cut when conducting piecemeal resections of larger lesions [10, 14, 17, 19].

12.2.3 Multiple-Band-Assisted EMR

For the multiband-assisted method too, specialized mucosectomy devices are now manufactured. A multiband ligator device containing bands mounted over a transparent cap (typically 6 or 7 bands depending on manufacturer) is attached to the distal part of the endoscope. The cap is placed over the target lesion (Fig. 12.1a). The lesion is completely suctioned into the cap, and a band is deployed creating a pseudopolyp (Fig. 12.1b). These unique bands are designed specifically to not have enough strength to catch and hold the rigid muscle layer. This is a safeguard against damage to the muscularis propria layer during electrocautery, so in theory this method can be performed without making a submucosal cushion. A hexagonal snare is then used to cauterize the specimen either above or below the band to ensure complete resection of lesion based on previously marked borders. Multiple

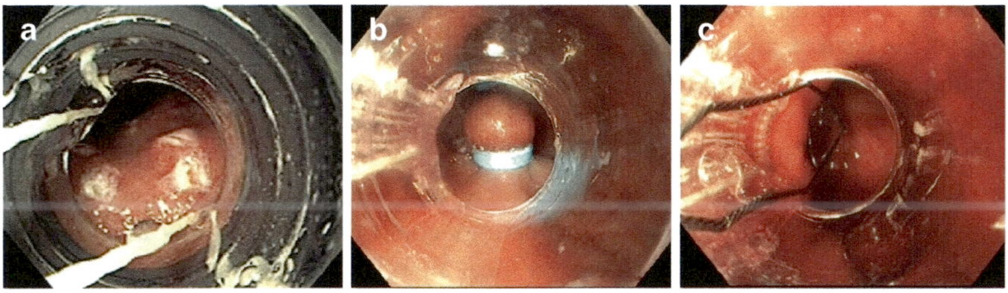

Fig. 12.1 Multiband assisted EMR. (**a**) Visualization of target lesion after demarcation 2 mm from lateral margins with cautery. (**b**) "Pseudopolyp" created by suctioning lesion into cap and placing specialized mucosectomy band around lesion. (**c**) Introduction and opening of hexagonal snare with band ligator remaining in place before strangulation and removal of target lesion

resections can be performed during a single session in this method as multiband ligator stays in place while the snare is passed through the working channel (Fig. 12.1c). Resected specimens can be retrieved at the completion of therapy using a net or suction alone.

Comparatively, both methods carry similar risk of perforation. The multiband method may be preferred for larger regions requiring piecemeal resection. Ultimately, choice of method should be based on patient-specific pathology, the endoscopists' expertise, and safety and cost to patient.

12.3 Use of EMR for Esophageal Cancers

12.3.1 Use in Esophageal Squamous Cell Cancer (ESCC)

SCC remains the most common pathology of esophageal cancer worldwide. Risk factors include tobacco and alcohol use (both independently and with compounding effects), achalasia, nutritional deficiencies including iron that are associated with lower socioeconomic status, and history of mediastinal radiation therapy usually in the setting of breast, head, or neck cancer [2]. Absolute indications for EMR in ESCC are T1a superficial lesions (m1 and m2 limited to mucosal epithelium and lamina propria), no lymph node, or vascular involvement, and <3/4th circumferential involvement. The reasoning for these indications is that these superficial lesions have very low risk of lymph node metastasis, resection of >3/4th circumference cannot be achieved en bloc and is associated with increased risk of stenosis as a long-term complication [4, 20, 21].

When doing EMR for ESCC, identification and characterization of dysplasia using NBI with magnification is distinctly useful with regard to the pattern of intrapapillary capillary loops (IPCL). The Japanese Esophageal Society established a system to classify IPCL patterns as Type A, if there is no change in microvascular pattern, or B, if specific abnormalities are present. Type B is further subcategorized as B1–B3 based on the size of abnormal IPCL, and if there is preservation of a loop pattern. NBI with magnification allows accurate classification of B1 vessels, which are appropriate for EMR, with a sensitivity of 97.5% and overall accuracy of >90% [10]. This is an exceptionally valuable diagnostic tool for ESCC. Both cap and multiband methods have been used extensively in these patients internationally, particularly in Japan.

A major limitation to the successful eradication of ESCC with EMR is inability to achieve complete removal of cancerous lesions, especially when en bloc excisions are not possible. Piecemeal resections could distort histology and it might become nearly impossible to confirm clear margins. Comparatively, endoscopic submucosal dissection (ESD) has better success with en bloc resection and R0 resection rates particularly in most cases of larger lesions >20 mm [10, 19]. ESD has been found to achieve significantly higher rates of both curative resection and 5-year recurrence-free survival in comparison to EMR in various studies across the world [21]. However, ESD also has higher risk of adverse effects including perforation and stricture formation [10, 22]. Currently, both ESD and EMR are first-line therapy options for m1 and m2 localized SCC with EMR used for smaller lesions. Given the risks and benefits between these endoscopic therapies, treatment options should be discussed at length with patients to determine the best individualized plan of care [10, 11, 21, 22]. Recurrence can occur at rates >20% after more than 1 year follow-up, making surveillance a fundamental aspect of treatment [13]. There are currently no standardized guidelines directing surveillance intervals and protocols.

12.3.2 Use in Esophageal Adenocarcinoma (EAC)

EAC has surpassed SCC as the most common type of esophageal cancer in the United States. The reasons for this epidemiological shift are not entirely understood, but multiple factors including national trends in central obesity, nutritional intake, smoking, and medications may all contribute. Barrett's esophagus (BE) is the precursor lesion for EAC. Incidence rates of cancer increase with higher degrees of dysplasia and once there is nodal involvement, the 5-year survival rate is <20% [2, 6, 7, 23, 24]. Notably, >90% of EAC is diagnosed in patients without a prior diagnosis of BE. The American College of Gastroenterology (ACG) and American Society of Gastrointestinal Endoscopy (ASGE) have published recommendations for endoscopic surveillance of BE and treatment based on degree of dysplasia with the ultimate goal of preventing progression to or early detection of EAC [24, 25].

If any mucosal abnormality (i.e., nodularity, ulceration, irregular contour etc.) is noted on surveillance endoscopy for patients with BE, EMR is used for diagnosis and treatment of such lesions. EMR resections encompass sufficient lateral margins and complete mucosal depth which allows for improved histological staging over standard endoscopic biopsies and changes the diagnosis in almost half of these patients [15]. Adjunctive NBI during upper endoscopy improves detection of subtle mucosal abnormalities. In the case that mucosal lift is not achieved during EMR, and histology shows dysplasia in deep margins or lesions are large (>15 mm), submucosal invasion is likely and ESD should be considered [7, 14]. If EAC is diagnosed on EMR resected specimen and has clean margins, cancer is limited to the mucosa (T1a) with low risk of lymph node metastasis and is also treated first line with endoscopic eradication therapy. Subsequent ablative therapy of remaining BE to achieve complete eradication of intestinal metaplasia markedly decreases risk of recurrent dysplasia or EAC [4, 17, 23, 24].

The likelihood of nodal involvement in T1b EAC depends on the depth of submucosal invasion. Further, deeper invasion increases possibility of lymphovascular spread, another predictor of lymph node spread and overall prognosis. Superficial (T1b sm1) submucosal EAC has lower likelihood of metastasis. Optimally, a multidisciplinary team, including surgery and oncology, should discuss the treatment plan for any T1b or more advanced EAC. Mid or deep submucosal invasion (sm2 and sm3) carries higher risk of metastasis, but in high-risk patients it can be treated with endoscopic therapy over surgery if benefits outweigh risks of complications [4, 13, 15, 16, 19, 26].

12.3.3 EMR for Early Gastric Adenocarcinoma (EGC)

Adenocarcinoma of the stomach especially gastric cardia began to rise in the United States at the same time as EAC incidence [27]. Both cancers also share similar epidemiological characteristics such as a predisposition for white males. As one might expect, with many pathological similarities to EAC, treatment is also similar but more restrictive [9, 19]. In 2001, the Japanese Gastric Cancer Association first published treatment guidelines for gastric cancer. Guidelines have since been updated with the advancement of EMR techniques as well as the enhancement of therapy with ESD and en bloc resection of larger lesions [5]. As with esophageal cancers, depth of invasion and lymphovascular spread are major predictors for metastasis of gastric cancer [5, 8, 19]. As of 2014, the absolute indication for EMR or ESD as standard treatment is a well-differentiated lesion, without ulcerations, T1a depth limited to the mucosa with a diameter of ≤ 2 cm in stomach. There are also expanded guidelines that allow for EMR, or recommended ESD for greater potential of complete en bloc removal, with tumors considered "very low possibility" of lymph node metastasis. These are T1a lesions without lymphovascular invasions and a combination of well/poor differentiation, presence or absence of ulcers, and diameter lesser or greater than 2–3 cm. Follow-up with annual or biannual endoscopies is recommended after curative resection. If EMR/ESD intervention is not curative with margins positive for carcinoma or there is recurrence, repeat ESD, surgical resection, or chemotherapy should be discussed [5].

ESD has a lower recurrence rate than EMR in early gastric cancer, so is the recommended method for endoscopic resection in Asia. EMR should be considered especially in patients with severe comorbidities including liver cirrhosis and cardiovascular disease due to its shorter procedure time and lower risk of adverse events such as perforation [14, 17]. The Japanese Gastric Cancer Society does instruct that both endoscopic treatment methods should be considered investigational until positive outcomes are established from ongoing trials [5]. Ultimately, determining

Table 12.1 Summary of indications for EMR in ESCC, EAC, and EGC

	ESCC	EAC	EGC
Stage	T1a	T1a	T1a
Diameter, mm	≤20	≤20	≤20
Depth of invasion	m1, m2 (m3 or sm1 ≤200 μm)	m1, m2, m3 (sm1)	m1, m2, m3
Histological differentiation	Low-grade or high-grade intraepithelial dysplasia (carcinoma in situ)	Low-grade dysplasia, high-grade dysplasia, adenocarcinoma	Well differentiated
Circumferential involvement of lumen	<3/4		
Surface morphology	Flat lesions (Paris Classification 0-IIb)	Any visible abnormality (Paris Classification I, IIa, IIb, IIc)	No ulcerations

between these two methods in early gastric cancer treatment should be based primarily on the experience of the endoscopist (Table 12.1).

12.4 Adverse Events

Complications with EMR include minor bleeding, strictures, and perforation. Rates reported vary based on numbers of cases in high-volume hospitals and are associated with the number of resections performed and extent of circumferential treatment. Immediate minor bleeding not affecting measured hemoglobin is the most common acute complication, with studies reporting rates ranging from 1 to 13% of cases [13, 17, 20, 26]. Esophageal strictures are the most common overall complication, occurring in approximately 3–20% and are usually treated with balloon dilatation [13, 17, 20, 26, 28]. Reported perforation rates with EMR vary but are very rare at about 1% [4, 20, 28]. ESD has been repeatedly shown to have a significantly higher rate of perforation than EMR [10, 17]. Endoscopist expertise has a significant impact on the outcome of these endoscopic procedures. Inoue et al. remarked, during the early establishment of EMR, that sufficient fluid for submucosal lift is important to decreased risk of perforation. He also noted that in the stomach, due to limited stretch, smaller caps and less suction may help protect against muscle involvement and lower the risk of perforation [18].

Overall, morbidity and cause-specific mortality with EMR are far less than that of the number of surgical treatments for esophageal and gastric cancer. Long-term survival studies after endoscopic resection are showing excellent results and survival rates similar to the general population [11].

12.5 Future of Endoscopic Mucosal Resection

While EMR therapy is very promising, there are areas for improvement. Regarding the procedure itself, defining an optimal injection fluid both in composition and quantity may help ensure consistent saline blebs and mucosal lift. Standardizing electrocautery settings to achieve optimal cut and coagulation would achieve faster bleeding control and may limit the obliteration of important histology at borders.

Studies have shown a difference in ESD versus EMR in terms of safety and efficacy. ESD is advantageous in its capacity for en bloc resections >2 cm or deeper lesions with m3 submucosal invasion or greater [5, 10, 19, 28]. However, ESD is a more complex procedure requiring an experienced endoscopist and carries higher risk of perforation. Currently there are only recommendations for use of ESD over EMR, chiefly for resection of larger lesions with preservation of histology at margins. Absolute indications for each procedure should be outlined in future guidelines for its positioning in each type of upper GI cancers.

Surveillance and follow-up is an important aspect of treatment in all cancers. Defined surveillance intervals and protocols for esophageal SCC, like those established for EAC, is necessary to address recurrence. Similarly, for early gastric cancer, we should establish surveillance protocol to monitor recurrence post-curative resection or track progression of active cancer to appropriately treat patients as soon as changes occur. Finally, for more radical resections in the esophagus, research should focus on reducing the rates of strictures.

References

1. Bray F, Ferlay J, Soerjomataram I, Siegel RL, Torre LA, Jemal A. Global cancer statistics 2018: GLOBOCAN estimates of incidence and mortality worldwide for 36 cancers in 185 countries. CA Cancer J Clin [Internet]. 2018 [cited 2020 Jul 6];68(6):394–424. http://doi.wiley.com/10.3322/caac.21492
2. Enzinger PC, Mayer RJ. Esophageal cancer. N Engl J Med [Internet]. 2003 [cited 2020 Jul 6];349(23):2241–52. http://www.nejm.org/doi/abs/10.1056/NEJMra035010
3. Howlander N, Noone A, Karpcho M, Miller D. SEER cancer statistics review, 1975–2017 [Internet]. Bethesda: National Cancer Institute; 2020. https://seer.cancer.gov/csr/1975_2017/
4. Kitagawa Y, Uno T, Oyama T, Kato K, Kato H, Kawakubo H, et al. Esophageal cancer practice guidelines 2017 edited by the Japan esophageal society: part 2. Esophagus [Internet]. 2019 [cited 2020 Jul 6];16(1):25–43. http://link.springer.com/10.1007/s10388-018-0642-8
5. Japanese Gastric Cancer Association. Japanese gastric cancer treatment guidelines 2014 (ver. 4). Gastric Cancer [Internet]. 2017 [cited 2020 Jul 6];20(1):1–19. http://link.springer.com/10.1007/s10120-016-0622-4
6. Rubenstein JH, Shaheen NJ. Epidemiology, diagnosis, and management of esophageal adenocarcinoma. Gastroenterology [Internet]. 2015 [cited 2020 Jul 6];149(2):302–317.e1. https://linkinghub.elsevier.com/retrieve/pii/S0016508515006423

7. Mansour NM, Groth SS, Anandasabapathy S. Esophageal adenocarcinoma: screening, surveillance, and management. Annu Rev Med [Internet]. 2017 [cited 2020 Jul 6];68(1):213–27. http://www.annualreviews.org/doi/10.1146/annurev-med-050715-104218
8. Abe N, Sugiyama M, Masaki T, Ueki H, Yanagida O, Mori T, et al. Predictive factors for lymph node metastasis of differentiated submucosally invasive gastric cancer. Gastrointest Endosc [Internet]. 2004 [cited 2020 Jul 9];60(2):242–5. https://linkinghub.elsevier.com/retrieve/pii/S0016510704016827
9. Takahashi T, Saikawa Y, Kitagawa Y. Gastric cancer: current status of diagnosis and treatment. Cancers [Internet]. 2013 [cited 2020 Jul 9];5(4):48–63. http://www.mdpi.com/2072-6694/5/1/48
10. Yip H-C, Chiu PW-Y. Endoscopic diagnosis and management of early squamous cell carcinoma of esophagus. J Thorac Dis [Internet]. 2017 [cited 2020 Jul 6];9(S8):S689–96. http://jtd.amegroups.com/article/view/14477/11819
11. Ishihara R, Tanaka H, Iishi H, Takeuchi Y, Higashino K, Uedo N, et al. Long-term outcome of esophageal mucosal squamous cell carcinoma without lymphovascular involvement after endoscopic resection. Cancer [Internet]. 2008 [cited 2020 Jul 6];112(10):2166–72. http://doi.wiley.com/10.1002/cncr.23418
12. Yao K, Anagnostopoulos G, Ragunath K. Magnifying endoscopy for diagnosing and delineating early gastric cancer. Endoscopy [Internet]. 2009 [cited 2020 Jul 6];41(05):462–7. http://www.thieme-connect.de/DOI/DOI?10.1055/s-0029-1214594
13. Namasivayam V, Wang KK, Prasad GA. Endoscopic mucosal resection in the management of esophageal neoplasia: current status and future directions. Clin Gastroenterol Hepatol [Internet]. 2010 [cited 2020 Jul 6];8(9):743–54. https://linkinghub.elsevier.com/retrieve/pii/S1542356510005628
14. Larghi A, Waxman I. State of the art on endoscopic mucosal resection and endoscopic submucosal dissection. Gastrointest Endosc Clin N Am [Internet]. 2007 [cited 2020 Jul 6];17(3):441–69. https://linkinghub.elsevier.com/retrieve/pii/S1052515707000669
15. Moss A, Bourke MJ, Hourigan LF, Gupta S, Williams SJ, Tran K, et al. Endoscopic resection for Barrett's high-grade dysplasia and early esophageal adenocarcinoma: an essential staging procedure with long-term therapeutic benefit. Am J Gastroenterol [Internet]. 2010 [cited 2020 Jul 6];105(6):1276–83. http://journals.lww.com/00000434-201006000-00013
16. Barnes JA, Willingham FF. Endoscopic management of early esophageal cancer. J Clin Gastroenterol [Internet]. 2015 [cited 2020 Jul 6];49(8):638–46. http://journals.lww.com/00004836-201509000-00005
17. Hwang JH, Konda V, Abu Dayyeh BK, Chauhan SS, Enestvedt BK, Fujii-Lau LL, et al. Endoscopic mucosal resection. Gastrointest Endosc [Internet]. 2015 [cited 2020 Jul 6];82(2):215–26. https://linkinghub.elsevier.com/retrieve/pii/S0016510715024050
18. Inoue H, Kawano T, Tani M, Takeshita K, Iwai T. Endoscopic mucosal resection using a cap: techniques for use and preventing perforation. Can J Gastroenterol [Internet]. 1999 [cited 2020 Jul 6];13(6):477–80. http://www.hindawi.com/journals/cjgh/1999/198230/abs/
19. Pouw RE, Bergman JJGHM. Endoscopic resection of early oesophageal and gastric neoplasia. Best Pract Res Clin Gastroenterol [Internet]. 2008 [cited 2020 Jul 6];22(5):929–43. https://linkinghub.elsevier.com/retrieve/pii/S1521691808000668
20. Malik S, Sharma G, Sanaka MR, Thota PN. Role of endoscopic therapy in early esophageal cancer. World J Gastroenterol [Internet]. 2018 [cited 2020 Jul 13];24(35):3965–73. http://www.wjgnet.com/1007-9327/full/v24/i35/3965.htm
21. Berger A, Rahmi G, Perrod G, Pioche M, Canard J-M, Cesbron-Métivier E, et al. Long-term follow-up after endoscopic resection for superficial esophageal squamous cell carcinoma: a multicenter Western study. Endoscopy [Internet]. 2019 [cited 2020 Jul 6];51(04):298–306. http://www.thieme-connect.de/DOI/DOI?10.1055/a-0732-5317
22. Ono S, Fujishiro M, Niimi K, Goto O, Kodashima S, Yamamichi N, et al. Long-term outcomes of endoscopic submucosal dissection for superficial esophageal squamous cell neoplasms. Gastrointest Endosc [Internet]. 2009 [cited 2020 Jul 6];70(5):860–6. https://linkinghub.elsevier.com/retrieve/pii/S0016510709018343

23. Singh T, Sanghi V, Thota PN. Current management of Barrett esophagus and esophageal adenocarcinoma. Cleve Clin J Med [Internet]. 2019 [cited 2020 Jul 6];86(11):724–32. https://www.ccjm.org//lookup/doi/10.3949/ccjm.86a.18106
24. Shaheen NJ, Falk GW, Iyer PG, Gerson LB. ACG clinical guideline: diagnosis and management of Barrett's esophagus: Am J Gastroenterol [Internet]. 2016 [cited 2020 Jul 6];111(1):30–50. http://journals.lww.com/00000434-201601000-00017
25. ASGE Standards of Practice Committee, Qumseya B, Sultan S, Bain P, Jamil L, Jacobson B, et al. ASGE guideline on screening and surveillance of Barrett's esophagus. Gastrointest Endosc. 2019;90(3):335–359.e2.
26. Barr H. Endoscopic therapy for Barrett's oesophagus. Gut [Internet]. 2005 [cited 2020 Jul 12];54(6):875–84. http://gut.bmj.com/cgi/doi/10.1136/gut.2004.047118
27. Blot WJ. Rising incidence of adenocarcinoma of the esophagus and ngastric cardia. JAMA J Am Med Assoc [Internet]. 1991 [cited 2020 Jul 6];265(10):1287. http://jama.jamanetwork.com/article.aspx?doi=10.1001/jama.1991.03460100089030
28. Ge PS, Muthusamy VR. Endoscopic mucosal resection for Barrett's esophagus. J Laparoendosc Adv Surg Tech [Internet]. 2017 [cited 2020 Jul 6];27(4):404–11. http://www.liebertpub.com/doi/10.1089/lap.2016.0532

Endoscopic Duodenal Mucosal Resurfacing: A Potential Therapeutic Treatment for Metabolic Disease

13

Alia Hadefi and Jacques Devière

13.1 Introduction

Type 2 diabetes mellitus (T2DM) and nonalcoholic fatty liver disease (NAFLD) are pandemic metabolic disorders [1, 2] that are closely linked to the prevalence of obesity [3] and affect 8.5% and 24%, respectively, of patients worldwide. These metabolic diseases present a large and growing public health issue and can lead to life-threatening complications. T2DM is related to cardiovascular disease and renal failure, whereas NAFLD may potentially evolve to a more aggressive necro-inflammatory form, nonalcoholic steatohepatitis (NASH), which may evolve to cirrhosis and hepatocellular carcinoma. In addition, mortality and advanced liver disease associated with NAFLD are expected to double by 2030 [4] and, consequently, NAFLD/NASH is expected to be, in the next decades, the first indication for liver transplantation in the Western world [5].

Insulin resistance is a pivotal pathogenic factor involved in the development of metabolic disease, not only due to its implication in glycemic control but also due to its pleiotropic actions in the modulation of lipid and protein metabolism [6–8]. Currently, the only effective strategy for reducing insulin resistance is weight loss. Although several pharmacological medications, such as metformin and thiazolidinedione, are recognized to exhibit insulin-sensitizing properties, their effect is somewhat limited. Furthermore, despite the many drugs available for treating T2DM,

A. Hadefi (✉)
Department of Gastroenterology, Hepatopancreatology, and Digestive Oncology, Erasmus Hospital, Université Libre de Bruxelles, Brussels, Belgium
e-mail: alia.hadefi@erasme.ulb.ac.be

J. Devière
Laboratory of Experimental Gastroenterology, Université Libre de Bruxelles, Brussels, Belgium
e-mail: jacques.deviere@erasme.ulb.ac.be

P. Sharma, N. Reddy (eds.), *Innovations in Gastrointestinal Endoscopy*,
https://doi.org/10.1007/978-981-15-9247-8_13

nearly 50% of patients are poorly controlled due to progressive beta cell loss and poor adherence to drug therapy.

Thus, existing treatment strategies for T2DM have been unable to slow the progressive course of the disease, and weight loss improving insulin sensitivity is currently the only validated treatment for NASH [9]. However, only a few patients achieve the significant and sustained weight loss required for an effect on liver damage and T2DM. Beyond lifestyle modifications, bariatric surgery, which involves bypass of the upper intestine (Roux en Y gastric bypass: RYGB), has been shown to have powerful corrective effects on histological lesions in NASH subjects [10]. Moreover, this procedure, and a less-invasive variant known as mini-bypass, is included among current treatment guidelines for patients with type 2 diabetes [11]. Notably, the metabolic improvement is observed acutely, within days after surgery, independently of significant weight loss, a feature which suggests that avoiding the contact of food with the duodenum and the proximal jejunum may elicit insulin-sensitizing effects [12, 13]. Nevertheless, bariatric surgery remains an invasive approach with a risk of significant complications and is still considered only for morbidly obese patients.

Experimental evidence showed that exposure to high levels of dietary fat and sugar induces pathological changes in the duodenum of both animals and humans including abnormal hypertrophy of the duodenal mucosa [14], changes in enteroendocrine cell density and number [15], endocrine hyperplasia [15], and alterations in gut hormone signaling [16].

Therefore, based on these considerations, the duodenal mucosa may become a potential therapeutic target for metabolic disease using a minimally invasive endoscopic approach. This review aims to discuss the existing evidence regarding the effectiveness and safety of a minimally invasive endoscopic procedure using thermoablation, the duodenal mucosal resurfacing (DMR).

13.2 Endoscopic Duodenal Mucosal Resurfacing

The findings described above support an approach that targets the duodenal mucosa, given its involvement in metabolic homeostasis, with the purpose of treating metabolic disorders. Duodenal mucosal resurfacing (DMR) is a novel, minimally invasive procedure that uses a trans-oral catheter (Fig. 13.1) and involves hydrothermal ablation of the duodenal mucosa, resulting in its replacement by new epithelium. The efficacy and safety of ablative therapies are well described, and these procedures are commonly used, most notably in Barrett's esophagus with dysplasia [17–19], through either radiofrequency or argon plasma coagulation.

13.2.1 Proof-of-Concept Study in Animal Models

Preclinical testing of DMR was achieved on Goto-Kakizaki rats, a model of insulin resistance, compared to sham-treated diabetic controls. Thermoablation of duodenal mucosa in Goto-Kakizaki rats improved oral glucose tolerance test results

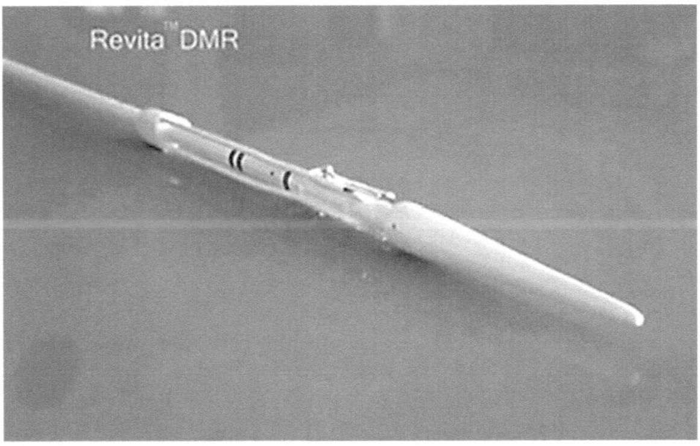

Fig. 13.1 The second-generation Revita™ catheter. DMR, duodenal mucosal resurfacing. (Courtesy of Fractyl laboratories, Inc., Lexington, MA)

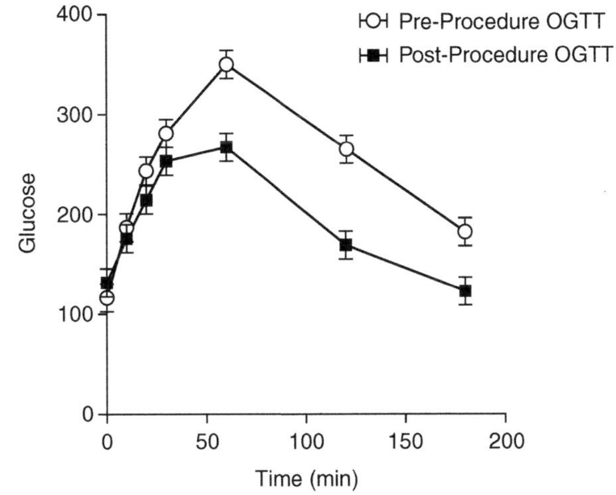

Fig. 13.2 Oral glucose tolerance test (OGTT) results in the Goto-Kakizaki rat (n = 9) before and after duodenal abrasion. Duodenal abrasion was associated with a 25% improvement in area under the curve for OGTT. (Reproduced from Cherrington et al. 2017)

compared to pre-procedure (Fig. 13.2) [20], whereas non-diabetic rodents (Sprague-Dawley) who have received the same intervention, no improvement in glucose tolerance was observed. The safety and the feasibility of this procedure was also assessed in a porcine model in which the absence of deeper damage in the underlying muscularis propria was demonstrated [20].

13.2.2 Duodenal Mucosal Resurfacing Procedure

The DMR device (RevitaSystem™; Fractyl Laboratories Inc., Lexington, MA, USA) is composed of a single-use catheter (Fig. 13.1) that allows submucosal expansion (to separate the mucosa from the muscle layer) and hot fluid ablation. The device includes three saline delivery needles located into catheters fixed around an inflatable balloon. This is connected to a console via a tubing set. Under fluoroscopic guidance, a guidewire is placed beyond the Treitz ligament allowing to position and maneuver the catheter. Before ablation, a hemoclip is fixed on the opposite side of the papilla enabling fluoroscopic visualization of the

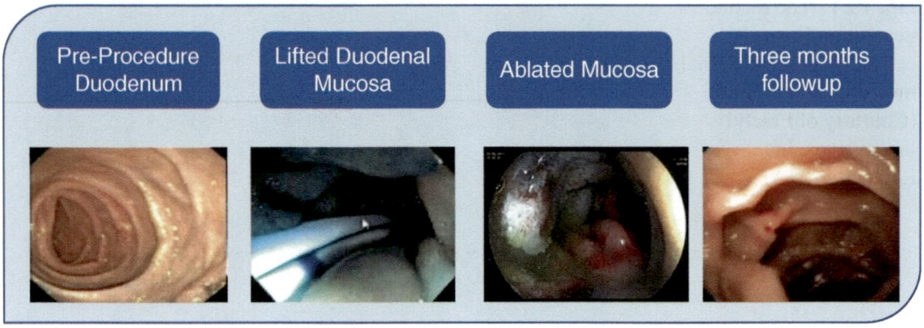

Fig. 13.3 Endoscopic aspect before and after duodenal mucosal resurfacing procedure

initial balloon's position in order to prevent any ablation at this level. The balloon is then inflated and, through suction applied in the side catheters, the three injection needles are inserted through the mucosa. Under endoscopic guidance (using a pediatric colonoscope), a circumferential submucosal expansion (Fig. 13.3) is performed with more than 200 mL of 0.9% saline solution and methylene blue. The same balloon catheter delivers a hot fluid (up to 90 °C; 10-s application with pre- and post-cooling) in order to perform circumferential hydrothermal ablation limited to the mucosa. Five to ten longitudinally adjacent injections/ablations are achieved from the genu inferius to the Treitz ligament. The sequence includes two submucosal injections, followed by one ablation and repeated proximally to distally. The catheter is then removed, and the necrosis of the superficial layer duodenal mucosa is inspected before withdrawing the endoscope (Fig. 13.3). Patients are discharged at day 1, and they are kept on a liquid diet for 3 days after the procedure and returned to a solid food within 14 days. Three months after DMR, an upper endoscopy is performed in order to assess any adverse events related to the device and observe the regeneration of the new epithelium (Fig. 13.3).

13.2.3 Safety and Effectiveness of Duodenal Mucosal Resurfacing Using the Revita TM System in Treatment of Type 2 Diabetes and Wider Effects on Fatty Liver Disease

A first human monocentric clinical study [21] was conducted including 44 patients with poorly controlled T2DM using oral antidiabetic drugs. Patients underwent a single DMR procedure over 3–12 cm of duodenum. Enrolled patients were obese, had T2DM for less than 10 years, and were on at least one oral antidiabetic drug. Patients with type 1 diabetes currently managed with injectable drugs or previous gastrointestinal surgery or anatomical alterations were excluded.

The procedure was well tolerated. The most common side effects being abdominal pain and three cases of duodenal stenosis, the latter were treated by a single endoscopic dilation. DMR was, at this time, realized with two separated balloon catheters for submucosal injection and ablation. Further improvements were implemented to ensure proper mucosal lifting before ablation avoiding the aforementioned device-related adverse events.

HbA1c was reduced significantly by 1.2% at 6 months (Fig. 13.4). Body weight was reduced by 3.9 kg at 3 months and by 2.5 kg at 6 months.

Recently, the DMR procedure was performed in an open-label, multicenter study in 46 obese patients with T2DM, mean age of 55 years (range 31–69), mean T2DM duration of 6 years (range 0.1–12) [22]. There were no duodenal stenosis. After 12 months, HbA1c was reduced by a mean of 1.0% ± 0.2% ($p \leq 0.001$), the homeostatic model assessment of insulin resistance (HOMA-IR) was decreased by a mean of −3.6 ± 0.9 ($p = 0.005$). Additionally, transaminases decreased significantly with a mean of 10 ± 2 ($p = 0.005$) for ALT. There was a modest weight loss (mean 2.7 ± 0.6 kg).

A multicenter, randomized, prospective, double-blinded trial of T2DM patients sub-optimally controlled on two oral antidiabetic medications comparing DMR to a sham procedure is currently ongoing in Europe and the United States (NCT02879383/NCT03653091). Two other pilot studies are also ongoing, one assessing the DMR procedure in patients with biopsy-proven NASH (NCT03536650) and the other one evaluating the potential benefit in patients with T2DM treated by insulin. Finally, the application of DMR might prove to be as pleiotropic as insulin activity, and a protocol is currently ongoing in infertility management in women.

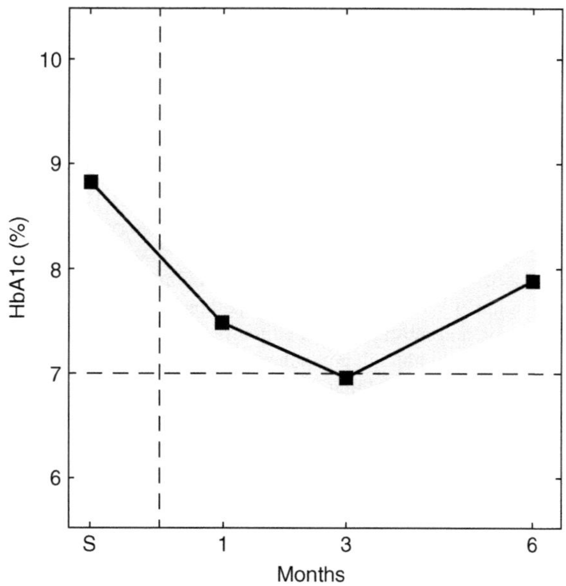

Fig. 13.4 Effect of DMR on HbA1C level. HbA1C levels at baseline, 1, 3, and 6 months in patients with pre-procedure levels of HbA1c of 7.5–10% and three or more ablations ($n = 19$). (Reproduced from Cherrington et al. 2017)

13.3 Conclusion and Perspectives

Collectively, clinical trial data available so far show that endoscopic duodenal mucosal resurfacing has an acceptable safety profile and elicits positive metabolic improvements in the setting of T2DM, and possibly in NAFLD.

With increasing prevalence of serious metabolic disorders such as T2DM and NAFLD, novel therapeutic approaches are needed. So far, approved therapies include weight loss, which is difficult to achieve and maintain, and currently available drugs, which only provide a transient effect. Bariatric surgery is currently considered to be the only approach able to halt progression and might even lead to complete remission of T2DM and NASH.

DMR promises to provide a minimally invasive alternative to bariatric surgery, leading to a regeneration of the pathological mucosa observed in metabolic diseases.

Further studies, and mostly large controlled trials, are needed to determine the place of this procedure in the treatment of T2DM and NAFLD.

References

1. Younossi Z, Anstee QM, Marietti M, Hardy T, Henry L, Eslam M, et al. Global burden of NAFLD and NASH: trends, predictions, risk factors and prevention. Nat Rev Gastroenterol Hepatol [Internet]. 2017. http://www.nature.com/doifinder/10.1038/nrgastro.2017.109.
2. NCD Risk Factor Collaboration (NCD-RisC). Worldwide trends in diabetes since 1980: a pooled analysis of 751 population-based studies with 4.4 million participants. Lancet (London, England) [Internet]. 2016 [cited 2018 Aug 4];387(10027):1513–30. http://linkinghub.elsevier.com/retrieve/pii/S0140673616006188.
3. Pimpin L, Cortez-Pinto H, Negro F, Corbould E, Lazarus J V, Webber L, et al. Burden of liver disease in Europe: epidemiology and analysis of risk factors to identify prevention policies. J Hepatol [Internet]. 2018 [cited 2018 Oct 29];69(3):718–35. https://linkinghub.elsevier.com/retrieve/pii/S0168827818320579.
4. Estes C, Anstee QM, Arias-Loste MT, Bantel H, Bellentani S, Caballeria J, et al. Modeling NAFLD disease burden in China, France, Germany, Italy, Japan, Spain, United Kingdom, and United States for the period 2016–2030. J Hepatol [Internet]. 2018 [cited 2018 Oct 29];69(4):896–904. https://linkinghub.elsevier.com/retrieve/pii/S0168827818321214.
5. Wong RJ, Aguilar M, Cheung R, Perumpail RB, Harrison SA, Younossi ZM, et al. Nonalcoholic steatohepatitis is the second leading etiology of liver disease among adults awaiting liver transplantation in the United States. Gastroenterology [Internet]. 2015 [cited 2018 Oct 29];148(3):547–55. http://www.ncbi.nlm.nih.gov/pubmed/25461851.
6. Samuel VT, Shulman GI. The pathogenesis of insulin resistance: integrating signaling pathways and substrate flux. J Clin Invest [Internet]. 2016 [cited 2018 Oct 31];126(1):12–22. http://www.ncbi.nlm.nih.gov/pubmed/26727229.
7. Shulman GI. Cellular mechanisms of insulin resistance in humans. Am J Cardiol [Internet]. 1999 [cited 2018 Oct 31];84(1A):3J–10J. http://www.ncbi.nlm.nih.gov/pubmed/10418851.
8. Saltiel AR, Kahn CR. Insulin signalling and the regulation of glucose and lipid metabolism. Nature [Internet]. 2001 [cited 2018 Oct 31];414(6865):799–806. http://www.ncbi.nlm.nih.gov/pubmed/11742412.
9. Vilar-Gomez E, Martinez-Perez Y, Calzadilla-Bertot L, Torres-Gonzalez A, Gra-Oramas B, Gonzalez-Fabian L, et al. Weight loss through lifestyle modification significantly reduces features of nonalcoholic steatohepatitis. Gastroenterology. 2015;149(2):367–378.e5.

10. Lassailly G, Caiazzo R, Buob D, Pigeyre M, Verkindt H, Labreuche J, et al. Bariatric surgery reduces features of nonalcoholic steatohepatitis in morbidly obese patients. Gastroenterology [Internet]. 2015;149(2):379–88. https://doi.org/10.1053/j.gastro.2015.04.014.
11. Rubino F, Nathan DM, Eckel RH, Schauer PR, Alberti KGMM, Zimmet PZ, et al. Metabolic surgery in the treatment algorithm for type 2 diabetes: a joint statement by International Diabetes Organizations. Diabetes Care [Internet]. 2016 [cited 2018 Jan 24];39(6):861–77. http://www.ncbi.nlm.nih.gov/pubmed/27222544.
12. Jørgensen NB, Jacobsen SH, Dirksen C, Bojsen-Møller KN, Naver L, Hvolris L, et al. Acute and long-term effects of Roux-en-Y gastric bypass on glucose metabolism in subjects with type 2 diabetes and normal glucose tolerance. Am J Physiol Metab [Internet]. 2012 [cited 2018 Aug 4];303(1):E122–31. http://www.physiology.org/doi/10.1152/ajpendo.00073.2012.
13. Bojsen-Møller KN, Dirksen C, Jørgensen NB, Jacobsen SH, Serup AK, Albers PH, et al. Early enhancements of hepatic and later of peripheral insulin sensitivity combined with increased postprandial insulin secretion contribute to improved glycemic control after Roux-en-Y gastric bypass. Diabetes [Internet]. 2014 [cited 2018 Oct 30];63(5):1725–37. http://www.ncbi.nlm.nih.gov/pubmed/24241533.
14. Verdam FJ, Greve JWM, Roosta S, Van Eijk H, Bouvy N, Buurman WA, et al. Small intestinal alterations in severely obese hyperglycemic subjects. J Clin Endocrinol Metab. 2011;96(2):379–83.
15. Theodorakis MJ. Human duodenal enteroendocrine cells: source of both incretin peptides, GLP-1 and GIP. AJP Endocrinol Metab [Internet]. 2005;290(3):E550–9. http://ajpendo.physiology.org/cgi/doi/10.1152/ajpendo.00326.2004.
16. Cherrington AD, Rajagopalan H, Maggs D, Devière J. Hydrothermal duodenal mucosal resurfacing: role in the treatment of metabolic disease. Gastrointest Endosc Clin N Am [Internet]. 2017;27(2):299–311. https://doi.org/10.1016/j.giec.2016.12.002.
17. Peter S, Mönkemüller K. Ablative endoscopic therapies for Barrett's-esophagus-related neoplasia. Gastroenterol Clin North Am [Internet]. 2015 [cited 2018 Jan 2];44(2):337–53. http://linkinghub.elsevier.com/retrieve/pii/S088985531500031X.
18. O'Connell K, Velanovich V. Effects of Nissen fundoplication on endoscopic endoluminal radiofrequency ablation of Barrett's esophagus. Surg Endosc Other Interv Tech. 2011;25(3):830–4.
19. Fleischer DE, Sharma VK. Endoscopic ablation of Barrett's esophagus using the Halo® system. Dig Dis. 2008;26(4):280–4.
20. Haidry R, Van Baar AC, Neto MG, Caplan J, Bergman JJ, Rodriguez L, Thompson CC, Deviere J. Duodenal mucosal resurfacing: proof-of-concept, procedural development, and initial implementation in the clinical setting. Gastrointest Endosc. 2019;90(4):673–681.e2.
21. Rajagopalan H, Cherrington AD, Thompson CC, Kaplan LM, Rubino F, Mingrone G, et al. Endoscopic duodenal mucosal resurfacing for the treatment of type 2 diabetes: 6-month interim analysis from the first-in-human proof-of-concept study. Diabetes Care. 2016;39(12):2254–61.
22. van Baar ACG, Nieuwdorp M, Holleman F, Deviere J, Crenier L, Haidry R, Batterham RL, Hopkins D, Rodriguez Grunert L, Galvao Neto M, Vignolo P, Costamagna G. BJJGHM. Single duodenal mucosal resurfacing elicits improvements in glycaemic and hepatic parameters in type 2 diabetes mellitus: complete 1 year results from the first prospective multicenter study. In: P1242, UEGW 2018 [Internet]. http://journals.sagepub.com/doi/pdf/10.1177/2050640617725676.

Electronic (Virtual) Chromoendoscopy 14

Ejaz Hossain, Mohamed Abdelrahim, Asma Alkandari,
and Pradeep Bhandari

14.1 Overview of Currently Available Techniques for Virtual Chromoendoscopy

14.1.1 Introduction

Ever since the advent of flexible endoscopy, one of the main aims has been to detect and characterize gastrointestinal neoplasia. Japanese colleagues introduced dye spray called 'conventional chromoendoscopy' in the seventies and found it very effective [1]. However, the conventional dye spray has not been widely adopted in the west. This has led to the development of various push button technologies called virtual chromoendoscopy. This includes narrow-band imaging (NBI) from Olympus, Flexible spectral imaging colour enhancement, blue light imaging (BLI) and linked colour imaging (LCI) from Fujifilm and I-scan from Pentax. All these technologies exploit the differences in the penetration ability of different wavelengths of light. Visible white light has a broad wavelength between 400 and 700 nm. The blue light has a short wavelength and if diffuses in a shallow and small range in contrast to red light which has long wavelength and diffuses deep and in a wide range. Furthermore, blue light is highly absorbed by haemoglobin, and this allows it to enhance the superficial microvessels. Neo-angiogenesis is a characteristic feature of neoplasia, and the pattern of distribution of these surface microvessels varies with the type of neoplasia and the stage of neoplasia. Light in blue spectrum could be used to enhance these surface vessel patterns, and this can help in detection and characterization of the neoplasia.

E. Hossain · M. Abdelrahim · P. Bhandari (✉)
Portsmouth University Hospital, Portsmouth, UK

A. Alkandari
Al Jahra Hospital, Kuwait City, Kuwait

P. Sharma, N. Reddy (eds.), *Innovations in Gastrointestinal Endoscopy*,
https://doi.org/10.1007/978-981-15-9247-8_14

14.1.2 Narrow-Band Imaging (NBI)

NBI (Olympus Medical System, Tokyo, Japan) was the first of the commercially available narrow-band technology. It is an optical filter technology which works by filtering the white light. NBI utilizes red-green-blue filters to modify white light endoscopy (WLE). The red component (650 nm) of the standard white light is filtered out, and a narrow spectral bandwidth of the blue and green light at 415 nm and 540 nm, respectively, is allowed through by the filter.

Blue light enhances the superficial capillary networks of the mucosal vessels which appear brownish, whilst green light highlights sub-epithelial vessels which appear cyan in colour. This results in greater clarity of mucosa and superficial vessels [1–4]. This is an excellent way of enhancing the surface vessel patterns, but the down side of the original version was the overall darkness of the image due to filtering out of light. However, this issue has been addressed in the newer version of NBI processors.

14.1.3 Flexible Spectral Imaging Colour Enhancement (FICE)

The major difference between FICE and NBI is the lack of real-time filter with FICE. FICE (Fujifilm, Tokyo, Japan) is a post-processor technology based on spectral estimation, which takes an ordinary white light endoscopic image from the video processor and produces an image of a given, dedicated wavelength of light after digital reconstruction. FICE selects specific wavelengths from digitized information and assigns them red, green and blue to display a composite colour enhanced multiband image in real time. This can be used like NBI to remove data from the red part of the waveband and to narrow to the green and blue spectra and produce an image very similar to NBI image. However, the system is flexible and has 10 pre-set digital filter settings with the ability to programme more [5, 6], making it very flexible. However, the wide range of these settings and lack of standardization of any one setting over the other could be very confusing for an endoscopist.

14.1.4 Blue Light Imaging (BLI), Linked Colour Imaging (LCI)

Fujifilm recently launched ELUXEO 7000 (FUJIFILM, Tokyo, Japan) a new-generation endoscopy system that is equipped with four high-intensity LED excitation and megapixel CMOS technology to enable full high-definition display.

These four LED sources produce light at different wavelengths and by altering the intensity of these wavelengths, new modes BLI and LCI are created. This is a non-filter technology which uses a dedicated laser at 410 nm instead of the conventional Xenon lamp to produce BLI. LCI is a new image-enhancing technology that acquires images by simultaneously using narrow-band short-wavelength light and WL in an appropriate balance to enhance slight colour differences in the red region of the mucosa. As most GI neoplasia are red in colour so it makes them look redder than the background mucosa [7–9].

14.1.5 I-Scan Digital Contrast (Pentax)

I-scan (Pentax, Tokyo, Japan) is another post-processing technology based on the post-image acquisition software with real-time mapping technology embedded in the endoscopic processor (EPKi). The computer-controlled digital processing provides resolution of 1.25 megapixels per image, which allows for analysis and modification of the pixel luminosity data. This consists of three modes of image enhancement. Surface enhancement (SE) can help visualize the edges of anatomical structure, improve light/dark contrast, making dark areas appear darker and light appear lighter to better delineate edges and lesion borders. Contrast enhancement (CE) slightly suppresses red and green wavelength components of the white light, whilst adding a minute blue hue to darker or more depressed area of mucosa to allow for detailed observation of subtle mucosa irregularities. This help defines 'peaks and valleys' within the mucosal surface. Tone enhancement (TE) can help tailor enhancement by modifying the colourization of each pixel that analyse all three components (R-G-B) of the white light image, and then dissects out and supresses most of the dominant red, creating an image with an elevated blue/green contrast for detecting subtler mucosal abnormalities [10–12].

14.1.6 I-Scan OE Technology (Pentax)

This is the latest development from Pentax. It incorporates a combination of bandwidth limiting light with digital image processing which enables the display of the surface structures of the blood vessels, glandular ducts, and mucosal membranes in higher contrasts than white light. The innovative optical filters achieve higher overall transmittance by connecting the peaks of the haemoglobin absorption spectrum (415 nm, 540 nm and 570 nm) creating a continuous wavelength spectrum; there are two modes with different OE filters. Mode 1—the optical filter used in this mode has a feature that enhances the contrast of blood vessels. There are two large absorption bands around 415 nm and around 540 nm similar to NBI. Mode 2—the filter used here transmits long –wavelength light (red) as well as light that has the characteristics suitable for highlighting blood vessels [12].

14.1.7 Auto-Fluorescence Imaging (Olympus)

AFI is based on tissue fluorescence emitted by endogenous fluorophores such as collagen, flavin and porphyrins when excited by short-wavelength light. AFI is altered by changes in mucosal thickness, in mucosal blood flow, and endogenous fluorophores. Normal, inflamed and neoplastic tissue have different auto-fluorescence characteristics. Differences in fluorescence between neoplastic and non-neoplastic tissue is detected by an additional CCD image sensor equipped with a filter that cuts out the blue excitation light. The video processor combines the auto-fluorescence signal with some mucosal reflectance of the green light used for illumination to produce a false-colour image where tissues area visualized in real time as purple, violet or green colour. A neoplastic lesion would then be highlighted as a purple/magenta lesion on a green background of normal mucosa [13].

14.1.8 Storz Professional Image Enhancement Software (SPIES)

This is another post-processing technology that allows for the recognition of the finest tissue details. The red colour of the visible spectrum is filtered out, and the remaining colour waves are expanded. The light/dark contrast is enhanced by obtaining luminance intensity data for each pixel and applying algorithm for each structure details. SPIES CLARA allows clear display of details in both the light and dark areas, whereas SPIES CHROMA intensifies the colour contrast [14].

14.2 Electronic Chromoendoscopy in the Upper GI Tract

In this section, we will discuss the use of these technologies to improve detection of Barrett's, as well as squamous neoplasia. It is important to highlight that oesophageal cancer is the eighth most common cancer worldwide, and although the incidence of oesophageal adenocarcinoma has been rapidly increasing in the West during the last few decades, squamous cell cancer (SCC) is still the most common type of oesophageal malignancy in other parts of the world.

The American Society for Gastrointestinal Endoscopy ASGE has developed a set of standards to be met for the clinical adoption of these technologies for Barrett's oesophagus; these were outlined by the ASGE Preservation and Incorporation of Valuable Endoscopic Innovations (PIVI) document on imaging in Barrett's oesophagus [15]. This document addressed the clinical issues related to real-time imaging of Barrett's oesophagus including the effectiveness, cost and compliance of the currently available surveillance protocols. This has set the following thresholds to be met by an imaging technology with targeted biopsies to replace the need for random mucosal biopsies during the endoscopic surveillance of non-dysplastic Barrett's oesophagus, a per-patient sensitivity of 90% or more, negative predictive value (NPV) of 98% or more for detecting high-grade dysplasia (HGD) or early oesophageal adenocarcinoma and a specificity of 80% or more [16].

14.2.1 Narrow-Band Imaging NBI for Barrett's Neoplasia

NBI, being the first commercially available narrowed-spectrum technology, is the most studied of these virtual chromoendoscopy techniques. In Barrett's oesophagus, it has been used to improve detection and targeting of both intestinal metaplasia (IM) and dysplasia.

In a prospective, controlled, tandem endoscopy study by Wolfsen et al. on patients evaluated for Barrett's oesophagus with dysplasia, HD-NBI without magnification detected significantly more patients with dysplasia and higher grades of dysplasia ($P < 0.001$), with fewer biopsy samples ($P < 0.001$) compared with standard resolution endoscopy [17]. It is difficult, however, to determine whether the improved results in this study were due to HD or NBI. More recently, a prospective international RCT by Sharma et al. comparing HD-WLE and HD-NBI has shown similar IM detection rate, but fewer biopsies per patient (3.6 vs 7.6, $P < 0.0001$), and more areas with dysplasia detected (30% vs 21%, $p = 0.01$) in the NBI group [18]. A meta-analysis by Mannath et al. of 8 studies and 446 patients have concluded that NBI with magnification is accurate for diagnosing HGD in Barrett's oesophagus based on vascular and mucosal pattern [19]. However, NBI had high sensitivity but poor specificity for characterizing specialized intestinal metaplasia SIM [18].

All these data have been produced in expert centres using an enriched/referred population with very high prevalence of neoplasia. There is no RCT data from surveillance population, so the role of NBI in Barrett's surveillance still remains to be established.

Different NBI-based classification systems have been proposed (Table 14.1). A study by Silva et al. has compared three of these classification systems and found accuracy between 57% and 63% for non-dysplastic IM, and 75% for neoplasia [20]. The Barrett's international NBI group BING have more recently developed and validated a simplified classification system with improved accuracy of 85–92% [21].

It is important to note that most of these classifications are validated by experts on static images with very high prevalence of neoplasia. Therefore, routine

Table 14.1 Classification systems for Barrett's oesophagus using narrow-band Imaging NBI

	Normal	Intestinal metaplasia	Neoplasia
Kansas	Mucosal pattern: circular Vascular pattern: normal	Mucosal pattern: ridged/villous Vascular pattern: normal	Mucosal pattern: irregular distorted Vascular pattern: abnormal
Amsterdam	Mucosal pattern: regular Vascular pattern: regular Abnormal blood vessels: absent	Mucosal pattern: regular Vascular pattern: regular (villous/gyrus) Abnormal blood vessels: absent	Mucosal pattern: irregular Vascular pattern: irregular Abnormal blood vessels: present
Nottingham	Type A: round/oval pits with regular microvasculature	Type B: villous/ridge/linear pits with regular microvasculature Type C: absent pits with regular microvasculature	Type D: distorted pits with irregular microvasculature
BING	Mucosal pattern: circular, ridged/villous, or tubular Vascular pattern: blood vessels situated regularly along or between mucosal ridges and/or those showing normal, long, branching patterns		Mucosal pattern: absent or irregular patterns Vascular pattern: focally or diffusely distributed vessels not following normal architecture of the mucosa

application of them in daily surveillance population by non-expert endoscopists remains to be proven. However, the simplicity of most of these classifications should make its applicability very easy as neoplasia is described by most classifications as areas with abnormal surface and vessel patterns.

14.2.2 NBI for Squamous Neoplasia

In a randomized controlled multicenter trial by Muto et al., NBI was able to detect superficial cancer more frequently than white light imaging in the oesophagus (97% vs. 55%, $P < 0.01$), with a sensitivity of 97.2% and accuracy of 88.9%. The sensitivity and accuracy were significantly higher using NBI than WL ($P < 0.001$ for both measures) [22]. In an another randomized trial by Chai et al. of 113 patients, NBI was also shown to significantly improve the detection of squamous cell carcinoma and HGD in the oesophagus compared to HD-WLE [23]. More recently, Morita et al. conducted a systematic review (18 studies) and meta-analysis (12 studies) to evaluate the diagnostic ability of NBI in comparison with Lugol's iodine solution for a total of 1911 patients [24]. They found the per-patient (and per-lesion) sensitivity, specificity and positive and negative predictive values with NBI were 88 (and 94%), 88 (and 65%), 8.32 (and 2.62) and 0.16 (and 0.12), respectively, compared with 92 and 98%, 82 and 37%, 5.42 and 1.4 and 0.13 and 0.39 in Lugol's iodine, respectively [24] (Fig. 14.1).

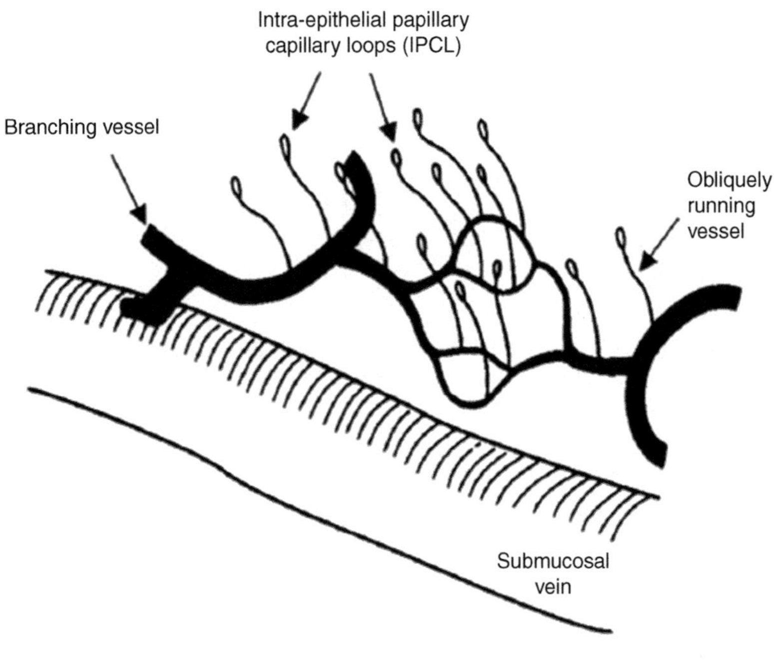

Fig. 14.1 A schematic illustration of superficial vascular structure of the squamous oesophagus (Inoue H, Honda T, Yoshida T, et al. Ultrahigh magnification endoscopy of the normal oesophageal mucosa. Dig Endosc. 1996;8:134–138)

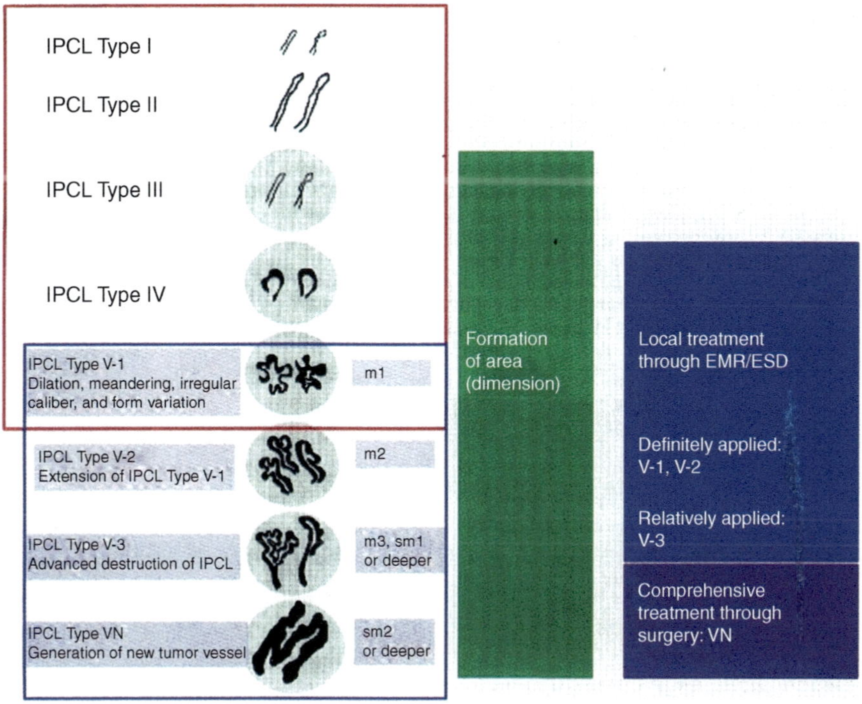

Fig. 14.2 The original intrapapillary capillary loop (IPCL) pattern classification by Inoue et al. [22]

Moreover, using the intrapapillary capillary loop (IPCL) classification (Inoue classification Fig. 14.2), NBI could also be used to assess the invasiveness of lesions [25]. This is a very detailed classification but has not been widely adopted in the west. Recently, The Japan Oesophageal Society in 2016 proposed a more simplified classification system using NBI and magnifying endoscopy ME [26], with an overall accuracy of 90.5%. The sensitivity, specificity and negative predictive value (NPV) for B1 tumours limited to epithelial layer (m1) or involving lamina propria (m2) was 97.5, 72.9 and 89.7%, and for B2 involving muscularis mucosa (m3) or superficial submucosa (sm1) was 75.0, 96.2 and 96.2%, and for B3 (involving deep submucosa (sm2)) was 55.0, 100 and 95.5%. This classification is a simplified version of Inoue classification and is more likely to be adopted by western endoscopists (Table 14.2).

14.2.3 Flexible Spectral Imaging Colour Enhancement FICE

A prospective study by Osawa et al. has compared trans-nasal FICE and WLE in patients with Barrett's oesophagus. FICE was shown to provide significantly clearer visualization of palisade vessels and better contrasting images of the demarcation between Barrett's and gastric mucosa ($P < 0.0001$) [27]. In another study by Pohl

Table 14.2 Summary and schema of the criteria of the JES magnifying endoscopic classification

Type of vessels	Schema	Definitions	
A	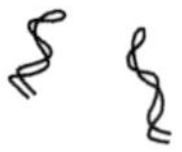	Normal IPCL or abnormal microvessels without severe irregularity[a]	
B1	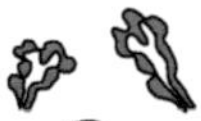	Abnormal microvessels with severe irregularity or highly dilated abnormal vessels	Type B vessels with a loop-like formation[b]
B2	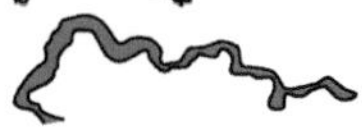		Type B vessels without a loop-like formation[b]
B3	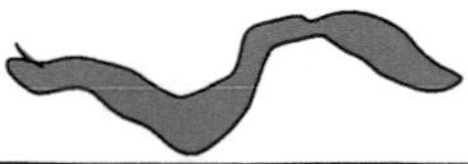		Highly dilated vessels which calibers appear to be more than three times that of usual B2 vessels[c]

et al., involving 57 patients with Barrett's, FICE has demonstrated a per-lesion sensitivity of 87%, which is comparable to conventional chromoendoscopy using acetic acid [28]. Furthermore, FICE was similar to Lugol's chromoendoscopy in the early detection of squamous cell neoplasia in the oesophagus [29].

14.2.4 Blue Light Imaging BLI

A recent international multicentre prospective cohort study by De Groof et al. has compared BLI and white light endoscopy WLE in 40 Barrett's lesions for macroscopic appearance, surface relief, and delineation of lesions [30]. They found that BLI was appreciated significantly better than WLE for visualization of macroscopic appearance (median 8.0 vs 7.0, $P < 0.001$), surface relief (8.0 vs 6.0, $P < 0.001$) and ability to delineate lesions on both overview and magnification images (8.0 vs 6.0, $P < 0.001$ and 8.0 vs 5.0, $P < 0.001$ respectively). Subramaniam et al. have developed and validated a classification system to identify Barrett's neoplasia using BLI [31]. The BLINC criteria included pit pattern, vascular pattern and colour, with an overall sensitivity, specificity, PPV and NPPV of 96.7%, 96.7%, 97.3% and 95.9%, respectively (Tables 14.3, 14.4, 14.5, and 14.6).

14.2.5 i-Scan

A small randomized trial (Hoffman et al) has shown that i-scan was comparable to acetic acid in targeting specialized intestinal metaplasia in patients with Barrett's oesophagus, compared to random biopsies (66% vs. 21% for I-SCAN-targeted vs. random biopsies) [32]. However, the absence of any dysplastic lesions in this study does limit its outcome. Moreover, Lipman et al. developed and validated a new classification based on mucosal and vascular pattern [33]. When used in combination

Table 14.3 BLINC criteria for diagnosing Barrett's neoplasia using BLI

Criteria	Non-neoplastic	Neoplastic
Pit pattern	Circular, tubular or branching with normal density	Irregular, crowded with increased density
Vessel pattern	Regular, peri-cryptal, non-dilated vessels with normal density	Irregular, non-cryptal, dilated vessels with increased density
Colour	Pale	Focal darkness

Table 14.4 Validation of BLINC criteria for diagnosing Barrett's neoplasia, among general endoscopists

	At baseline (prior to training on BLINC)	Following training on BLINC	Significance
Sensitivity (95% confidence interval)	85.2 (78.1–90.7) %	96.8 (92.0–99.1) %	$p = 0.001$
Specificity (95% confidence interval)	85.2 (77.4–91.2)%	82.4 (74.6–88.6)%	$p > 0.05$
NPV (95% confidence interval)	83.1 (76.5–88.1) %	96.3 (90.7–98.6) %	$p = 0.001$

Table 14.5 *i*-Scan magnification classification system for the detection of dysplasia in BE

Mucosal pattern	M1	Regular circular or villous pits
	M2	Distorted or irregular pits OR featureless mucosa
Vascular pattern	V1	Regular and uniform vessels
	V2	Irregular, dilated corkscrew vessels

Table 14.6 Interpretation of M and V scores

MV classification	Diagnosis
M1 V1	**No dysplasia**
M1 V2	**Dysplasia**
M2 V1	**Dysplasia**
M2 V2	**Dysplasia**

with i-scan magnification and acetic acid, this classification system showed good accuracy when used in routine clinical practice.

There is very limited data published on the use of i-Scan in detecting and assessing squamous cell neoplasia in the oesophagus. A single-centre prospective non-inferiority trial showed a detection rate of early ESCC of 10.4% in the i-scan group, compared to 12.9% with Lugol's chromoendoscopy ($P < 0.01$ for non-inferiority) [34].

More recently, Pentax Medicals has developed i-scan OE (Optical Enhancement), to further improve the diagnostic accuracy of this technology; this is yet to be tested through larger-scale clinical studies.

It is worth mentioning here that out of the several virtual chromoendoscopy technologies currently available, only narrow-band imaging (NBI) and confocal laser endomicroscopy (CLE) were found to meet thresholds set by ASGE PIVI standards.

In summary, the electronic chromoendoscopy (EC) has shown its potential in improving the neoplasia detection rate in Barrett's and assessing the depth on invasion in squamous neoplasia. However, all these studies have been performed by experts in highly enriched population, and the data is still not enough to give up protocol-guided biopsies in favour of EC-guided targeted biopsies. We urgently need more well-designed, multicentre trials with average risk patients for EC to replace protocol-guided non-targeted biopsies.

14.3 Electronic Chromoendoscopy in the Lower GI Tract

With the advancement of imaging technologies as described above, the current need would be the application of these technologies in the characterization of detected lesions, thereby guiding us regarding decisions about endoscopic resection and surveillance. This will best be achieved by real-time endoscopic diagnosis, a sort of an 'optical biopsy', which may allow for an in vivo assessment and management plan.

Currently the role of advanced endoscopic imaging is both in the detection as well as in characterization of colorectal polyps. ESGE guidelines currently suggest the use of HDWL in the detection of polyps in the average risk population; however, they do advocate the use of chromoendoscopy (conventional or virtual) in detection of polyps in patients with hereditary syndromes (Lynch/serrated polyposis syndrome) and patients with ulcerative colitis [35].

In this chapter we will be focusing on the aspects of virtual or electronic chromoendoscopy in the detection and characterization of colorectal lesions. As described above, a few techniques of virtual chromoendoscopy have been developed so far, but for practical reasons, we will be discussing the three techniques with the most evidence behind it—namely NBI, I-Scan and FICE.

14.3.1 EC in Detection of Colorectal Polyps

Early adenoma detection is shown to reduce mortality from colorectal cancers. Advances in endoscopy are aimed at improving adenoma detection. Contrast enhancement using dye spray has historically been used to improve detection of subtle mucosal changes especially in colitic patients.

Initial studies showed an improvement in detecting colorectal polyps with NBI compared to HDWL. However, recent meta-analysis has shown no significant difference between NBI and WL in the detection of colorectal polyps [36].

A summary of studies comparing White Light and NBI in detection of colorectal polyps is shown in Table 14.7.

We can therefore conclude that although initial studies from enthusiasts showed an increased detection rate, subsequent and most recent studies showed no improvement in detection rates. This suggests some sort of retrospective learning curve

Table 14.7 NBI vs WL in colorectal polyp detection

Year	Study	No. of polyps	Polyp/Adenoma detection rate
2007	Rex et al.	434	WL: 65% NBI: 67%
2009	Adler et al.	658	WL: 36.9% NBI: 33.4%
2009	East et al.	214	WL: 67% NBI: 73%
2009	Paggi et al.	41	WL: 58.3%. NBI: 57.3%
2010	Rastogi et al.	630	WL: 45.7% NBI: 46.2%

related to EC. As the endoscopist experience with EC increases, then they can start seeing those polyps with EC on simple WL. Alternatively, it could be that with time quality of colonoscopy has improved, quality of white light has improved and finally enthusiasm-related bias for a new technology has gone down.

14.3.2 EC for Differentiation between Neoplastic and Non-neoplastic Diminutive Colorectal Polyps

Approximately 60% of all polyps detected at primary screening colonoscopy are diminutive polyps (<5 mm in size). Currently, all these polyps are removed and sent for histopathology. This is an expensive, time-consuming strategy which increases the work burden of the pathology department, thus delaying the important cancer reporting. EC technologies have been evaluated for in vivo optical diagnosis. This would enable the endoscopists to either 'resect and discard' diminutive polyps without histological assessment or 'diagnose and leave' diminutive hyperplastic polyps in the recto-sigmoid after sufficient photo documentation [37].

The American Society of Gastrointestinal Endoscopy has set criteria in its Preservation and Incorporation of Valuable endoscopic Innovations [PIVI] statement against which a technology can be used to 'resect and discard' colorectal polyps <5 mm without pathological assessment or leave suspected recto-sigmoid hyperplastic polyps 5 mm or smaller in place [38].

This was based on a systematic review and meta-analysis calculating the pooled negative predictive value (NPV) for narrow-band imaging (NBI), I-SCAN and Fujinon Intelligent Colour Enhancement (FICE)-assisted optical biopsy for predicting adenomatous polyp histology of diminutive colorectal polyps.

After excluding citations for duplication, paediatric patients, patients with hereditary polyposis syndromes and citations not in English, 19 studies were reported to have enabled calculation of NPV of optical biopsy performed by using NBI for predicting adenomatous polyp histology of diminutive colorectal polyps. The pooled NPV using the random effects model was 91% and was noted to have a higher NPV with experienced operators and when operators made an assessment with high confidence (Table 14.8).

We can therefore conclude that in the hands of EC experts, NBI has been shown to meet the PIVI criterion and based on that, bodies like NICE have advocated its clinical application in routine practice [39]. However, more recent multicentre

Table 14.8 Studies done on NBI

Year	Study	No of polyps	Sensitivity	Specificity	Accuracy	NPV
2008	East et al.	116	0.88	0.91	89.6	94
2008	Rogart et al.	265	0.80		80	81
2009	Ignjatovic et al.	363	0.94	0.89	93	82.3
2009	Rex et al.	451	0.80		91	95.4
2009	Sano et al.	150	0.96	0.92	95.3	90
2009	Van den Broek et al.	50	0.90	0.70	79	90.2
2010	Henry et al.	126	0.93	0.88	90	90.7
2011	Lee et al.	296	0.88	0.87	87.8	92
2012	Gupta et al.	410			86	95.4
2012	Paggi et al.	511	0.95	0.66	85.7	86.4
2012	Hewett et al.	235	0.94	0.98	97.7	95
2012	Shahid et al.	130	0.64	0.92	79	75
2012	Kuiper et al.	281	0.77	0.79	83	86.6
2013	Repici et al.	574	0.9	0.88	89	92
2013	Singh et al.	149	0.91		97	100
2014	Wallace et al.	927			97	91
2017	Visovan et al.	505	0.91	0.95	91.1	
2018	Tsuji et al.	501	0.99	0.46	88.9	92.1
2019	Bae et al.*	7294			77.1	92.5

studies performed with endoscopists in non-academic centres have shown very disappointing results and NBI failed to meet PIVI [40].

Both I-SCAN and FICE had eight studies reporting their use in optical biopsy of small polyps. The pooled NPV for I-SCAN was 84% compared with 80% that for FICE, whereas in I-SCAN there was a significant improvement in results obtained with experienced endoscopists, the FICE analysis showed improvement in optical diagnoses with the use of magnification (Tables 14.9 and 14.10).

Both I-SCAN and FICE have shown promising results; however, given the limited data available for these technologies, further studies would need to be performed before their widespread application.

Other new technologies which have been introduced include BLI (Blue Light Imaging) and LCI (Linked Colour Imaging). Studies are still awaited with regard to the above technologies although initial evidence looks promising (Table 14.11).

Whereas the PIVI commented on the pooled NPV for various electronic chromoendoscopy techniques, other studies have been done comparing sensitivity and specificity. All three techniques (NBI, I-Scan, FICE) described above showed similar sensitivity (90%) and specificity (~85%) for differentiation between neoplastic and non-neoplastic polyps [40]. The results obtained by electronic chromoendoscopy in differentiating between neoplastic and non-neoplastic lesions are similar to that of conventional chromoendoscopy using dye spray; however, it spares the inconvenience and costs associated with the use of dyes and would be more.

Table 14.9 Studies done on I-scan

Year	Study	No of polyps	Sensitivity	Specificity	Accuracy	NPV
2011	Lee et al.	296	0.95	0.86	90.7	94.7
2010	Hoffman et al.	220			98.6	97
2012	Chan et al.	103	0.74	0.69	71.8	70
2012	Hong et al.	432	0.86	0.91	79.3	76.2
2013	Pigo et al.	150	0.95	0.82	92	93
2014	Schachschal et al.	675	78.1	73.4	76.6	72.3
2014	Basford et al.	209	0.97	0.91	94.7	100
2016	Kim et al.	501			89	
2017	Bisschops et al.	61			88	
2018	Klenske et al.	230	0.91	0.90	90	94
2018	Iacucci et al.		0.97	0.88	83	91

Table 14.10 Studies done on FICE

Year	Study	No of polyps	Sensitivity	Specificity	Accuracy	NPV
2008	Pohl et al.					77
2009	Togashi et al.	107	0.9	0.74	86	76
2010	Buchner et al.	119	0.73	0.68	78	50
2011	Longcroft et al.	232			88	78
2011	Kim et al.	525	0.89		87	83
2012	Dos Santos et al.	215	0.91	0.96	92.6	92
2012	Longcroft et al.	237	0.96	0.84	92	84
2015	Kang et al.	955	0.75	0.86	81.4	
2017	Akarsu et al.	217	0.95	0.51	74.2	89.6
2018	Cassinotti et al.	205	0.91	0.76		

Table 14.11 Studies done on BLI

Year	Study	No. of polyps	Accuracy	NPV
2014	Yoshida et al.	314	WL: 83.2% BLI: 95.2%	
2019	Rondonotti et al.	483	WL: 84% BLI: 92%	88%

ESGE concludes that the diagnostic performance of NBI, I-SCAN and FICE would be acceptable for clinical use, and it should be possible to estimate surveillance intervals with a fair degree of accuracy.

In conclusion, we feel that in expert hands EC can deliver optical biopsy as good as pathology but in the hands of general endoscopists with no research or technology bias; it has failed to deliver the required outcome. This suggests that technology certainly has the ability to deliver, but outcome is very subjective depending on the expertise of the endoscopist and the quality of training of the endoscopist. It is also worth noting that the general endoscopist might have a complete lack of appetite to change the conventional histology-based practice to an optical biopsy-based practice which shifts the responsibility from pathologist to endoscopist with no additional gain for the endoscopist. We wonder if some financial or other initiatives for the endoscopists could help in a general role out of EC-assisted optical biopsy. Policymakers should try and think about barriers and facilitators to improve the implementation of such a strategy.

An exciting new development in the field of advanced endoscopy is the emergence of Artificial Intelligence. New data suggests that AI could potentially take over this field in the near future [41]. However, the endoscopists still will need to have the knowledge to accept or reject the decision made by AI as the ultimate responsibility will still lie on the endoscopist.

14.3.3 Examination of Post-polypectomy Scar Site

Another application of EC in lower GI endoscopy has been examination of post-polypectomy scar site. Recurrence at the site of a previous polypectomy or endoscopic mucosal resection is a known occurrence. Recurrence rates have differed in different studies, but what has been proved is that rates of recurrence are higher for larger lesions and for lesions removed in a piecemeal fashion compared to an en bloc method [42]. Most gastroenterology societies recommend an endoscopic follow-up at 3–6 months after piecemeal resection of colorectal polyps to look at residual neoplasia. Initial studies have suggested higher detection rates of neoplastic lesions in post-polypectomy scars with virtual chromoendoscopy compared with high-definition white light (HDWL) alone [43, 44]. Lesions examined with white light appeared more extensive when examined with NBI as well as higher sensitivity to detect neoplastic lesions with NBI compared to WL (88% vs 69%) [43].

More studies are required to prove if EC-assisted optical biopsy can replace the biopsy and histopathology in this group of patients.

References

1. Tada M, Katoh S, Kohli Y, et al. On the dye spraying method in colonofiberscopy. Endoscopy. 1977;8:70–4.
2. East JE, Vleugels JL, Roelandt P, Bhandari P, Bisschops R, Dekker E, Hassan C, et al. Advanced endoscopic imaging: European Society of Gastrointestinal Endoscopy (ESGE) technology review. Endoscopy. 2016;48:1029–45.
3. Gono K, Obi T, Yamaguchi M, Ohyama N, Machida H, Sano Y, Yoshida S, Hamamoto Y, Endo T. Appearance of enhanced tissue features in narrow-band endoscopic imaging. J Biomed Opt. 2004;9:568–77.
4. Tajiri H, Niwa H. Recent advances in electronic endoscopes: image-enhanced endoscopy. JMAJ. 2008;51(3):199–203.
5. Teixeira CR, et al. FICE (Fuji Intelligent Color Enhancement) digital chromoendoscopy in the differentiation of neoplastic and non-neoplastic colorectal lesions. Gastrointest Endosc. 65(5):AB336.
6. Burgos H, et al. Correlation of Fujinon FICE endoscopic imaging and histopathological findings in colorectal adenomas. Gastrointest Endosc. 67(5):AB133.

7. Rondonotti E, Paggi S, Amato A, et al. Blue-light imaging compared with high-definition white light for real-time histology prediction of colorectal polyps less than 1 centimeter: a prospective randomized study. Gastrointest Endosc. 2019;89(3):554–64.
8. Togashi K, et al. Blue laser imaging endoscopy system for the early detection and characterization of colorectal lesions: a guide for the endoscopist. Therap Adv Gastroenterol. 2016;9(1):50–5.
9. Kanzaki H, et al. Linked colour imaging (LCI), a novel image-enhanced endoscopy technology, emphasizes the colour of early gastric cancer. Endosc Int Open. 2017;5(10):E1005–13.
10. Hancock S, Bowman E, Prabakaran J, et al. Use of I-scan endoscopic image enhancement technology in clinical practice to assist in diagnostic and therapeutic endoscopy: a case series and review of the literature. Diagn Therap Endosc. 2012;2012:193570.
11. Kodashima S, Fujishiro M. Novel image-enhanced endoscopy with I-scan technology. World J Gastroenterol. 2010;16(9):1043–9.
12. Neumann H, Fujishiro M, Wilcox CM, Mönkemüller K. Present and future perspectives of virtual chromo endoscopy with I-scan and optical enhancement technology. Dig Endosc. 2014;26(Suppl 1):43–51.
13. Filip M, Iordache S, Saftoiu A, Ciurea T. Autofluorescence imaging and magnification endoscopy. World J Gastroenterol. 2011;17(1):9–14.
14. Ko WJ, An P, Ko KH, et al. Image quality analysis of various gastrointestinal endoscopes: why image quality is a prerequisite for proper diagnostic and therapeutic endoscopy. Clin Endosc. 2015;48(5):374–9.
15. Sharma P, Savides TJ, Canto MI, Corley DA, Falk GW, et al. The American Society for Gastrointestinal Endoscopy PIVI (preservation and incorporation of valuable endoscopic innovations) on imaging in Barrett's oesophagus. Gastrointest Endosc. 2012;76:252–4.
16. Thosani N, et al. ASGE Technology Committee systematic review and meta-analysis assessing the ASGE preservation and incorporation of valuable endoscopic innovations thresholds for adopting real-time imaging–assisted endoscopic targeted biopsy during endoscopic surveillance of Barrett's oesophagus. Gastrointest Endosc. 83(4):684–98.
17. Wolfsen HC, Crook JE, Krishna M, et al. Prospective, controlled tandem endoscopy study of narrow band imaging for dysplasia detection in Barrett's oesophagus. Gastroenterology. 2008;135:24–31.
18. Sharma P, Hawes RH, Bansal A, et al. Standard endoscopy with random biopsies versus narrow band imaging targeted biopsies in Barrett's oesophagus: a prospective, international, randomised controlled trial. Gut. 2013;62:15–21.
19. Mannath J, Subramanian V, Hawkey CJ, et al. Narrow band imaging for characterization of high grade dysplasia and specialized intestinal metaplasia in Barrett's oesophagus: a meta-analysis. Endoscopy. 2010;42:351–9.
20. Silva FB, Dinis-Ribeiro M, Vieth M, et al. Endoscopic assessment and grading of Barrett's oesophagus using magnification endoscopy and narrow-band imaging: accuracy and interobserver agreement of different classification systems (with videos). Gastrointest Endosc. 2011;73:7–14.
21. Sharma P, Bergman JJ, Goda K, et al. Development and validation of a classification system to identify high-grade dysplasia and oesophageal adenocarcinoma in Barrett's oesophagus using narrow-band imaging. Gastroenterology. 2016;150:591–8.
22. Muto M, Minashi K, Yano T, et al. Early detection of superficial squamous cell carcinoma in the head and neck region and esophagus by narrow band imaging: a multicenter randomized controlled trial. J Clin Oncol. 2010;28(9):1566–72. https://doi.org/10.1200/JCO.2009.25.4680.
23. Chai TH, Jin XF, Li SH, et al. A tandem trial of HD-NBI versus HD-WL to compare neoplasia miss rates in oesophageal squamous cell carcinoma. Hepatogastroenterology. 2014;61:120–4.
24. Morita FH, Bernardo WM, Ide E, et al. Narrow band imaging versus lugolchromoendoscopy to diagnose squamous cell carcinoma of the esophagus: a systematic review and meta-analysis. BMC Cancer. 2017;17(1):54.
25. Inoue H, Kaga M, Ikeda H, et al. Magnification endoscopy in oesophageal squamous cell carcinoma: a review of the intrapapillary capillary loop classification. Ann Gastroenterol. 2015;28:41–8.

26. Oyama T, Inoue H, Arima M, et al. Prediction of the invasion depth of superficial squamous cell carcinoma based on microvessel morphology: magnifying endoscopic classification of the Japan Esophageal Society. Esophagus. 2017;14(2):105–12. https://doi.org/10.1007/s10388-016-0527-7.
27. Osawa H, Yamamoto H, Yamada N, et al. Diagnosis of endoscopic Barrett's oesophagus by transnasal flexible spectral imaging colour enhancement. J Gastroenterol. 2009;44:1125–32.
28. Pohl J, May A, Rabenstein T, et al. Comparison of computed virtual chromoendoscopy and conventional chromoendoscopy with acetic acid for detection of neoplasia in Barrett's oesophagus. Endoscopy. 2007;39:594–8.
29. Li YX, Shen L, Yu HG, et al. Fujinon intelligent colour enhancement for the diagnosis of early oesophageal squamous cell carcinoma and precancerous lesion. Turk J Gastroenterol. 2014;25:365–9.
30. de Groof AJ, Swager A-F, Pouw RE, et al. Blue-light imaging has an additional value to white-light endoscopy in visualization of early Barrett's neoplasia: an international multicenter cohort study. Gastrointest Endosc. 2019;89(4):749–58. https://doi.org/10.1016/j.gie.2018.10.046.
31. Subramaniam S, Kandiah K, Chedgy F, et al. OC-068 blue light imaging for Barrett's neoplasia classification (blinc): the development and validation of a new endoscopic classification system to identify Barrett's neoplasia. Gut. 2017;66:A36–7.
32. Hoffman A, Korczynski O, Tresch A, et al. Acetic acid compared with I scan imaging for detecting Barrett's oesophagus: a randomized, comparative trial. Gastrointest Endosc. 2014;79:46–54.
33. Lipman G, Bisschops R, Sehgal V, et al. Systematic assessment with I-SCAN magnification endoscopy and acetic acid improves dysplasia detection in patients with Barrett's esophagus. Endoscopy. 2017;49(12):1219–28.
34. Guo J, Li CQ, Li M, Zuo XL, Yu T, Liu JW, et al. Diagnostic value of probe-based confocal laser endomicroscopy and high definition virtual chromoendoscopy in early oesophageal squamous neoplasia. Gastrointest Endosc. 2015;81:1346–54.
35. Kaminski MF, et al. Advanced imaging for detection and differentiation of colorectal neoplasia: European Society of Gastrointestinal Endoscopy (ESGE) guideline. Endoscopy. 2014;46:435–49.
36. Nagorni A, Bjelakovic G, Petrovic B. Narrow band imaging versus conventional white light colonoscopy for the detection of colorectal polyps. Cochrane Database Syst Rev. 2012;18:1.
37. Rees CJ, et al. Narrow band imaging optical diagnosis of small colorectal polyps in routine clinical practice: the Detect Inspect Characterise Resect and Discard 2 (DISCARD 2) study. Gut. 2017;66:887–95.
38. ASGE Technology Committee. ASGE Technology Committee systematic review and meta-analysis assessing the ASGE PIVI thresholds for adopting real-time endoscopic assessment of the histology of diminutive colorectal polyps. Gastrointest Endosc. 2015;81(3):502.e1–502.e16.
39. NICE Diagnostic Advisory Committee. Virtual chromoendoscopy to assess colorectal polyps during colonoscopy. NICE guidelines. 2017, DG28.
40. Wanders LK, East JE, Uitentuis SE, et al. Diagnostic performance of narrowed spectrum endoscopy, autofluorescence imaging, and confocal laser endomicroscopy for optical diagnosis of colonic polyps: a meta- analysis. Lancet Oncol. 2013;14:1337–47.
41. Misawa M, et al. Artificial intelligence-assisted polyp detection for colonoscopy: initial experience. Gastroenterology. 2018;154(8):2027–9.
42. Moss A, Bourke MJ, Williams SJ, et al. Endoscopic mucosal resection outcomes and prediction of submucosal cancer from advanced colonic mucosal neoplasia. Gastroenterology. 2011;140(7):1909–18.
43. Rogart JN, Aslanian HR, Siddiqui UD. Narrow band imaging to detect residual or recurrent neoplastic tissue during surveillance endoscopy. Dig Dis Sci. 2011;56:472–8.
44. Higaki S, Hashimoto S, Harada K, et al. Long-term follow-up of large flat colorectal tumours resected endoscopically. Endoscopy. 2003;35:845–9.

Stenting for Pancreatic Walled-Off Necrosis (WON)

15

Majidah Abdulfattah Bukhari and Mouen A. Khashab

Key Points

1. Endoscopic drainage is considered the standard of care in the management of symptomatic pancreatic walled-off necrosis (WON).
2. The choice of technique depends on the local expertise of the center.
3. An effective WON approach requires a multidisciplinary team approach.
4. The lumen-apposing metal stent (LAMS) is a specially designed stent used for endoscopic drainage and necrosectomy. The larger diameter stent may allow direct endoscopic necrosectomy at the index procedure.
5. The most common adverse events associated with endoscopic management are bleeding and perforation.
6. Double pigtail stents (DPSs) can be left permanently in situ to prevent recurrence of WON in patients with disrupted pancreatic duct syndrome.
7. The multiple transluminal gateway technique should be considered in patients with large WON who do not adequately respond to the initial endoscopic drainage.
8. Dual-modality drainage should be considered in patients with WON that extends to the paracolic gutter and in patients not responding to endoscopic drainage.

M. A. Bukhari (✉)
Division of Gastroenterology and Hepatology, Johns Hopkins Medical Institutions, Baltimore, MD, USA

Division of Medicine and Gastroenterology and Hepatology, International Medical Center, Jeddah, Saudi Arabia

M. A. Khashab
Division of Gastroenterology and Hepatology, Johns Hopkins Medical Institutions, Baltimore, MD, USA
e-mail: mkhasha1@jhmi.edu

P. Sharma, N. Reddy (eds.), *Innovations in Gastrointestinal Endoscopy*,
https://doi.org/10.1007/978-981-15-9247-8_15

15.1 Introduction

Pancreatic walled-off necrosis (WON) is a local complication of severe necrotizing pancreatitis occurring in 15–20% of patients, and it has been associated with high morbidity (34–95%) and mortality (2–39%) [1, 2]. It is characterized by well-defined, non-epithelialized, enhancing wall tissue containing necrotic material that involves pancreatic and/or peripancreatic tissue.

In recent decades, there has been a paradigm shift in the management of WON after acute pancreatitis. Despite surgical necrosectomy being the historic gold standard for management of WON, it is associated with significant morbidity (34–95%) and mortality (10–25%) [3]. Endoscopic drainage is a minimally invasive alternative technique for the management of WON, and it is associated with a higher success rate and lower morbidity and mortality rates compared to surgical necrosectomy. Because of this, endoscopic drainage has become the standard of care in the management of patients with pancreatic WON [4–6].

In this chapter, we highlight the endoscopic management of WON. We provide information regarding indications, timing of interventions, endoscopic techniques, periprocedural management, and follow-up.

15.2 Medical Management

Management of pancreatic WON can be challenging. All patients require supportive care, which includes fluid resuscitation and nutritional support. Some endoscopists prefer to stop proton pump inhibitors (PPIs) before necrosectomy to allow liquefaction of necrosis by gastric and bile acids. An in-depth discussion of medical therapy of necrotizing pancreatitis is beyond the scope of this chapter.

15.3 Drainage

Drainage of pancreatic WON is indicated only for symptomatic patients based on the current evidence-based data. Size alone is no longer an indication for drainage although collections larger than 6 cm tend to be symptomatic. Therapeutic options for drainage include endoscopic, percutaneous, and surgical drainage. The decision to choose one option over the other depends on the time, type of the collection, the goal of therapy (i.e., control the infection versus relieve the obstruction), the experience of the endoscopist, the local resources, and patient preference.

15.3.1 Indication for Drainage of Pancreatic WON

- Infected WON
- Gastric outlet obstruction (GOO)
- Biliary obstruction

- Refractory abdominal pain attributed to the collection
- Anorexia and weight loss
- Pancreatic duct leak (manifests with ascites or pleural effusion with high amylase)

15.3.2 Contraindication for Endoscopic Drainage

- Absolute
  - Immature collection (<4 weeks)
  - The collection is away from the gastrointestinal wall (> 1 cm)
  - Collection with pseudoaneurysm
- Relative
  - Presence of neovascularization by portal hypertension
  - Significant coagulopathy (INR > 1.5)
  - Significant thrombocytopenia (platelets <50,000)
  - Patients with hemodynamic instability

15.3.3 Timing of Intervention

The optimal timing of intervention has been debated over the past few decades. Drainage of necrosis within the first few weeks is associated with higher adverse events, poorer outcomes, and longer hospital stays [7, 8]. Early intervention is typically reserved for severely ill patients with infected necrosis [9, 10].

Based on the current guidelines, intervention should be delayed if possible until at least 4 weeks after the onset of pancreatitis to allow liquefaction of the necrosis and maturation of the wall ("walled–off"), thereby preserving viable pancreatic tissue and reducing the risk of pancreatic insufficiency [9, 11, 12].

15.3.4 Pre-drainage Patient Evaluation

Patient preparation before endoscopic drainage is crucial, and it includes the following (Table 15.1):

- **Review of imaging**

  Review of imaging is essential before any intervention (Fig. 15.1). Three main criteria should be met before endoscopic drainage:
  - The fluid collection should be mature, usually >4 weeks
  - Wall of the collection should be adjacent to the gut wall (<1 cm)
  - No large intervening vessels or collaterals
- **Multidisciplinary approach**

  Endoscopic drainage of pancreatic WON is more technically challenging, carries a higher rate of adverse events, and tends to involve more severely ill patients

Table 15.1 Pre-drainage patient evaluation

Diagnostic checklist
• Review abdominal imaging to assess the precise location of the collection in relation to the stomach and duodenum, to determine whether the wall is mature, and to look for the presence of a pseudoaneurysm
• Indication and contraindication for drainage
• Time of the intervention
• EUS assessment
1. Size
2. Location
3. Contents of the collection (liquid or a significant amount of solid debris)
4. The extent of the collection
5. Evaluate the vascular structures within or close to the collection and rule out a pseudoaneurysm
6. Rule out other causes of cystic lesion in the pancreas
• Multidisciplinary meeting
• Laboratory test (CBC, INR, type, and screen)
• NPO at midnight
• Consent
• Anesthesia and nursing support
• Position of patient
• Use of CO_2 during endoscopic drainage

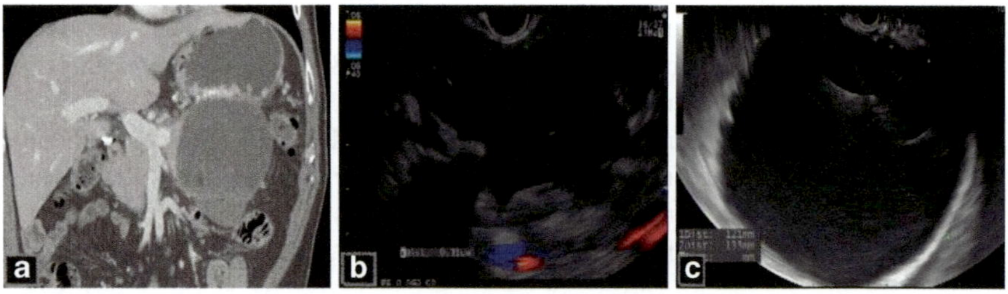

Fig. 15.1 (**a**) Contrast-enhanced CT scan obtained 4 weeks after the onset of acute necrotizing pancreatitis revealing a pancreatic walled-off necrosis with solid necrotic debris. (**b** and **c**) EUS images of large walled-off pancreatic necrosis with solid and liquid contents

as compared to drainage of pseudocysts. Thus, the effective management of WON requires a multidisciplinary team approach, including dedicated advanced gastrointestinal endoscopists, interventional radiologists, and expert hepatopancreatic surgeons working in tandem to minimize morbidity and mortality [9]. Multidisciplinary teams need to be involved from the onset of the disease to establish the diagnosis and to determine the appropriate therapeutic approach—endoscopic or percutaneous drainage, or both. An adequate surgical back up is mandatory. Endoscopic drainage should be performed by endoscopists experienced in both endoscopic ultrasound (EUS) and endoscopic retrograde cholangiopancreatography (ERCP) procedures. Adequate communication among the teams is essential for optimal management of these complex patient populations.

- **Laboratory**

  Routine laboratory testing is needed, and as a general rule, endoscopic drainage should be avoided in patients with significant coagulopathy (INR > 1.5 or platelets <50,000). Endoscopic drainage with debridement may lead to early or delayed bleeding. Therefore, routine blood analysis and screening before endoscopic drainage are recommended.
- **Discontinue anticoagulation and antiplatelet agents before the procedure**

  The approach of discontinuing anticoagulant and antiplatelet agents is based on the patient's risk of a thromboembolic event based on the American Society for Gastrointestinal Endoscopy (ASGE) guidelines for the management of antithrombotic agents for patients undergoing gastrointestinal (GI) endoscopy [13].
- **Nil per Os (NPO) after midnight before the procedure**
- **Antibiotic periprocedural**

  To reduce the risk of periprocedural bacteremia, most experts recommend routine use of broad-spectrum antibiotics before endoscopic interventions for those not already receiving antibiotics for infected WON. The current practice is to use a single 1–2 g dose of ceftriaxone or cefotetan administered intravenously before the procedure, whereas others recommend ciprofloxacin 500 mg administered orally before the procedure.
- **Consent**

  Before endoscopic drainage, it is mandatory to undertake a discussion with the patient and family about the risks, benefits, and alternative techniques. It is also important to discuss with the patient the potential need for additional procedures (e.g., direct endoscopic necrosectomy).
- **Anesthesia support**

  Patients undergoing endoscopic drainage almost always require deep sedation/general anesthesia. The duration of the procedure can be lengthy, especially when performing endoscopic necrosectomy at the index procedure. Therefore, enough time needs to be allocated in the endoscopy suite when the procedure starts. General anesthesia is preferable to decrease the risk of aspiration during transmural drainage. In general, an endoscopic necrosectomy procedure takes between 60 and 120 min.
- **The position of the patient**

  The patient's position during endoscopic drainage is determined based on the clinical situation of the patient and the endoscopist's preferences. In general, the supine position is more comfortable for the patient and allows easy monitoring and access to cardiorespiratory systems. The prone position allows better posterior drainage collection by gravity and may decrease the risk of fluid reflux and aspiration [14].
- **Carbon dioxide (CO_2)**

  All procedures should be performed using CO_2 insufflation to reduce the risk of air embolism, which is a rare adverse event that occurs when air enters the systemic venous circulation. Gas embolism can develop even with the use of CO_2 [15, 16].

15.3.5 Drainage Techniques

There are several interventional options for the management of pancreatic WON. In the past few decades, minimally invasive drainage techniques, including transmural endoscopic drainage with direct endoscopic necrosectomy (DEN), percutaneous drainage, and video-assisted retroperitoneal debridement (VARD), have been used as step-up approaches in several multicenter studies and have replaced the traditional open necrosectomy surgery [12, 17–19]. The advantages and disadvantages of the different interventions are described in Table 15.2.

A "step-up" approach begins with a minimally invasive method, and a surgical intervention should be performed when the initial procedure has failed. Step-up approaches can be either surgical or endoscopic. A surgical step-up approach consists of percutaneous drainage followed by minimally invasive necrosectomy with retroperitoneal debridement, if necessary. An endoscopic step-up approach is a less invasive approach consisting of endoscopic transmural drainage followed by DEN if there is no clinical improvement after endoscopic drainage.

Two randomized controlled trials undertaken by the Dutch Pancreatitis Study Group (DPSG) showed that the endoscopic step-up approach is a potentially less invasive alternative to step-up surgery. The PENGUIN trial was the first RCT to compare the proinflammatory response and clinical outcomes of endoscopic necrosectomy and open surgical debridement. The trial involved 22 patients with infected pancreatic necrosis. The study demonstrated that patients who underwent endoscopic necrosectomy had significantly less inflammatory responses, fewer occurrences of new multi-organ failure (0 versus 50%, RD, 0.50; 95% CI, 0.12–0.69, $P = 0.03$), and less pancreatic fistulas (10% versus 70%; RD, 0.60; 95% CI, 0.17–0.81; $P = 0.02$) [20]. A recent large multicenter randomized superiority trial by Brunschot et al. compared an endoscopic step-up approach with the surgical step-up approach in 98 patients with infected necrotizing pancreatitis (TENSION Trial). The endoscopic step-up approach included placement of two 7-Fr double pigtail stents (DPSs) and an 8.5-Fr nasocystic tube as the first step, followed by endoscopic transmural necrosectomy if there was no clinical improvement with transmural drainage. The study showed no difference in mortality (18% versus 13%, RR 1.38, 95% CI 0.53–3.59, $p = 0.50$) or major morbidity (43% versus 45%, $p = 0.88$) in the endoscopic step-up group versus the surgical step-up group. However, the hospital stay was shorter with the endoscopic approach (mean 53 days versus 69 days, $P = 0.014$). The rate of external pancreatic fistula was also significantly lower with the endoscopic approach (5% versus 32%, $P = 0.0011$). This study showed that the endoscopic step-up approach is superior to the surgical step-up approach in the reduction of indirect medical costs due to the shorter hospital stay [21].

Endoscopic drainage of a pancreatic WON is different from drainage of a pancreatic pseudocyst. Drainage of the pancreatic WON requires the creation of a large access point to allow spontaneous drainage of the necrotic materials and allow DEN if there is no clinical/radiologic improvement. There are three endoscopic approaches used to drain pancreatic WON: transmural, trans-papillary, or both. The transmural approach is the most commonly used nowadays.

Table 15.2 Comparison of endoscopic, percutaneous, and surgical approaches

Drainage type	Advantages	Disadvantages
Endoscopic drainage		
EUS-guided drainage	• Allows both diagnosis and therapeutic drainage • Allows accurate assessment of the location and the distance between the collection and the digestive wall • Identifies possible pseudoaneurysm and intervening blood vessel • Allows real-time visualization of the needle and other instruments • Can be performed in a non-bulging collection • Less invasive • Can be performed with conscious sedation • Can be performed in an outpatient setting • Shorter hospital stay as compared to surgical drainage	• Tangential access through the gut wall • Needs expertise in EUS • Challenging in altered anatomy • Small scope channel renders placement of 10-Fr stent challenging
Conventional transmural drainage	• Direct visualization of puncture endoscopically • Large instrument channel allows for adequate suction of fluid and solid debris	• Feasible only if the collection is adjacent to the gastroduodenal wall and causing luminal compression/bulging • Inability to visualize the interposed vessel which may cause bleeding • The potential for misdiagnosed cystic neoplasm • Longer procedure time • Risk of guidewire misplacement
Percutaneous drainage	• Less invasive • Can be performed in an acute setting	• Risk of cutaneous infection and bleeding • Risk of pancreaticocutaneous fistula formation
Surgical drainage	• Effective therapy • Salvage therapy following failed endoscopic and radiological drainage	• Invasive • Associated with high morbidity and mortality • Longer hospital stay • Expensive

The transmural approach requires the creation of a fistula between the collection and the gut by placing plastic or metal stents into the cavity through a single or several access sites, whereas the trans-papillary approach requires placement of a pancreatic stent to drain the collection that is communicating with the main pancreatic duct.

15.3.6 Endoscopic Techniques

15.3.6.1 Trans-Papillary Drainage

- **Disconnected pancreatic duct syndrome**

  Disconnected pancreatic duct syndrome (DPDS) results from necrosis in the center of the pancreas and is characterized by complete disruption of the main pancreatic duct (MPD).

  It occurs in 30–50% of patients with necrotizing pancreatitis [22, 23]. Disruption of the duct leads to persistent leakage of pancreatic juice from the viable upstream pancreatic parenchyma and the formation of collections around the pancreas [24, 25]. When pancreatic duct disruption is present, recurrence of the collection may occur after complete resolution of WON and removal of transmural stents. Contrast-enhanced CT (CECT), MRCP with or without secretin, and ERCP are the most common modalities used to diagnose and confirm DPDS. CECT adequately visualizes the disruption in 75–100% of cases [26, 27]. Secretin injection increases the sensitivity of MRCP from 47.1 to 66.4% [28–30]. There are some limitations of cross-sectional imaging and these include the following: (1) unreliable assessment of the duct disruption if the collection overlies the MPD and (2) assessing the integrity of the duct can be challenging in the presence of endoprosthesis. ERCP is considered to be the most accurate method for the diagnosis of disconnected pancreatic duct syndrome with pancreatography showing non-visualization (filling) of the upstream disconnected segment.

  Endoscopic techniques for the treatment of DPDS include (1) trans-papillary stenting with pancreatic sphincterotomy if the disruption of the duct is partial, and the site of disruption can be bridged [31–33], (2) Permanent placement of transmural DPS during drainage of WON to allow permanent conduit into the digestive lumen, and (3) EUS-guided pancreaticogastrostomy between the stomach and the upstream disrupted segment.

- **Technique for trans-papillary pancreatic stent placement**

  ERCP is performed in a standard fashion and pancreatography is performed to identify the site of disruption. Pancreatic stents can be placed with or without pancreatic sphincterotomy. The diameter of the pancreatic stents used is dependent on the diameter of the duct, but 7-Fr stents are most commonly used. The aim is to use the largest diameter stent that fits comfortably within the pancreatic duct, and the length of the stent depends on the site of the leak that needs bridging.
- **Efficacy of the trans-papillary approach**

  In general, WON does not respond to trans-papillary drainage alone because the necrotic debris is unlikely to drain through the small diameter stent. There are several studies involving a small number of patients with WON that describe the effect of the trans-papillary approach alone or in combination with transmural drainage for the management of pancreatic fluid collections (PFCs) [34–36].

One meta-analysis showed that the combination of transmural drainage with trans-papillary drainage did not have additional benefits with regard to the rate of recurrent PFCs (OR 1.49, 95% CI 0.53–4.21, $P = 0.45$) or a reduction in complications (OR 1.15, 95% CI 0.61–2.18, $P = 0.67$) as compared to transmural drainage alone [37]. Therefore, a combined trans-papillary and transmural approach is not routinely recommended [38].

Transmural drainage usually works better in cases of complete disruption of the MPD. The currently accepted practice is to leave the transmural stent in permanently after transmural drainage of the WON in patients with DPDS to prevent recurrence of the collection [38, 39].

15.3.7 Endoscopic Transmural Drainage

The transmural drainage technique requires the creation of a conduit between the cavity and the gut lumen (cyst-gastrostomy or cyst-duodenostomy) either through an echo-endoscope (EUS-guided drainage) or direct endoscopic guidance (non-EUS-guided or conventional drainage). A prospective comparative trial showed no difference in efficacy or safety between conventional transmural ($n = 53$) and EUS-guided ($n = 46$) drainage for patients with PFCs. The success rate and complication rates were similar in the two groups (94% versus 93% and 18% versus 19%, respectively) [40].

However, in two randomized controlled trials, EUS-guided transmural drainage was superior to conventional drainage. The technical success rates were 94% versus 72% and 100% versus 33%. There was no difference in the rate of complications between the groups [41, 42]. Over the last several decades, EUS-guided transmural endoscopic drainage has become the mainstay of treatment for pancreatic WON and has replaced the conventional transmural approach.

(a) ***Conventional transmural drainage***

Conventional transmural drainage relies on endoscopic visualization of a bulge within the stomach or duodenum caused by the pancreatic collection with the aid of the most recent cross-sectional imaging techniques. Conventional drainage can be challenging when targeting the ideal puncture site in the absence of a bulging sign or when there is peristalsis, respiratory motion, or difficulty in instrument position due to edema and distortion of the GI tract.

(b) ***EUS-guided transmural drainage***

EUS-guided drainage allows visualization of the collection even if there is no bulge into the gut wall, determines the contents of the collection, assesses the distance from the gut wall, and determines an optimal trajectory that avoids intervening blood vessels with the aid of a color Doppler technique to avoid hemorrhagic complications.

Table 15.3 Equipment for EUS-guided drainage

Equipment required for EUS-guided drainage of WON
• Therapeutic linear echo-endoscope (3.7 mm or 3.8 mm channel) • 19-G FNA needle • 0.035-inch guidewire • Tract dilation device (4-Fr or 5-Fr ERCP cannula), 10-Fr Soehendra dilation catheter, over the wire needle knife catheter, or 10-Fr cystotome) • Balloon dilator (CRE balloon dilator) • Double pigtail stents or SEMS or LAMS

15.3.8 Equipment for EUS-Guided Transmural Drainage (Table 15.3)

(a) **Therapeutic echo-endoscope:** This is a linear therapeutic echo-endoscope with large working channels of 3.7 mm or 3.8 mm, which allows the placement of an 8.5–10Fr plastic stents, metallic stents, and nasocystic drain.

Linear EUS has an oblique axis, resulting in a tangential puncture of the collection, which may lead to inadequate transmission of force during stent insertion and renders placements of multiple stents challenging at times. Recently, a forward-viewing echo-endoscope has become available, which allows puncturing and insertion of stents along the direction of the scanning plane. However, a multicenter randomized controlled trial compared the forward-viewing echo-endoscope and linear echo-endoscope in 52 patients with PFCs, and did not show differences in outcomes [43].

(b) **Accessories**

- ***Puncture device:***
  - **19-gauge fine needle aspiration (FNA) needle:**

    A 19-G needle is used to puncture the collection under EUS guidance, allowing passage of the guidewire.
  - **Guidewires:**

    A 0.035 or 0.025-inch guidewire is used to advance and coil within the cavity of the collection under fluoroscopic guidance. A stiff wire improves the push ability of accessories across the transmural track.
- ***Tract dilation device***
  - ***Electrocautery device***

    Over the wire needle knife sphincterotome:

    A needle knife is used, and it has a single or double lumen. It is a sub-optimal device for cyst access because the difference in size between the cutting wire and catheter creates a step-off that can increase the risk of vascular and mural injuries if excessive force results in the displacement of the needle. The exposed wire can be bent back along the catheter to create a more tapered cutting surface.

    Specialized fistulotomy device:

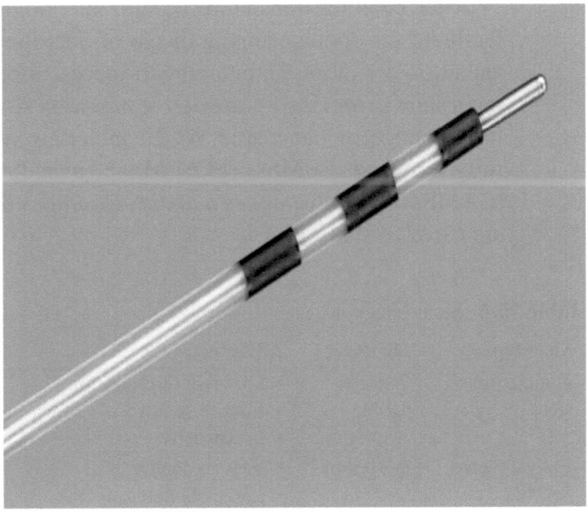

Fig. 15.2 Cystotome (Wilson Cook, Winston-Salem, NC, USA)

Cystotome: The only commercially available cystotome in the USA is a 10-Fr cystotome (Fig. 15.2). A Cremeric cystotome is a 5-Fr device with a retractable needle knife catheter with a distal end electrocautery ring and an outer 10-Fr sheath. It is used to create a 10-Fr fistula tract at the initial puncture site. The inner needle knife is used to puncture the collection. The outer sheath with a metal tip is advanced through the gut wall while applying a diathermy current to create a 10-Fr cyst enterostomy. After puncture, the needle knife wire is withdrawn while keeping the outer sheath in place within the cavity, followed by the insertion of the guidewire within the cavity.

- ***Non-electrocautery dilation device***

  ERCP cannula (4-Fr to 5 Fr)

  Soehendra biliary dilation catheter (6-Fr to 10-Fr)

  Biliary balloon dilator 6–10 mm or controlled radial expansion (CRE) balloon

  The extent of fistula dilation is dependent upon the size and number of stents or the size of the endoscope for direct endoscopic necrosectomy. For a transmural gastric approach dilation, up to 15 mm is safe [44]. Placement of a large bore fully covered self-expandable metal stent (SEMS) allows advancement of the gastroscope through the stent for necrosectomy, and it can reduce the size of fistula dilation to 4–6 mm. When DEN is planned, progressive dilation of the tract is recommended using a CRE balloon. The extent of the fistula dilation has not been adequately studied and has not been standardized.

- ***Stent placement***

After creating transmural access, maintaining the access is essential to facilitate the spontaneous drainage of necrotic material into the gut lumen and allow for DEN. Maintaining the access for drainage is achieved by placing a stent across the *cystoenterostomy* wall. A variety of stents are available for drainage of pancreatic WON, including double pigtail stents (DPSs), fully covered SEMSs (FCSEMSs), and lumen-apposing metal stents (LAMSs). *The advantages and disadvantages* of the different types of *stents* are *listed in* Table 15.4.

Table 15.4 Stent selection

Stent type	Diameter	Advantages	Disadvantages
Double pigtail stent	7-Fr to 10-Fr	• Low risk of migration • Easy to remove • Inexpensive	• Difficult to place • High risk of occlusion due to small diameter
Fully covered SEMS	6–10 mm	• Easy to deploy • Large diameter	• Risk of leakage around the stent • Risk of migration • Possible risk of delayed bleeding (if the length of the stent exceeds the anatomical requirement, there will be a risk of erosion of the wall by the stent end when the collection is resolved, which can lead to perforation or bleeding) • Expensive
LAMS • AXIOS stent • NAGI stent • SPAXUS • AIX stent	10 mm, 15 mm, 20 mm 10 mm, 12 mm, 14 mm, 16 mm 8 mm, 10 mm, 16 mm 10 mm, 14 mm	• Large lumen diameter allows better drainage with a low risk of stent blockage • May reduce the risk of leakage • Tamponade effect may reduce the risk of bleeding • Easy to deploy • No need for dilation before insertion • Deployment under EUS and endoscopic guidance • LAMS delivery system has electrocautery enabled access catheter that provides the ability for over the wire or freehand thermal puncture and stent delivery using the same sheath • DEN can be performed through the stent • Low risk of migration	• Expensive • Long-term safety has not been established

- **Plastic stents:**

  Double pigtail stents (DPSs):

  Short length (3–5 cm) 7-Fr or 10-Fr DPSs are commonly used. The straight stents are more prone to migration and may cause bleeding due to irritation of the wall of the collection. The resolution rate of WON with DPS without endoscopic necrosectomy is suboptimal due to their small caliber, which is insufficient for spontaneous drainage of solid debris. The downside of placing a DPS is the risk of stent occlusion by necrotic debris, which occurs in 40% of patients and leads to secondary infection [16, 45, 46]. Furthermore, if necrosectomy is required after placement of a DPS, the stent has to be removed, and the tract has to be dilated up to 15–18 mm to allow the passage of the scope into the cavity. Excessive dilation of the tract may lead to bleeding or perforation.

  Single or multiple stents

  Placement of multiple short DPSs to maintain adequate drainage in WON is commonly performed in clinical practice, despite the lack of studies documenting the superiority of multiple stent use over single stent use. It has been postulated that placement of multiple stents provides drainage alongside the stent and through the stent [45, 47]. However, the disadvantage of placing multiple stents is a significant increase in the procedure time, and it can be challenging to place the second or the third stent alongside the previously placed stent(s). When placing multiple stents, multiple wires are advanced into the cyst through the established fistula tract alongside an existing wire or stent. This technique can be challenging in some cases as the wire may dissect between the digestive tract and the cyst wall. To overcome this issue, different options have been developed, including the use of a dedicated multi-wire catheter (Haber ramp, cook endoscopy). The Haber ramp is 200 cm long with a diameter of 8-Fr and a 6-Fr taper tip. It has three wire ports, which can accommodate a 0.035-inch guidewire. The wire sites are on the distal tip of the catheter at 1.5 cm and 2.5 cm from the distal tip (Fig. 15.3). The Haber ramp is advanced into the cyst over the guidewire after subsequent tract dilation where the second and/or the third wire is easily advanced and coiled into the cyst for subsequent multi-stent deployment. A 10-Fr stent pusher or a wire-guided cytology brush (with brush removed) can also be for the multiple wire technique. They are advanced over the first wire after accessing the cyst followed by advancement of the second wire. The 10-Fr cystotome also has larger lumen to accommodate two wires after removal of the needle and the internal catheter. For the placement of multiple stents, placing multiple guidewires through the working channel can compromise the placement of the larger 10-Fr plastic stents. Therefore, as a rule, the first stent inserted alongside the one or two guidewires cannot be larger than 7-Fr.
- **Metallic stents:**

  Conventional tubular metal stents have a larger lumen diameter and theoretically facilitate spontaneous drainage of necrotic tissue, which reduces the rate of stent occlusion and secondary infection. Insertion of metallic stents without prior tract dilation may eliminate the risks of leakage and perforation when the cyst and gut lumen are inadequately adherent. Furthermore, a tamponade effect created by the stent may reduce the bleeding risk. The treatment success rate ranges from 78 to 100% in studies using biliary or esophageal stents, but the adverse events are high, ranging from 15 to 33% [48–51]. These stents are long, which may increase the chance of erosion or ulceration over the gastric or retroperitoneal side. The stent can erode the pancreatic bed and cause severe bleeding.

– **Lumen-apposing metal stent (LAMS)**

  LAMS were specifically designed for the transmural drainage of pancreatic fluid collections to overcome the limitations of the conventional SEMS (Figs. 15.4 and 15.5). There are four types of LAMS (Table 15.5).

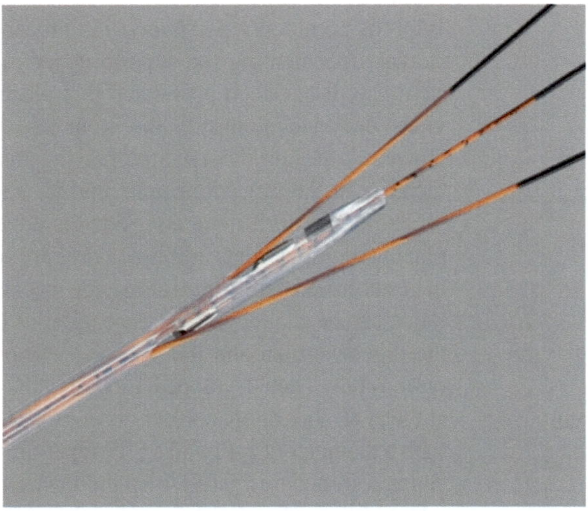

Fig. 15.3 The multi-wire catheter (Haber ramp, cook endoscopy)

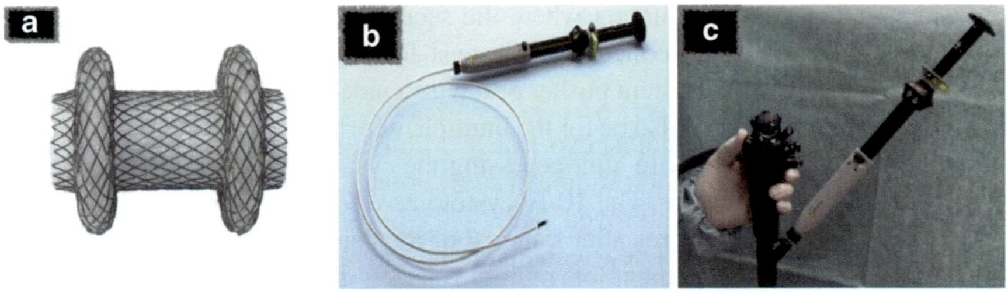

Fig. 15.4 (**a**) The AXIOS stent consists of double-walled flanges that are perpendicular to the lumen and hold the tissue walls in apposition. (**b**) The delivery system of AXIOS stent is a 0.8-Fr catheter. (**c**) The handle of the delivery system is Luer locked onto the echo-endoscope instrumentation channel inlet port. The handle consists of a distal portion (black hub) for catheter control and a proximal portion (gray hub) for stent control

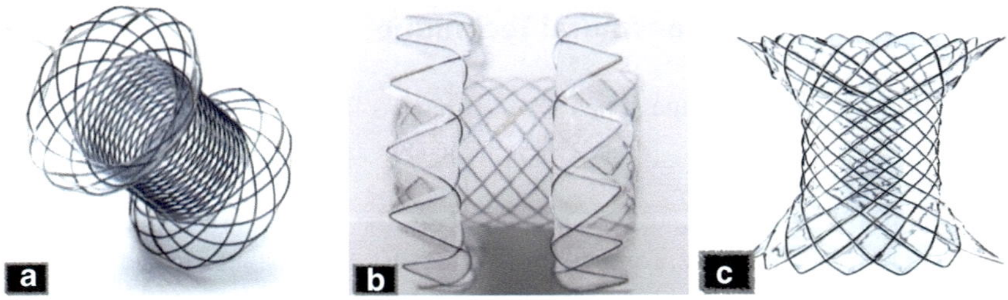

Fig. 15.5 (**a**) NAGI Stent has two flanges end to prevent migration. A suture is attached at the distal flange to remove the stent. (**b**) Niti-S Spaxus stent has folding back anchoring flanges for lumen apposition. (**c**) AIX stent has a diabolo-design to prevent migration

Table 15.5 Different types of lumen-apposing metal stent (LAMS)

Name of stent	Design of the stent
1. AXIOS (Boston Scientific, Marlborough, MA, USA) (107)	The stent consists of double-walled flanges that are perpendicular to the lumen and hold the tissue walls in opposition to create an anastomosis (Fig. 15.4) The two flanges on both ends are designed to decrease stent migration and reduce the risk of leakage and perforation The flanges are short in length, and therefore have limited extension into the gut lumen and the cavity wall, which potentially reduces the risk of stent erosion The stent is a fully covered made of braided nitinol wire to prevent tissue ingrowth and tract leakage Flange diameter: 20 mm and 24 mm Lumen diameter: 10 mm, 15 mm and 20 mm Saddle length: 10 mm
2. Niti-S NAGI (Taewoong Medical, Korea) (108)	The short stent is made of nitinol material covered with a silicon sheath and has a 10.5-Fr delivery system (Fig. 15.5a) The wide flares at both ends of the stent were designed to prevent stent migration The stent has drawstrings along the gastric flare of the stent to facilitate stent removal Length: 10 mm, 20 mm and 30 mm Diameters: 10 mm, 12 mm, 14 mm, and 16 mm
3. Niti-S Spaxus stent (Taewoong Medical, Korea) (109)	The stent is made of nitinol wire and entirely covered with a silicone membrane, and has a 10-Fr delivery system (Fig. 15.5b) The stent has a blue marker on the outer sheath to confirm the complete deployment of the distal flange Length: 20 mm Lumen diameters: 8 mm, 10 mm, and 16 mm Flange diameter: 23 mm, 25 mm and 31 mm
4. AIX stent (Leufen Medical, Germany) (110)	The AIX stent is a fully covered metal stent with wide flanges on each end (Fig. 15.5c) The flanges have an atraumatic folded wire design to prevent tissue damage Length: 30 mm Lumen diameter: 10 mm or 15 mm Flange dimeter: 25 mm This stent is currently only commercially available in Europe

15.3.9 EUS-Guided Transmural Technique

EUS-guided transmural drainage has several steps as follows:

- **Identify the puncture site**
  Using a therapeutic linear echo-endoscope, the collection is visualized and assessed for location, size, contents, wall thickness, and distance from the gastrointestinal wall.
  A color Doppler ultrasound is used to identify any vascular structures and rule out pseudoaneurysm. The most optimal site of puncture is identified by EUS.
- **Puncturing the WON cavity**
  When the appropriate site is identified, the WON is targeted and punctured under direct EUS guidance. Most endoscopists use a 19-G FNA according to the Seldinger technique. The stylet is then removed. Fluid is aspirated to confirm the correct position of the needle. The aspirated fluid is sent for gram stain and culture at the discretion of the endoscopist. A bloody aspirate may suggest recent bleeding of a pseudoaneurysm. If the aspirated fluid is bloody, drainage should be delayed until CT angiogram is performed to exclude pseudoaneurysm. Contrast can be injected at the discretion of the endoscopist into the collection to delineate the cyst under fluoroscopy. Fluoroscopy is not mandatory for this procedure, but it has safety benefits.
- **Creation of the fistula tract**
  Once the collection is accessed, a 0.025/0.035-inch stiff guidewire is advanced through the 19-G needle and coiled about two times into the cavity under fluoroscopic guidance, after which the needle is removed over the guidewire and exchanged for dilating devices. The fistula tract can be established over the guidewire with cautery assistance or non-cautery devices at the discretion of the endoscopist.
- **Dilation of the fistula tract**
  The tract can be dilated using different dilating devices. In the non-electrocautery technique, the tract is sequentially dilated using either a 4.5-Fr or 5-Fr ERCP cannula, 6-Fr to 10-Fr Soehendra dilators, and/or an 8 mm or 10 mm biliary balloon dilation catheter over the guidewire. In the electrocautery technique, a modified wire-guided needle knife or a 10-Fr cystotome can be used to create and dilate the fistula tract. Dilation of the tract to 6–10 mm is typically needed for placement of two 10-Fr plastic stents. If a metal stent is used, the tract does not need to be dilated more than 4 mm to allow passage of the delivery system into the collection. If necrosectomy is planned, the tract must be dilated to at least 12–15 mm to enable easy passage of the endoscope into the collection (Fig. 15.6).
- **Stent placement**
  After dilation of the tract, at least two plastic DPSs, FCSEMSs, or LAMSs are inserted into the collection under fluoroscopic, endoscopic, and/or sonographic guidance (Fig. 15.7).

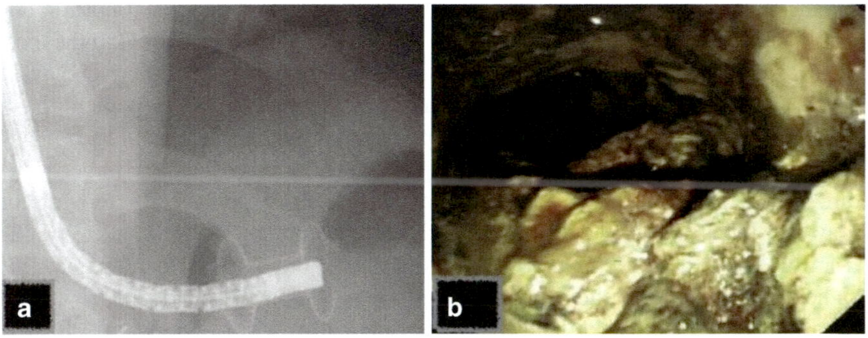

Fig. 15.6 (**a**) Fluoroscopic view showing endoscopic transgastric necrosectomy through LAMS. (**b**) Endoscopic image of pancreatic necrosis upon entry into the necrotic collection

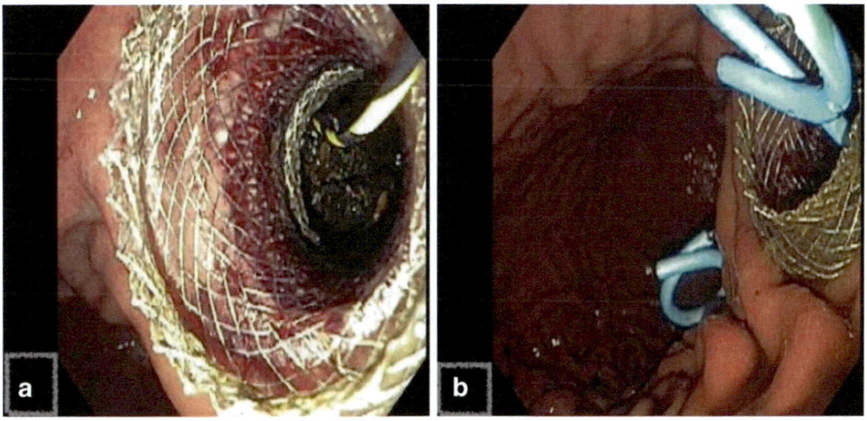

Fig. 15.7 (**a**) Endoscopic view of lumen-apposing metal stent immediately after deployment. Note solid debris through the stent. (**b**) Endoscopic view of plastic double pigtail stent coaxially deployed across the cystogastrostomy to maintain adequate drainage of WON

15.3.10 The Technique of EUS-Guided Drainage Using a LAMS

The cautery-enhanced LAMS (HOT AXIOS, Boston Scientific) has an electrocautery wire at the distal tip of the delivery system, which allows for a clean and sharp cut with minimal coagulation into the target lumen without the need for a prior needle puncture, guidewire insertion, or dilation of the tract. It can also be inserted over the guidewire after initial puncture of the cyst with a 19-G FNA needle. The delivery catheter is inserted into the working channel of the echo-endoscope and the Luer lock secured to the inlet port of the working channel. After unlocking, the 10.8-Fr catheter is advanced until contact is made with the gut wall by the advancement of the black hub (catheter control hub) along the distal portion and then locked into the desired position. The delivery system is connected to the electrosurgical generator (settings: pure-cut mode, 100 watts, ICC 200, AUTOCUT mode, effect 5) (ERBE Electrosurgery, Tübingen, Germany), and the penetration of the target structure is accomplished by applying a pure-cut current, while advancing the black hub further downwards. Once the catheter is fully inside the target structure, the distal flange of the stent is deployed under EUS guidance by moving the gray hub (stent deployment hub) upwards (after removing the yellow safety clip from the stent lock). Retraction of the gray hub to the halfway mark retracts the catheter sheath (unsheathing of the distal flange within the collection cavity for distal flange release). There is a full stop at the halfway position, and a "click" is heard as the gray hub is locked into place. When fully opened, the distal flange becomes visible inside the target structure and appears completely flat like a disc. Complete deployment of the distal flange is verified under EUS or fluoroscopic guidance. The black hub is then unlocked and retracted until the shape of the distal flange changes from flat to oval. Once this change in the shape of the distal flange occurs, the proximal flange can be deployed safely by moving the gray hub fully upwards. Deployment of the proximal flange occurs inside the working channel without the assistance of an endoscopic view. The scope is then gently withdrawn while the catheter control hub is slowly pushed downwards, to allow for the exit of the proximal flange from the working channel to complete the release of the stent. There are several features integrated into the catheter sheath for better control of the stent deployment. A 1 cm black band found at the distal end of the white catheter sheath indicates the position of the preload proximal flange compressed inside the catheter sheath. The proximal flange can be deployed under direct endoscopic visualization by pulling back the white catheter sheath until visualization of 2–3 mm of the black band. Once the catheter is pulled back sufficiently, fully retracting the gray hub deploys the proximal flange into the gut lumen. The catheter sheath also has two radiopaque markers indicating each end of the preloaded stent to enable fluoroscopic control of stent position. It should be noted, however, that the use of fluoroscopy for routine stent deployment is not needed because this change carries the risk of a shift in, and loss of, the optimal sonographic access plane. It also results in unnecessary radiation exposure.

15.3.10.1 Selection and Route of the Drainage (Cyst-Gastrostomy or Cyst-Duodenostomy)

The best site for endoscopic drainage should be identified on EUS considering three criteria:

(a) No intervening abnormal vessels or collateral vessels
(b) The distance between the WON and the gastric or duodenal wall should be <10 mm
(c) The puncture site and the access path should be at the center of the collection to decrease the risk of perforation

In general, the safest and most stable location should be selected for fistula creation before endoscopic necrosectomy to allow the advancement of the endoscope into the cavity for debridement without compromising the stent.

15.3.10.2 Efficacy of Transmural Endoscopic Drainage

The reported success rates for EUS-guided transmural drainage are between 84% and 94%, with collection recurrence rates ranging from 3 to 18% [40, 41, 52–54]. Over 30 retrospective studies, four prospective studies and one randomized control trial evaluated the effectiveness of LAMS for the drainage of PFCs. A recent randomized controlled trial compared the efficacy of LAMS versus plastic stents for the management of 60 patients with pancreatic WON (31 patients with LAMSs and 29 patients with plastic stents). That study showed that there was no significant difference in the number of procedures performed in terms of treatment success, clinical adverse events, readmissions, length of stay, and overall treatment costs between LAMS and plastic stent in the drainage of pancreatic WON. However, a significantly higher rate of stent-related adverse events was observed if LAMS was not removed within 3 weeks post intervention. The authors concluded that LAMS removal should be performed at 3 weeks if WON has been resolved [55]. A recently published retrospective study including 249 patients with PFCs, most of whom were treated with DPS and only 97 of whom received LAMS, showed similar technical and clinical success rates (90.1% versus 92.8%, $p = 0.67$, and 96.7% versus 97.6%, $p = 0.71$, respectively) and adverse events (17.8% versus 24.7%, $p = 0.67$). However, the rate of bleeding was much higher in the LAMS group, particularly that of serious pseudoaneurysm bleeding (OR 10; 95% CI: 1.19–84.6, $p = 0.009$) [56].

A large multicenter retrospective study compared FCSEMSs, LAMSs, and plastic stents in the management of 313 patients with pancreatic WON (121 with FCSEMSs, 106 with DPSs, and 86 with LAMSs). The study showed that transmural drainage of WON with FCSEMSs and LAMSs was superior to that with DPSs in terms of efficacy. However, no significant differences were observed when comparing LAMS and FCSEMS although the mean number of procedures required for WON resolution was significantly lower with LAMSs than with FCSEMSs (2.2 versus 3, $P = 0.04$). However, the rate of bleeding in the LAMS group was higher (7% versus 2% with DPSs and 0% with SEMSs) [57]. A recent meta-analysis evaluated the technical and clinical success rates and the percentage of adverse events with LAMS in 812 patients (608 WON and 204 pancreatic pseudocyst [21] patients) from 14 studies. The pooled technical success rate in patients with WON was 98.9%, and the clinical success rate was 90% [58].

15.3.11 Adjunctive Therapies to Optimize Endoscopic Drainage

In some cases (e.g., collections >12 cm, extension to paracolic gutters, and those with extensive necrosis), standard endoscopic drainage alone is maybe suboptimal for drainage of WON. Therefore, a complementary procedure is frequently required to improve the clinical result. This approach includes the use of a multiple transluminal gateway technique (MTGT), DEN, and percutaneous drainage. Combined endoscopic and percutaneous drainage is referred to as dual-modality drainage (DMD) [59–63].

- **Multiple transmural gateway technique (MTGT)**

  MTGT involves the creation of multiple transmural tracts under EUS guidance to facilitate adequate drainage of necrotic debris in patients with WON, with a goal to reduce the number of endoscopic necrosectomies and reduce the risk of infection [43, 59]. MTGT is performed in the same fashion as the EUS-guided transmural approach with the creation of multiple tracts.

  There are three retrospective case series comparing the MTGT drainage technique with conventional drainage. In total, 39 out of 204 patients were treated with MTGT when there was either no clinical response to conventional endoscopic drainage or if the WON exceeded 12 cm. The clinical success rate ranged between 92% and 100% in patients with MTGT, compared to 52–70% in patients who received a conventional drainage technique. The downside of placing MTGT is a significant increase in procedure time (37 min versus 22 min, $P = 0.0017$) [59, 61, 64].
- **MTGT technique**

  Initially, the most distal part of the WON is accessed under EUS guidance. The WON is punctured using a 19-G FNA needle, and the guidewire is coiled within the cavity. The transmural tract is then dilated sequentially by balloon or cannula up to 8 mm. A 7-Fr, 4 cm DPS is deployed within the necrotic cavity. Then, a second site in the same cavity distal from the first site is identified using EUS guidance, and the same process is repeated but with dilation of the tract to 15 mm, and multiple [2–4] DPSs are placed. The rationale behind dilation of the first tract to 8 mm and placement of a single stent at the first site is to avoid rapid evacuation of the necrotic fluid after multiple stent placements. Generally, if the WON is 6–12 cm in size, only one transmural tract is created. If the WON is between 12 and 15 cm in size, at least two transmural tracts can be created, and if the WON is >15 cm, three transmural gates can be created [7]. When needed, a nasocystic catheter is advanced over the guidewire into the gateway that drains the cranial part of the WON, which is usually at the level of the proximal stomach. The nasocystic catheter is used for irrigation and flushing of necrotic material throughout the multiple gateways in the gastric lumen.
- **Dual-modality drainage (DMD)**

  A percutaneous approach is usually used if the collection extends to the paracolic gutter or if the collection has multiple loculations. DMD involves combined percutaneous and endoscopic drainage. In a large retrospective study evaluating the long-term outcomes of DMD in 117 patients who underwent DMD for WON, 103 patients showed complete resolution of WON, and none of them needed additional therapy or developed pancreatocutaneous fistula after treatment with DMD, and the follow-up was 750 days [60].

A retrospective study that compared DMD with percutaneous drainage alone showed that the DMD was associated with shorter hospital stays (mean 24 versus 54 days, $P < 0.002$). In addition, patients who underwent DMD required fewer endoscopic procedures (1.9 versus 2.7, $P < 0.02$) and fewer CT scans (7.8 versus 14.0, $P < 0.001$) [63].

15.3.12 Complications and Management

The interventional nature of the endoscopic approach for WON and endoscopic necrosectomy does lend itself to potential complications. Complications occur in 10–40% of patients with WON who undergo endoscopic drainage [45]. Although endoscopic necrosectomy is an effective procedure, it can cause serious adverse events, including death. Therefore, it should not be performed unless clinically indicated. The rates of morbidity and mortality associated with endoscopic necrosectomy are 10.4–26% and 0–7.5%, respectively [4, 6, 65–67]. In a recent systematic review including 13 retrospective studies ($n = 455$) and the aforementioned RCTs (n = 98), the overall rate of adverse events was 36% with a 6% mortality rate [46]. It is important for endoscopists to recognize life-threatening complications and act accordingly.

(a) **Bleeding**

The most common complication of endoscopic drainage is bleeding, which occurs in 18% of patients based on a recent systematic review of endoscopic transmural necrosectomy [46]. The rate of bleeding has decreased dramatically with the use of EUS with Doppler flow guidance, which helps identify and thus avoid a vascular path [46]. Bleeding can be classified as early or late depending on the time of bleeding in relation to endoscopic intervention. Bleeding can occur during initial access and tract creation, which can cause injury to transmural or adjacent venous structures. The majority of bleeding is treated endoscopically by coagulation, epinephrine injection, clips, or tamponade with radial expansion balloon dilation or placement of a fully covered (FC) stent [46]. Bleeding during dilation is usually venous in origin. It rarely causes life-threatening bleeding unless the splenic vein, portal vein, or intra-abdominal varices are injured. In cases where the bleeding cannot be controlled endoscopically, interventional radiology for embolization is necessary. The most serious and possibly life-threatening cause of bleeding can be from an unrecognized pseudoaneurysm, but fortunately, this is rare. Three clinical features suggest the possibility of pseudoaneurysm—unexplained GI bleeding, a sudden expansion of PFCs, and an unexplained drop in hemoglobin and hematocrit [46]. Bleeding during necrosectomy can also occur and is often not endoscopically manageable due to limited visualization. Early or delayed bleeding within the cavity may require immediate referral to interventional radiology for angiographic embolization.

In a recent systematic review and meta-analysis by Bazerbachi et al. that included 41 studies with pancreatic WON, the rate of bleeding with a metal stent in a single arm study meta-analysis (total of 18 studies with 935 patients) was lower than that with plastic stent (19 studies with 1083 patients) (5.6% versus 12.6%; $p = 0.002$). The level of heterogeneity in the studies using metal stents was 38.3 ($p = 0.055$) and 52.6 in those using plastic stents ($p = 0.004$). A subanalysis assessing the amount of bleeding with LAMSs (total of 15 studies with 785 patients) showed that the event rate was 6.2% (95% CI, 3.9–9.6%; LAMS versus PS; $p = 0.007$ with a heterogeneity of 40.3; $p = 0.053$) [68]. However, the result of the randomized controlled trial by Bang et al. comparing LAMSs versus DPSs in patients with pancreatic WON has raised concerns about stent-related adverse events, with a reported incidence rate of 32.2% (10 out of 31 patients); the majority of adverse events were observed within the first 5 months and included major bleeding ($n = 3$), buried stent syndrome ($n = 2$), and biliary stricture ($n = 3$). Moreover, significant bleeding was observed in three patients who received LAMS, and blood transfusion and ICU admission were required. On EUS examination, interlacing vessels were noted within the distal flanges of LAMS. A CT angiogram confirmed pseudoaneurysms in all three patients, which were then managed with embolization. All bleeding events were delayed bleeding that occurred within 6 weeks after placement of LAMSs, requiring the authors to change their protocol to repeat CT imaging at 3 weeks after LAMS placement to assess the resolution of the collection. Following a change to the study protocol, only two stent-related adverse events were reported (stent migration and localized bleeding at the tip of the electrocautery enhanced delivery system) [55]. In a larger retrospective comparative study by Brimhall et al., the rate of bleeding was significantly higher in the LAMS group than in the DPSs group (15.5% versus 3.3%, $p = 0.0005$). There was also a higher risk of pseudoaneurysms in the LAMSs group (8.2% versus 7%, $p = 0.009$) [56].

(b) **Perforation**

The risk of perforation during endoscopic drainage is low and occurs in 0.05–4% of cases. It may occur during dilation of the tract when the cavity has not adhered to the gastroduodenal wall at the puncture site [46, 69–71]. In one comparative study between LAMSs, DPSs, and FCSEMSs, perforation occurred in three cases with LAMSs due to stent misdeployment. Two out of three required surgical intervention, while the third patient was managed endoscopically using an over-the-scope clip [57].

Perforation can occur during necrosectomy and usually requires surgical intervention. Patients can present with abdominal sepsis or worsening of hemodynamic status. Early suspicion and recognition of perforation are mandatory. If any doubt exists, an abdominal CT scan with oral contrast is needed. A small perforation/leak can occur during stent placement and may lead to peritonitis or pneumoperitoneum. In the majority of cases, it can be managed conservatively, although a surgical team should be on board to evaluate the role of surgical intervention. If perforation occurs during stent misdeployment outside the cavity or due to the separation of the two walls, the endoscopist should remove the stent, and the site should be closed endoscopically. Endoscopic treatment of a perforation includes endoscopic clips, over-the-scope clip placement, overstitch endoscopic suturing, or a combination of these approaches.

(c) **Stent occlusion**

Stent occlusion can occur due to solid debris or food. If this happens, the patient will present with worsening abdominal pain or sepsis due to inadequate drainage. Stent occlusion occurs more frequently in fully covered SEMS and DPSs than in LAMS (26 versus 23 versus 3, $p = 0.0006$) [57]. Some endoscopists prefer placing a DPS through the SEMS/LAMS to reduce the risk of stent occlusion. Stent occlusion requires endoscopic intervention to remove solid debris or food by forceps or retrieval net to reestablish tract patency.

(d) **Buried stent**

A buried stent means that the gastric or duodenal mucosa has grown over the flanged end of the LAMS. The mechanism and risk factors are not well understood, but a buried stent may occur due to tight apposition of the gut wall and the WON. It has been reported in up to 17% of cases [72–74]. Some authors propose that deployment of the stent across the gastric antrum may increase the risk of a buried stent due to high gastric peristalsis in the antrum [75]. The treatment of a buried stent includes the use of Aragon plasma coagulation (APC) and a needle knife device to uncover the enteric side of the stent and free the stent. Dilation of the stent may lead to stent retrieval. The other technique is to grasp the stent from the internal flange by entering the cavity [71, 74]. Care must be taken during retrieval of the stent as aggressive removal of the stent may lead to bleeding or potential disruption of the cystenterostomy.

(e) **Infection**

Infection can occur after endoscopic manipulation. The rate of infection is reported at 2.7% [76]. Infection may also result from inadequate drainage due to stent malfunction or due to the presence of necrosis. Infection can be managed with antibiotics and endoscopy to reestablish the patency of the fistula tract, upsizing of the stents, or placement of additional pigtail stents, and if necessary, endoscopic debridement. Peri- and post-procedure antibiotics are recommended to reduce the risk of secondary infection in the sterile WON.

(f) **Air embolism**

Air embolism is a rare but potentially fatal complication during DEN. It occurs in 0.9–2% of endoscopic necrosectomies when there is direct communication between the source of gas and the bloodstream [4, 66, 77, 78]. CO_2 does not reduce the risk of air embolism; however, CO_2 is absorbed about 150 times faster than air into the bloodstream, which makes the hemodynamic effect of an air embolism with CO_2 less dramatic. Therefore, it is recommended that CO_2 is used during endoscopic necrosectomy. Fatal gas embolism has been described with CO_2 insufflation [15, 16]. Prompt recognition of a gas embolism is important. Therefore, continuous monitoring of cardiorespiratory vitals during the procedure is essential as abrupt changes in these vital structures may indicate gas embolism [78].

15.3.13 Recurrence Rate

Recurrence of collection after successful endoscopic drainage has been reported in 10–15% of cases [79]. In a randomized controlled trial comparing patients in whom the stent was removed after complete resolution of the collection and patients in whom it was not, patients who underwent stent removal after clinical resolution had a higher rate of recurrence (38% versus 0%) compared to patients in whom the double pigtail stent remained in place [80]. Patients with recurrence were noted to have a DPDS [81].

The current practice in most institutions is to perform cross-sectional imaging with a CECT scan, MRCP with secretin to assess the resolution of the WON and to assess the integrity of the MPD, and/or ERCP before removal of transmural stents. If endoscopic drainage has been performed in patients with a DPDS, long-term placement of a transmural DPS is recommended [80, 82]. If endoscopic therapy fails and recurrence of collection occurs, a surgical approach with either distal pancreatectomy or Roux-en-Y drainage can be indicated with a success rate of 90% [31, 33].

15.4 Conclusion

Over the last few decades, EUS-guided transmural drainage has been considered the standard of care for the initial management of symptomatic WON in lieu of surgical necrosectomy. Effective management of WON requires a multidisciplinary team approach. The evolution of endoscopic techniques in the management of pancreatic WON has significantly improved the efficacy and safety of endoscopic drainage and reduced the use of other minimally invasive techniques. There is still no clear consensus regarding the optimal choice of stents for endoscopic drainage. LAMS is a specially designed EUS stent system with a large diameter that facilitates adequate transmural drainage and direct endoscopic necrosectomy. It has significantly simplified and shortened the procedure time itself. However, certain potential complications are associated with the use of LAMSs. The optimal time for stent removal has not been defined to date. Altogether, the removal of LAMS after a maximum of 4 weeks, if the WON has resolved, is recommended to prevent stent-related complications. Further multicenter randomized prospective studies are necessary to validate the benefits, cost, and safety of metal stents over plastic stents and to determine the optimal time for stent removal. Furthermore, dual-modality drainage should be considered in patients with large WON that extends to the paracolic gutter and in patients not responding to endoscopic drainage.

Financial Disclosures and Conflicts of Interest Mouen A. Khashab is a consultant and on medical advisory board for Boston Scientific and Olympus and a consultant for Medtronic.

References

1. Baron TH, Morgan DE. Acute necrotizing pancreatitis. N Engl J Med. 1999;340(18):1412–7.
2. Beger HG, Rau B, Mayer J, Pralle U. Natural course of acute pancreatitis. World J Surg. 1997;21(2):130–5.
3. Kourtesis G, Wilson SE, Williams RA. The clinical significance of fluid collections in acute pancreatitis. Am Surg. 1990;56(12):796–9.
4. Yasuda I, Nakashima M, Iwai T, Isayama H, Itoi T, Hisai H, et al. Japanese multicenter experience of endoscopic necrosectomy for infected walled-off pancreatic necrosis: the JENIPaN study. Endoscopy. 2013;45(8):627–34.
5. Varadarajulu S, Bang JY, Sutton BS, Trevino JM, Christein JD, Wilcox CM. Equal efficacy of endoscopic and surgical cystogastrostomy for pancreatic pseudocyst drainage in a randomized trial. Gastroenterology. 2013;145(3):583–90.e1.
6. Gardner TB, Coelho-Prabhu N, Gordon SR, Gelrud A, Maple JT, Papachristou GI, et al. Direct endoscopic necrosectomy for the treatment of walled-off pancreatic necrosis: results from a multicenter U.S. series. Gastrointest Endosc. 2011;73(4):718–26.
7. Giovannini M. Endoscopic ultrasound-guided drainage of pancreatic fluid collections. Gastrointest Endosc Clin N Am. 2018;28(2):157–69.
8. Takahashi N, Papachristou GI, Schmit GD, Chahal P, LeRoy AJ, Sarr MG, et al. CT findings of walled-off pancreatic necrosis (WOPN): differentiation from pseudocyst and prediction of outcome after endoscopic therapy. Eur Radiol. 2008;18(11):2522–9.
9. Freeman ML, Werner J, van Santvoort HC, Baron TH, Besselink MG, Windsor JA, et al. Interventions for necrotizing pancreatitis: summary of a multidisciplinary consensus conference. Pancreas. 2012;41(8):1176–94.
10. Besselink MG, Verwer TJ, Schoenmaeckers EJ, Buskens E, Ridwan BU, Visser MR, et al. Timing of surgical intervention in necrotizing pancreatitis. Arch Surg. 2007;142(12):1194–201.
11. Werner J, Hartwig W, Hackert T, Buchler MW. Surgery in the treatment of acute pancreatitis—open pancreatic necrosectomy. Scand J Surg. 2005;94(2):130–4.
12. Working Group IAPAPAAPG. IAP/APA evidence-based guidelines for the management of acute pancreatitis. Pancreatology. 2013;13(4 Suppl 2):e1–15.
13. ASGE Standards of Practice Committee, Acosta RD, Abraham NS, Chandrasekhara V, Chathadi KV, Early DS, et al. The management of antithrombotic agents for patients undergoing GI endoscopy. Gastrointest Endosc. 2016;83(1):3–16.
14. Fisher JM, Gardner TB. Endoscopic therapy of necrotizing pancreatitis and pseudocysts. Gastrointest Endosc Clin N Am. 2013;23(4):787–802.
15. Bonnot B, Nion-Larmurier I, Desaint B, Chafai N, Paye F, Beaussier M, et al. Fatal gas embolism after endoscopic transgastric necrosectomy for infected necrotizing pancreatitis. Am J Gastroenterol. 2014;109(4):607–8.
16. Gardner TB, Chahal P, Papachristou GI, Vege SS, Petersen BT, Gostout CJ, et al. A comparison of direct endoscopic necrosectomy with transmural endoscopic drainage for the treatment of walled-off pancreatic necrosis. Gastrointest Endosc. 2009;69(6):1085–94.
17. Steinberg WM. A step-up approach, or open necrosectomy for necrotizing pancreatitis. N Engl J Med. 2010;363(13):1286–7; author reply 7
18. van Santvoort HC, Besselink MG, Bakker OJ, Hofker HS, Boermeester MA, Dejong CH, et al. A step-up approach or open necrosectomy for necrotizing pancreatitis. N Engl J Med. 2010;362(16):1491–502.
19. van Baal MC, van Santvoort HC, Bollen TL, Bakker OJ, Besselink MG, Gooszen HG, et al. Systematic review of percutaneous catheter drainage as primary treatment for necrotizing pancreatitis. Br J Surg. 2011;98(1):18–27.
20. Bakker OJ, van Santvoort HC, van Brunschot S, Geskus RB, Besselink MG, Bollen TL, et al. Endoscopic transgastric vs surgical necrosectomy for infected necrotizing pancreatitis: a randomized trial. JAMA. 2012;307(10):1053–61.

21. van Brunschot S, van Grinsven J, van Santvoort HC, Bakker OJ, Besselink MG, Boermeester MA, et al. Endoscopic or surgical step-up approach for infected necrotising pancreatitis: a multicentre randomised trial. Lancet. 2018;391(10115):51–8.
22. Irani S, Gluck M, Ross A, Gan SI, Crane R, Brandabur JJ, et al. Resolving external pancreatic fistulas in patients with disconnected pancreatic duct syndrome: using rendezvous techniques to avoid surgery (with video). Gastrointest Endosc. 2012;76(3):586.e1–93.e3.
23. Bang JY, Navaneethan U, Hasan MK, Hawes RH, Varadarajulu S. EUS correlates of disconnected pancreatic duct syndrome in walled-off necrosis. Endosc Int Open. 2016;4(8):E883–9.
24. Deviere J, Antaki F. Disconnected pancreatic tail syndrome: a plea for multidisciplinarity. Gastrointest Endosc. 2008;67(4):680–2.
25. Abdo A, Jani N, Cunningham SC. Pancreatic duct disruption and nonoperative management: the SEALANTS approach. Hepatobiliary Pancreat Dis Int. 2013;12(3):239–43.
26. Wong YC, Wang LJ, Fang JF, Lin BC, Ng CJ, Chen RJ. Multidetector-row computed tomography (CT) of blunt pancreatic injuries: can contrast-enhanced multiphasic CT detect pancreatic duct injuries? J Trauma. 2008;64(3):666–72.
27. Itoh S, Ikeda M, Ota T, Satake H, Takai K, Ishigaki T. Assessment of the pancreatic and intrapancreatic bile ducts using 0.5-mm collimation and multiplanar reformatted images in multislice CT. Eur Radiol. 2003;13(2):277–85.
28. Gillams AR, Kurzawinski T, Lees WR. Diagnosis of duct disruption and assessment of pancreatic leak with dynamic secretin-stimulated MR cholangiopancreatography. AJR Am J Roentgenol. 2006;186(2):499–506.
29. Drake LM, Anis M, Lawrence C. Accuracy of magnetic resonance cholangiopancreatography in identifying pancreatic duct disruption. J Clin Gastroenterol. 2012;46(8):696–9.
30. Sherman S, Freeman ML, Tarnasky PR, Wilcox CM, Kulkarni A, Aisen AM, et al. Administration of secretin (RG1068) increases the sensitivity of detection of duct abnormalities by magnetic resonance cholangiopancreatography in patients with pancreatitis. Gastroenterology. 2014;147(3):646–54.e2.
31. Howard TJ, Rhodes GJ, Selzer DJ, Sherman S, Fogel E, Lehman GA. Roux-en-Y internal drainage is the best surgical option to treat patients with disconnected duct syndrome after severe acute pancreatitis. Surgery. 2001;130(4):714–9; discussion 9–21
32. Pearson EG, Scaife CL, Mulvihill SJ, Glasgow RE. Roux-en-Y drainage of a pancreatic fistula for disconnected pancreatic duct syndrome after acute necrotizing pancreatitis. HPB (Oxford). 2012;14(1):26–31.
33. Tann M, Maglinte D, Howard TJ, Sherman S, Fogel E, Madura JA, et al. Disconnected pancreatic duct syndrome: imaging findings and therapeutic implications in 26 surgically corrected patients. J Comput Assist Tomogr. 2003;27(4):577–82.
34. Hookey LC, Debroux S, Delhaye M, Arvanitakis M, Le Moine O, Deviere J. Endoscopic drainage of pancreatic-fluid collections in 116 patients: a comparison of etiologies, drainage techniques, and outcomes. Gastrointest Endosc. 2006;63(4):635–43.
35. Trevino JM, Tamhane A, Varadarajulu S. Successful stenting in ductal disruption favorably impacts treatment outcomes in patients undergoing transmural drainage of peripancreatic fluid collections. J Gastroenterol Hepatol. 2010;25(3):526–31.
36. Varadarajulu S, Noone TC, Tutuian R, Hawes RH, Cotton PB. Predictors of outcome in pancreatic duct disruption managed by endoscopic transpapillary stent placement. Gastrointest Endosc. 2005;61(4):568–75.
37. Amin S, Yang DJ, Lucas AL, Gonzalez S, DiMaio CJ. There is no advantage to transpapillary pancreatic duct stenting for the transmural endoscopic drainage of pancreatic fluid collections: a meta-analysis. Clin Endosc. 2017;50(4):388–94.
38. Arvanitakis M, Dumonceau JM, Albert J, Badaoui A, Bali MA, Barthet M, et al. Endoscopic management of acute necrotizing pancreatitis: European Society of Gastrointestinal Endoscopy (ESGE) evidence-based multidisciplinary guidelines. Endoscopy. 2018;50(5):524–46.
39. Shrode CW, Macdonough P, Gaidhane M, Northup PG, Sauer B, Ku J, et al. Multimodality endoscopic treatment of pancreatic duct disruption with stenting and pseudocyst drainage: how efficacious is it? Dig Liver Dis. 2013;45(2):129–33.

40. Kahaleh M, Shami VM, Conaway MR, Tokar J, Rockoff T, De La Rue SA, et al. Endoscopic ultrasound drainage of pancreatic pseudocyst: a prospective comparison with conventional endoscopic drainage. Endoscopy. 2006;38(4):355–9.
41. Park DH, Lee SS, Moon SH, Choi SY, Jung SW, Seo DW, et al. Endoscopic ultrasound-guided versus conventional transmural drainage for pancreatic pseudocysts: a prospective randomized trial. Endoscopy. 2009;41(10):842–8.
42. Varadarajulu S, Christein JD, Tamhane A, Drelichman ER, Wilcox CM. Prospective randomized trial comparing EUS and EGD for transmural drainage of pancreatic pseudocysts (with videos). Gastrointest Endosc. 2008;68(6):1102–11.
43. Voermans RP, Ponchon T, Schumacher B, Fumex F, Bergman JJ, Larghi A, et al. Forward-viewing versus oblique-viewing echoendoscopes in transluminal drainage of pancreatic fluid collections: a multicenter, randomized, controlled trial. Gastrointest Endosc. 2011;74(6):1285–93.
44. Prasad GA, Varadarajulu S. Endoscopic ultrasound-guided abscess drainage. Gastrointest Endosc Clin N Am. 2012;22(2):281–90, ix
45. Varadarajulu S, Bang JY, Phadnis MA, Christein JD, Wilcox CM. Endoscopic transmural drainage of peripancreatic fluid collections: outcomes and predictors of treatment success in 211 consecutive patients. J Gastrointest Surg. 2011;15(11):2080–8.
46. van Brunschot S, Fockens P, Bakker OJ, Besselink MG, Voermans RP, Poley JW, et al. Endoscopic transluminal necrosectomy in necrotising pancreatitis: a systematic review. Surg Endosc. 2014;28(5):1425–38.
47. Singhal S, Rotman SR, Gaidhane M, Kahaleh M. Pancreatic fluid collection drainage by endoscopic ultrasound: an update. Clin Endosc. 2013;46(5):506–14.
48. Antillon MR, Bechtold ML, Bartalos CR, Marshall JB. Transgastric endoscopic necrosectomy with temporary metallic esophageal stent placement for the treatment of infected pancreatic necrosis (with video). Gastrointest Endosc. 2009;69(1):178–80.
49. Tarantino I, Traina M, Barresi L, Volpes R, Gridelli B. Transgastric plus transduodenal necrosectomy with temporary metal stents placement for treatment of large pancreatic necrosis. Pancreas. 2010;39(2):269–70.
50. Krishnan A, Ramakrishnan R. EUS-guided endoscopic necrosectomy and temporary cystogastrostomy for infected pancreatic necrosis with self-expanding metallic stents. Surg Laparosc Endosc Percutan Tech. 2012;22(5):e319–21.
51. Sarkaria S, Sethi A, Rondon C, Lieberman M, Srinivasan I, Weaver K, et al. Pancreatic necrosectomy using covered esophageal stents: a novel approach. J Clin Gastroenterol. 2014;48(2):145–52.
52. Antillon MR, Shah RJ, Stiegmann G, Chen YK. Single-step EUS-guided transmural drainage of simple and complicated pancreatic pseudocysts. Gastrointest Endosc. 2006;63(6):797–803.
53. Kruger M, Schneider AS, Manns MP, Meier PN. Endoscopic management of pancreatic pseudocysts or abscesses after an EUS-guided 1-step procedure for initial access. Gastrointest Endosc. 2006;63(3):409–16.
54. Varadarajulu S, Lopes TL, Wilcox CM, Drelichman ER, Kilgore ML, Christein JD. EUS versus surgical cyst-gastrostomy for management of pancreatic pseudocysts. Gastrointest Endosc. 2008;68(4):649–55.
55. Bang JY, Navaneethan U, Hasan MK, Sutton B, Hawes R, Varadarajulu S. Non-superiority of lumen-apposing metal stents over plastic stents for drainage of walled-off necrosis in a randomised trial. Gut. 2018;68(7).
56. Brimhall B, Han S, Tatman PD, Clark TJ, Wani S, Brauer B, et al. Increased incidence of pseudoaneurysm bleeding with lumen-apposing metal stents compared to double-pigtail plastic stents in patients with peripancreatic fluid collections. Clin Gastroenterol Hepatol. 2018;16(9):1521–8.
57. Siddiqui AA, Kowalski TE, Loren DE, Khalid A, Soomro A, Mazhar SM, et al. Fully covered self-expanding metal stents versus lumen-apposing fully covered self-expanding metal stent versus plastic stents for endoscopic drainage of pancreatic walled-off necrosis: clinical outcomes and success. Gastrointest Endosc. 2017;85(4):758–65.

58. Han D, Inamdar S, Lee CW, Miller LS, Trindade AJ, Sejpal DV. Lumen apposing metal stents (LAMSs) for drainage of pancreatic and gallbladder collections: a meta-analysis. J Clin Gastroenterol. 2018;52(9):835–44.
59. Varadarajulu S, Phadnis MA, Christein JD, Wilcox CM. Multiple transluminal gateway technique for EUS-guided drainage of symptomatic walled-off pancreatic necrosis. Gastrointest Endosc. 2011;74(1):74–80.
60. Ross AS, Irani S, Gan SI, Rocha F, Siegal J, Fotoohi M, et al. Dual-modality drainage of infected and symptomatic walled-off pancreatic necrosis: long-term clinical outcomes. Gastrointest Endosc. 2014;79(6):929–35.
61. Bang JY, Wilcox CM, Trevino J, Ramesh J, Peter S, Hasan M, et al. Factors impacting treatment outcomes in the endoscopic management of walled-off pancreatic necrosis. J Gastroenterol Hepatol. 2013;28(11):1725–32.
62. Mukai S, Itoi T, Sofuni A, Itokawa F, Kurihara T, Tsuchiya T, et al. Novel single transluminal gateway transcystic multiple drainages after EUS-guided drainage for complicated multilocular walled-off necrosis (with videos). Gastrointest Endosc. 2014;79(3):531–5.
63. Gluck M, Ross A, Irani S, Lin O, Gan SI, Fotoohi M, et al. Dual modality drainage for symptomatic walled-off pancreatic necrosis reduces length of hospitalization, radiological procedures, and number of endoscopies compared to standard percutaneous drainage. J Gastrointest Surg. 2012;16(2):248–56; discussion 56–7
64. Minaga K, Kitano M, Imai H, Yamao K, Kamata K, Miyata T, et al. Modified single transluminal gateway transcystic multiple drainage technique for a huge infected walled-off pancreatic necrosis: a case report. World J Gastroenterol. 2016;22(21):5132–6.
65. Isayama H, Nakai Y, Rerknimitr R, Khor C, Lau J, Wang HP, et al. Asian consensus statements on endoscopic management of walled-off necrosis. Part 2: endoscopic management. J Gastroenterol Hepatol. 2016;31(9):1555–65.
66. Seifert H, Biermer M, Schmitt W, Jurgensen C, Will U, Gerlach R, et al. Transluminal endoscopic necrosectomy after acute pancreatitis: a multicentre study with long-term follow-up (the GEPARD study). Gut. 2009;58(9):1260–6.
67. Thompson CC, Kumar N, Slattery J, Clancy TE, Ryan MB, Ryou M, et al. A standardized method for endoscopic necrosectomy improves complication and mortality rates. Pancreatology. 2016;16(1):66–72.
68. Bazerbachi F, Sawas T, Vargas EJ, Prokop LJ, Chari ST, Gleeson FC, et al. Metal stents versus plastic stents for the management of pancreatic walled-off necrosis: a systematic review and meta-analysis. Gastrointest Endosc. 2018;87(1):30–42.e15.
69. ASGE Standards of Practice Committee, Ben-Menachem T, Decker GA, Early DS, Evans J, Fanelli RD, et al. Adverse events of upper GI endoscopy. Gastrointest Endosc. 2012;76(4):707–18.
70. Fabbri C, Luigiano C, Maimone A, Polifemo AM, Tarantino I, Cennamo V. Endoscopic ultrasound-guided drainage of pancreatic fluid collections. World J Gastrointest Endosc. 2012;4(11):479–88.
71. DeSimone ML, Asombang AW, Berzin TM. Lumen apposing metal stents for pancreatic fluid collections: recognition and management of complications. World J Gastrointest Endosc. 2017;9(9):456–63.
72. Fabbri C, Luigiano C, Marsico M, Cennamo V. A rare adverse event resulting from the use of a lumen-apposing metal stent for drainage of a pancreatic fluid collection: "the buried stent". Gastrointest Endosc. 2015;82(3):585–7.
73. Rodrigues-Pinto E, Grimm IS, Baron TH. Removal of buried gastroduodenal stents after drainage of pancreatic fluid collections: silence of the LAMS (with video). Gastrointest Endosc. 2016;83(4):853–4.
74. Seerden TC, Vleggaar FP. Endoscopic removal of buried lumen-apposing metal stents used for cystogastrostomy and cholecystogastrostomy. Endoscopy. 2016;48 Suppl 1:E179.
75. Irani S, Kozarek RA. The buried lumen-apposing metal stent: is this a stent problem, a location problem, or both? VideoGIE. 2016;1(1):25–6.

76. Varadarajulu S, Christein JD, Wilcox CM. Frequency of complications during EUS-guided drainage of pancreatic fluid collections in 148 consecutive patients. J Gastroenterol Hepatol. 2011;26(10):1504–8.
77. Gardner TB. Endoscopic management of necrotizing pancreatitis. Gastrointest Endosc. 2012;76(6):1214–23.
78. Donepudi S, Chavalitdhamrong D, Pu L, Draganov PV. Air embolism complicating gastrointestinal endoscopy: a systematic review. World J Gastrointest Endosc. 2013;5(8):359–65.
79. Deviere J, Bueso H, Baize M, Azar C, Love J, Moreno E, et al. Complete disruption of the main pancreatic duct: endoscopic management. Gastrointest Endosc. 1995;42(5):445–51.
80. Arvanitakis M, Delhaye M, Bali MA, Matos C, De Maertelaer V, Le Moine O, et al. Pancreatic-fluid collections: a randomized controlled trial regarding stent removal after endoscopic transmural drainage. Gastrointest Endosc. 2007;65(4):609–19.
81. Lawrence C, Howell DA, Stefan AM, Conklin DE, Lukens FJ, Martin RF, et al. Disconnected pancreatic tail syndrome: potential for endoscopic therapy and results of long-term follow-up. Gastrointest Endosc. 2008;67(4):673–9.
82. Rana SS, Bhasin DK, Rao C, Sharma R, Gupta R. Consequences of long term indwelling transmural stents in patients with walled off pancreatic necrosis & disconnected pancreatic duct syndrome. Pancreatology. 2013;13(5):486–90.

Radiofrequency Ablation

16

Kenneth K. Wang

Radiofrequency ablation has seen a widespread popularity in medical applications. As well as gastroenterology, applications in cardiology for ablation of conduction pathways, use in orthopedics for treatment of disc disease, pain clinic applications for destruction of nerve bundle, as well as tumor ablation in endocrine organs have become widespread. In gastroenterology, the primary uses have been an ablation of Barrett's esophagus, treatment of gastric antral ectasias, therapy of cholangiocarcinoma, as well as ablation of hepatomas. Radiofrequency ablation has become an important treatment modality in therapeutic endoscopy.

16.1 What Is Radiofrequency Ablation?

Energy can be delivered in multiple different forms. The most common form from an electrosurgical generator is an alternating current. By varying the frequency and the voltage of the alternating current, the function of the electrical generator can be altered from primarily a cutting current to coagulation current. Moreover, if the frequency is increased, there is less tissue penetration and more control of the depth of injury from the energy. This is the primary reason that radiofrequency ablation is performed at a frequency of about 400,000 cycles a second. The amount of energy applied is dependent on the application. For luminal gastrointestinal tissue ablation, the generator produces energy at a frequency of 460.8 KHz using a quasi-sinusoidal waveform for all type of catheters (Fig. 16.1). The maximum power delivered is 300 W which is used only for the 360-degree balloon unit [1]. The focal ablation catheters use less power depending on the size of the catheter; for example, the 90-degree focal catheter has a

K. K. Wang (✉)
Russ and Kathy Van Cleve Professor of Gastroenterology Research, Mayo Clinic, Rochester, MN, USA
e-mail: wang.kenneth@mayo.edu

P. Sharma, N. Reddy (eds.), *Innovations in Gastrointestinal Endoscopy*,
https://doi.org/10.1007/978-981-15-9247-8_16

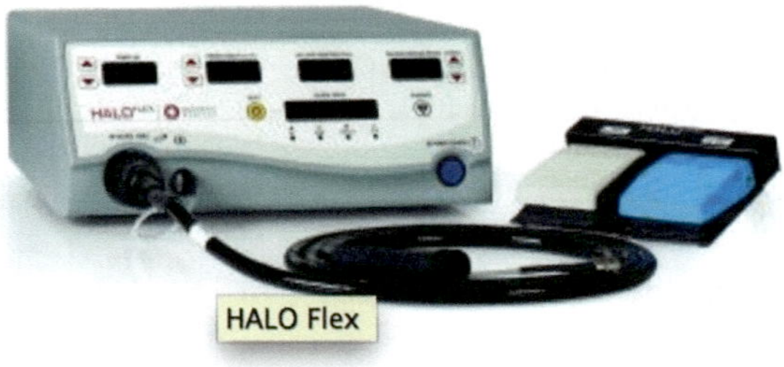

Fig. 16.1 This is the radiofrequency ablation generator that can power both focal and circumferential ablation devices. The device has auto-inflation capabilities to inflate the balloon for circumferential ablation. This is controlled by a foot pedal. The delivery of radiofrequency energy is also initiated by the use of the foot pedal

power output of 104 W which is adjusted by the generator upon recognition of the catheter that is placed into the device. The maximum voltage procedure by the generator is 40 V RMS (root mean square) as the voltage will fluctuate throughout the sinusoidal wave form. The current is produced at a maximum of 24 Amperes RMS. The delivery of this energy is controlled by a computer processing unit that regulates the outputs dependent on the device attached. These devices are relatively stable with a power variation of up to 15% (3 W) depending on the amount of resistance encountered. The generator used in gastroenterology is a Class A device by CISPR 11 standards for radiofrequency emissions and can affect sensitive devices in medical hospital areas.

Electrical generators for ablation of hepatic or pancreatic masses are generally much lower in power since the energy is delivered by a needle device that can be inserted into tissue so that the current density is much higher despite the smaller amount of power. The delivery devices surface area is so much smaller than the requirement for widespread tissue ablation. There are a number of devices available for use at this point, and their individual characteristics vary although they all are usually regulated using a CPU with smart and precise delivery of targeted energy.

16.2 Why Was Radiofrequency Ablation Used for Mucosal Ablation?

The prior therapies for mucosal ablation were generally all developed for other applications and then ported to gastrointestinal use. The first among these was thermal laser therapy and then thermal therapy with either bipolar coagulation or argon plasma coagulation. The difficulty with these therapies is that the amount of surface contacted by these probes was very small, and it was often easy to miss small areas of Barrett's mucosa. The small probes also had variable contact so the treatment depth was less certain. Subsequently, photodynamic therapy was used that was much easier to apply and could treat up to 7 cm lengths of Barrett's esophagus with a single application. This was only limited by the length of the diffusing fiber and the power of the laser. Unfortunately, the penetration depth of this therapy was probably deep, and strictures (18%) were common as was an unfortunate side effect of photosensitivity that caused patients remain in darkness for about a month.

Radiofrequency ablation was specifically targeted for Barrett's esophagus because of its superficial therapy that could decrease the stricture rate and the lack of systemic effects. Initial studies done in pre-esophagectomy patients and in non-dysplastic Barrett's esophagus demonstrated a fairly uniform and superficial tissue destruction that could eliminate specialized mucosa.

16.3 Who Are the Best Candidates for Radiofrequency Ablation in Barrett's Esophagus?

Patient selection is key in performing endoscopic ablation therapy in Barrett's esophagus. The consensus agreement is that patients with reasonable survival and the presence of high-grade dysplasia or low-grade dysplasia that is confirmed by expert pathologists are eligible for ablation therapy. This patient population has been demonstrated to be at the highest risk of progression in randomized prospective studies. Due to the superficial nature of the therapy, patients need to have nodular lesions within the Barrett's esophagus removed using endoscopic resection techniques prior to RFA. Patients with strictures that cannot be dilated are also a problem with radiofrequency ablation since the diameter of the catheters can be difficult to pass although the newest through the scope catheter eliminates this need. However, this catheter cannot be used to treat large areas of tissue due to the limited size of the probe and the need to reclean this frequently. There has also been a small study that examined the use of resection in the same session as circumferential radiofrequency ablation. Though it was feasible, the performance of resection was more difficult though it resulted in elimination of 95% of the Barrett's segment. The problem was complications including perforation in 4%, 16% bleeding rate, and 21% stenosis rate in this group [2]. Use of radiofrequency ablation has been compared to stepwise resection for the treatment of Barrett's esophagus. Though both were efficacious in eliminating dysplasia and Barrett's metaplasia, the group treated with stepwise endoscopic resection had an 88% stricture rate as compared to 18% in the combined resection with radiofrequency ablation group [3]. This was despite the use of stepwise resection being only 50% resection of the circumference of the esophagus.

The prospective randomized trials have all involved segment lengths less than 7–8 cm, but retrospective cohort studies have found that even ultra-long segment Barrett's segments (<14 cm) can be treated with radiofrequency ablation with response rates similar to shorter segments though recurrence rates at 3 years were higher in the ultra-long segments [4].

16.4 How Is Radiofrequency Ablation Applied to Barrett's Esophagus?

It is important to realize that radiofrequency ablation has evolved a great deal since its original development. The technique involves first carefully visualizing the entire Barrett's segment with careful notation as to the maximum height of the segment as well as the distribution of the columnar mucosa. Shorter eccentric tongues of columnar mucosa in the esophagus can easily be treated with focal devices, while the longer circumferential lengths of Barrett's esophagus can be treated with a circumferential device. Biopsies are generally not encouraged at the time of therapy as bleeding from the sites of biopsy can interfere with the delivery of radiofrequency energy. The mucosal surface should be cleaned of mucous using n-acetylcysteine sprayed onto the mucosa. The mucous layer tends to inhibit conduction of the radiofrequency energy and can carbonize further inhibiting conduction. The generator does feedback on the conduction ability of the treatment catheters, and the user receives digital feedback regarding the amount of energy delivered with every application. The entire surface should be sprayed, and the n-acetyl cysteine suctioned away to prevent aspiration.

Ablation therapy needs to be commenced at the proximal portion of the Barrett's segment with some overlap 1 cm or so with the normal squamous tissue to ensure that the Barrett's mucosa is totally ablated. The treatment catheters can be advanced distally toward the stomach with an overlap of about 1 cm with the treated region. The generator is automatically set to produce an energy dose of 10 J per square centimeter for the circumferential treatment balloon. In the past, sizing of the esophagus was required to determine the size of treatment catheter required, but currently the treatment catheter adjusts to fit the diameter of the esophagus. The circumferential device is applied only once per segment. This cauterizes the surface of the mucosa which can then be removed by mechanical application of a cap fitted to the end of the endoscope. The circumferential device is then applied again once through the entire treated area. The generator actually measures the resistance from the mucosa, and if there is lack of contact or high resistance, the catheter can be re-positioned or if there is a great deal of eschar on the ablation electrodes, this can be removed and cleaned (See Fig. 16.2). The current circumferential catheter must be carefully turned in a counter-clockwise direction as it is withdrawn to decrease the stiffness of the probe and to prevent the RF coil from folding and potentially cutting the surface of the mucosa.

If a focal device is used, the energy is set to be 12 J per centimeter squared. This is applied twice and then the mucosal surface can be cleaned before applying the focal device twice again. There is an assortment of focal devices that are attached to the tip of the endoscope and have a pivot point to allow greater opposition to the surface of the esophageal wall. The focal devices primarily vary in length with the standard being about 2 cm in length going up to 4 cm. The most commonly used are a 90-degree of the circumference focal device that has a treatment area of 20 mm by 13 mm in size and can fit over endoscopes between 8.6 and 12.8 mm in diameter (Fig. 16.3). In addition, there are smaller width devices for treatment of small residuals Barrett's esophageal islands that cover perhaps a sixth of the diameter and are termed 60-degree focal

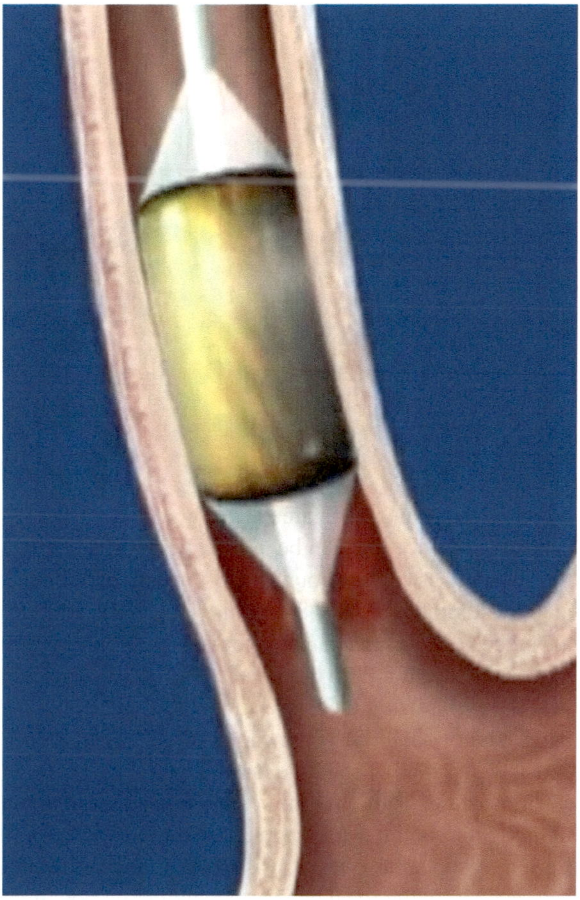

Fig. 16.2 Circumferential balloon inflated in the esophagus. The 3-cm-long treatment catheter contacts the surface of the Barrett's mucosa. The positioning is controlled under direct endoscopic visualization

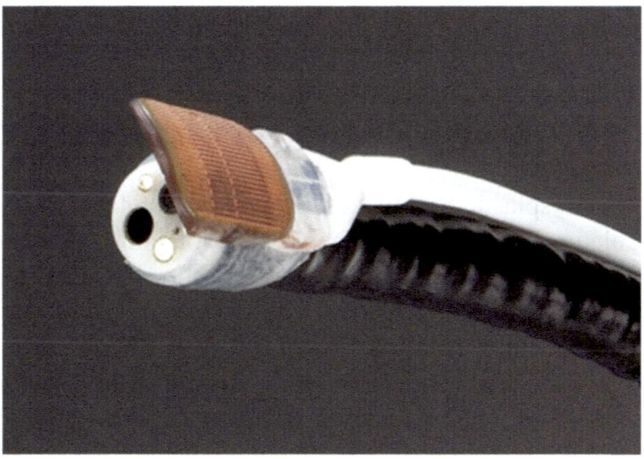

Fig. 16.3 The focal ablation catheters are friction fitted onto the end of a standard endoscope. The ablation surface can pivot to allow opposition to the esophageal wall. The illustrated focal device covers approximately a quarter of the circumference and is termed a 90-degree device. There are smaller focal devices that cover 60°

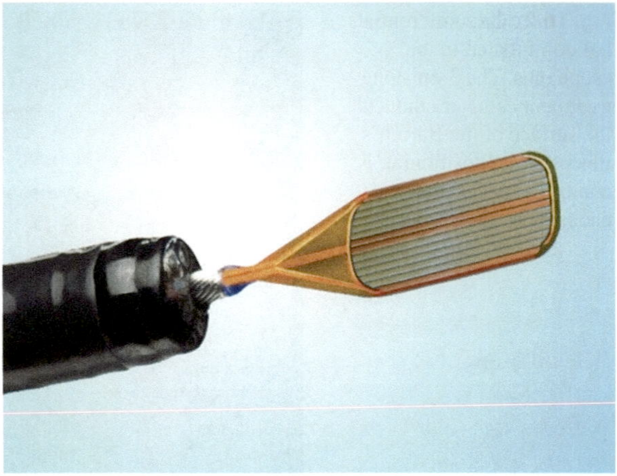

Fig. 16.4 An ablation catheter that actually can be rolled up and passed through a standard 2.8 mm biopsy channel which then unrolls once it is in the lumen. This device can only be used for small lesions

catheters that can treat an area of 10 by 15 mm in size. The smallest is a through - the-endoscope device that can be used in very difficult situations and is termed a channel RFA device. It will fit through a 2.8-mm standard biopsy channel and delivers a treatment paddle of 15.7 by 7.8 mm in width. After a first round of ablation is applied to the mucosa, the eschar can be removed by an endoscope equipped with a cleaning cap that can be friction fit to the tip of the endoscope and is made of soft plastic to gently peel the eschar from the tissue so that this eschar tissue does not interfere with a second round of ablation. These caps vary in size from small to medium and accommodate a wide range of standard endoscopes (Fig. 16.4).

In a patient with circumferential Barrett's esophagus, the balloon probe is used initially to treat the entire segment. However, after the initial ablation, the remaining Barrett's esophagus often consists of tongues and islands of columnar tissue that can be treated with the focal devices depending on how much columnar mucosa remains. Repeated treatments with the circumferential balloon were done in the initial studies of RFA, but with the development of the focal devices, this is much less common.

16.5 Treatment of Non-dysplastic Barrett's Esophagus

Non-dysplastic Barrett's esophagus was the first lesion treated with radiofrequency ablation as a proof of principal that ablation would cause re-epithelialization with squamous mucosa [5]. This lesion responded well to ablation therapy, and it was clearly shown that ablation with RFA could cause intestinal metaplasia to regress. Subsequently, there has been debate over the need to treat non-dysplastic tissue that has never been previously treated. The difficulty has been that since Barrett's esophagus does not have a very high rate of progression, it has been difficult to create a study that can confirm the benefit of ablation. Hypothetically, if the lifetime risk of progression to cancer is 8% and radiofrequency ablation is 100% effective, the study would need about 1500 patients followed over an average of 10 years to have 80% power to detect this small difference.

There has been some discussion that the absolutely risk of progression is similar to that of a colon polyp evolving into cancer. However, polyps are discrete and easier to resect than trying to ablate an entire mucosal surface. In addition, given the low risk of progression, it is uncertain if more aggressive ablation or resection methods should be applied if the Barrett's segment is resistant to ablation.

16.6 Role of Radiofrequency Ablation of Low-Grade Dysplasia Barrett's Esophagus

The ablation of low-grade dysplasia was feasible as demonstrated in the initial pivotal trial of 127 patients for radiofrequency ablation [6]. Though the number of patients was relatively small, over 90% of those treated had elimination of dysplasia versus 23% in the control group. However, despite the statistically significant decrease in dysplasia, it remained unclear if this actually changed outcomes, given the low risk of progression in patients with low-grade dysplasia. A study was conducted in the Netherlands that prospectively evaluated 136 patients randomized 1:1 to either RFA ablation or observation in 9 European centers. It was found that 1.5% progressed in the ablated group to either high-grade dysplasia or carcinoma versus 26.5% in the control group. This was statistically significant and the follow-up was 3 years. This study was controversial initially as the control rate of progression was much higher than that reported in the United States though progression rates in European studies were also much higher than previously thought.

Subsequent studies have varied these results including retrospective multicenter studies as well as several retrospective histological studies that utilized low-grade dysplasia that had been confirmed by at least two experienced pathologists [7–9]. It appears that ablation of low-grade dysplasia does appear to decrease its progression in the near term. However, retrospective studies also suggest that overall progression is not affected by radiofrequency ablation as opposed to surveillance [10]. Nonetheless, when meta-analysis and systematic reviews are performed in patients with low-grade dysplasia, there is still lower risk of progression when studies are summarized with those receiving radiofrequency ablation having a 0.77% rate of progression versus 6.6% in those receiving only surveillance [11].

16.7 Radiofrequency Ablation for GAVE

Radiofrequency ablation using focal ablation catheters has been reported with success in small clinical series for decreasing or eliminating transfusion requirements in patients with gastric antral vascular ectasias (GAVE) [12]. This series of 21 patients had an 86% response rate in patients who were still transfusion-dependent after therapy with argon plasma coagulation. This indicates that RFA may be beneficial in patients with GAVE as a second-line therapy in those patients who do not do well. Other series have reported successful therapies though the patient population were less well characterized [13].

16.8 Radiofrequency Ablation for Cholangiocarcinoma

Radiofrequency ablation has been applied to bile duct cancers by applying percutaneous catheters originally used for hepatocellular carcinomas [14]. ERCP-directed radiofrequency was developed to provide palliation for cholangiocarcinoma, given the relatively poor results from stenting. ERCP-directed RFA required new probes that were more flexible to be passed into the bile duct. The catheters developed so far are about the size of an 8F catheter and require introduction over a 0.035-inch 450-cm-long wire. These flexible probes generally require a therapeutic duodenoscope to be employed with at least a 3.2-mm-diameter channel. The probes themselves have a 5 mm leading tip with 8 mm electrodes separated by 8 mm allowing for treatment of 25 mm of tissue with a single application. The energy is usually applied using electrosurgical generators in soft coagulation mode using effect 8. These catheters can also be used in bipolar coagulation mode. Smaller catheters are also available and can be passed using echoendoscopes to their target. These catheters have a 1 Fr diameter and can fit into either a 19 or 22 Fr Fine Needle Aspiration needle. The electrode is about 20 mm long at the tip of this probe. Energy applied at EUS is typically soft coagulation mode at an effect 4 with 10 W power (Fig. 16.5).

RFA for cholangiocarcinoma in small retrospective cohort studies indicate that this thermal treatment appears to be at least as effective as photodynamic therapy in palliation of the tumor by relieving jaundice [15, 16]. Lesions including intraductal pancreatic mucinous neoplasia and neuroendocrine tumors have been treated with RFA with reported success [17].

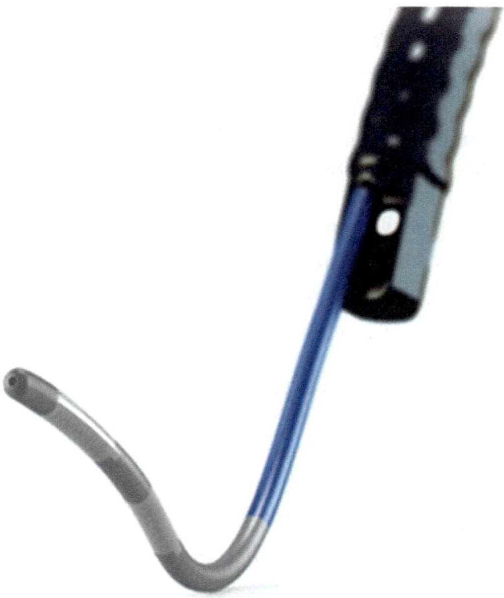

Fig. 16.5 This is a cartoon of a radiofrequency probe that can be passed through a duodenoscope with a channel diameter of at least 3.2 mm. The probe itself is 8 Fr in dimeter and can be used to treat a 8-mm length tumor with a single application

References

1. Sharma VK, Wang KK, Overholt BF, et al. Balloon-based, circumferential, endoscopic radiofrequency ablation of Barrett's esophagus: 1-year follow-up of 100 patients.[see comment]. Gastrointest Endosc. 2007;65:185–95.
2. van Vilsteren FG, Alvarez Herrero L, Pouw RE, et al. Radiofrequency ablation and endoscopic resection in a single session for Barrett's esophagus containing early neoplasia: a feasibility study. Endoscopy. 2012;44:1096–104.
3. van Vilsteren FG, Pouw RE, Seewald S, et al. Stepwise radical endoscopic resection versus radiofrequency ablation for Barrett's oesophagus with high-grade dysplasia or early cancer: a multicentre randomised trial. Gut. 2011;60:765–73.
4. Dulai PS, Pohl H, Levenick JM, Gordon SR, MacKenzie TA, Rothstein RI. Radiofrequency ablation for long-and ultralong-segment Barrett's esophagus: a comparative long-term follow-up study. Gastrointest Endosc. 2013;77:534–41.
5. Sharma VK, Wang KK, Overholt BF, et al. Balloon-based, circumferential, endoscopic radiofrequency ablation of Barrett's esophagus: 1-year follow-up of 100 patients. Gastrointest Endosc. 2007;65:185–95.
6. Shaheen NJ, Sharma P, Overholt BF, et al. Radiofrequency ablation in Barrett's esophagus with dysplasia. N Engl J Med. 2009;360:2277–88.
7. Duits LC, Phoa KN, Curvers WL, et al. Barrett's oesophagus patients with low-grade dysplasia can be accurately risk-stratified after histological review by an expert pathology panel. Gut. 2015;64:700–6.
8. Mitlyng BL, Leon S, Ganz RA. Esophageal adenocarcinoma in Barrett's esophagus with low-grade dysplasia. Gastrointest Endosc. 2015;81:484.
9. Thota PN, Lee H-J, Goldblum JR, et al. Risk stratification of patients with Barrett's esophagus and low-grade dysplasia or indefinite for dysplasia. Clin Gastroenterol Hepatol. 2015;13:459–65.e1.
10. Kahn A, Al-Qaisi M, Kommineni V, et al. Longitudinal outcomes of radiofrequency ablation versus surveillance endoscopy for Barrett's esophagus with low-grade dysplasia. Dis Esophagus. 2018;31(4).
11. Small AJ, Araujo JL, Leggett CL, et al. Radiofrequency ablation is associated with decreased neoplastic progression in patients with Barrett's esophagus and confirmed low-grade dysplasia. Gastroenterology. 2015;149:567–576.e3; quiz e13–4.
12. McGorisk T, Krishnan K, Keefer L, Komanduri S. Radiofrequency ablation for refractory gastric antral vascular ectasia (with video). Gastrointest Endosc. 2013;78:584–8.
13. Dray X, Repici A, Gonzalez P, et al. Radiofrequency ablation for the treatment of gastric antral vascular ectasia. Endoscopy. 2014;46:963–9.
14. Carrafiello G, Lagana D, Cotta E, et al. Radiofrequency ablation of intrahepatic cholangiocarcinoma: preliminary experience. Cardiovasc Intervent Radiol. 2010;33:835–9.
15. Strand DS, Cosgrove ND, Patrie JT, et al. ERCP-directed radiofrequency ablation and photodynamic therapy are associated with comparable survival in the treatment of unresectable cholangiocarcinoma. Gastrointest Endosc. 2014;80:794–804.
16. Schmidt A, Bloechinger M, Weber A, et al. Short-term effects and adverse events of endoscopically applied radiofrequency ablation appear to be comparable with photodynamic therapy in hilar cholangiocarcinoma. United European Gastroenterol J. 2016;4:570–9.
17. Barthet M, Giovannini M, Lesavre N. UEG week 2017 oral presentations-OP 315: EUS-guided radiofrequency ablation (RFA) for pancreatic neuroendocrine tumor (NET) and pre-malignant intraductal pancreatic mucinous tumor (IPMN): first results of prospective multicenter study. United European Gastroenterol J. 2017;5:A1–A160.

Peroral Endoscopic Myotomy

17

Xiaocen Zhang, Rani J. Modayil,
and Stavros N. Stavropoulos

17.1 Introduction

Idiopathic achalasia is an esophageal motility disorder that has an annual incidence of roughly 1 in 100,000 and a prevalence of about 10 in 100,000 [1]. It is thought to be caused by a loss of inhibitory ganglion cells in the myenteric plexus of the esophagus, characterized by failure of the lower esophageal sphincter (LES) to relax and aperistalsis of the esophageal body [2]. Currently there is no treatment that can reverse the loss of the neurons, and all treatments are palliative in nature, aiming to weaken the LES and thus allow passive emptying of the esophagus by gravity and relieve the usual symptoms of dysphagia, regurgitation, and chest pain. The classic treatments for achalasia, forceful dilation, and surgical myotomy have been performed for over 100 years [3, 4] and have robust efficacy data. An attempt at performing a myotomy endoscopically was first reported in a 1980 publication by three Venezuela gastroenterologists [5]. They described using a self-made needle knife to cut the LES in a retrograde fashion first in a dog model and then in 17 patients. A reduction of LES pressure and relief of symptoms were seen in all 17 patients and there was no adverse event. There was no further publication on this technique possibly due to concerns regarding the risk of perforation and leak. Interest in endoscopic myotomy was revived with the emergence of the NOTES (Natural Orifice Transluminal Endoscopic Surgery) concept in the early 2000s. In 2007 two publications from the USA reported use of a submucosal tunnel technique to perform mediastinoscopy [6] and esophageal myotomy [7], in pigs. In 2010 Inoue published his landmark study on endoscopic myotomy using this submucosal tunnel technique in

X. Zhang
Department of Medicine, Mount Sinai St Luke's-West Hospital Center, New York, NY, USA

R. J. Modayil · S. N. Stavropoulos (✉)
Division of Gastroenterology, Hepatology and Nutrition, NYU-Winthrop Hospital, Mineola, NY, USA

P. Sharma, N. Reddy (eds.), *Innovations in Gastrointestinal Endoscopy*,
https://doi.org/10.1007/978-981-15-9247-8_17

17 achalasia patients and coined the now established name for this procedure, Peroral Endoscopic Myotomy (POEM) [8]. This study re-invigorated the languishing NOTES field spurring development of a host of "New-NOTES" "third-space endoscopy" procedures, where endoscopists venture out of the gastrointestinal lumen but stay in close proximity to the GI wall (unlike the ambitious long-range excursions in the abdominal cavity and organ resections envisioned in the early NOTES era). The procedure was rapidly adopted by gastroenterologists and surgeons worldwide. In 2010, our group (Winthrop University Hospital, USA) reported the first POEM case in the West performed in October of 2009 [9]. To date, there are an estimated >6000 POEMs performed worldwide. Despite early data reporting outstanding POEM outcomes on prospective series from pioneers and early adopters, various technical aspects, applications in special populations, comparison with dilation or surgical myotomy, and post-POEM acid reflux, a crucial concern, are still short on high-quality evidence and some fine-tuning is probably needed to achieve the best possible outcomes for this versatile, non-invasive NOTES evolution of the Heller myotomy. In this chapter we will address some of these issues in addition to reviewing the status of POEM.

17.2 Poem Technique [Fig. 17.1]

POEM achieves a surgical myotomy in an innovative way by creating a working space in the submucosa and preserving the mucosal layer to achieve easy and secure closure. The small mucosal incision that allows endoscope entry into the submucosal space is sealed securely at the end of the procedure achieving secure closure and minimizing any risk of leakage of luminal contents into the mediastinum. The steps of POEM are well described in the literature and include (1) mucosa incision, (2) submucosal tunneling, (3) myotomy, and (4) mucosa closure. The International Per Oral Endoscopic Myotomy Survey (IPOEMS) [11] conducted as part of the 2012 NOSCAR meeting took a "snapshot" of the practice of 16 pioneer centers and highlighted a few technical variations which are still under debate today.

17.2.1 Short vs. Long Myotomy

Conventionally myotomy is carried out for a total of 6–8 cm including at least 1.5–2 cm on the gastric cardia in Heller myotomy [12, 13]. Extended gastric myotomy up to 3 cm was proposed by some groups based on the observation that incomplete cardiomyotomy was a common reason for treatment failure [14, 15]. Incomplete esophageal myotomy, in comparison, is rarely the cause of treatment failure [16], and the optimal length of myotomy on the esophageal side is unknown. We should also bear in mind that the majority of the surgical myotomy studies were performed prior to the advent of high-resolution manometry (HRM) when achalasia was broadly categorized as "vigorous" vs. "non-vigorous," which by today's knowledge does not correlate to distinctive disease entities [17]. Based on HRM and the

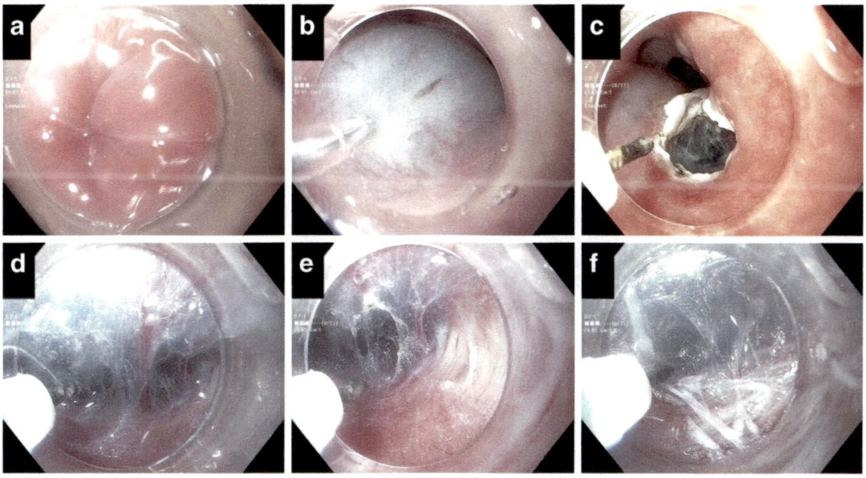

Fig. 17.1 Current Winthrop POEM technique. (**a**) Tight EGJ with the classic "puckered" appearance seen in untreated achalasia patients. (**b**) Submucosal injection to expand the submucosal space. A posterior location at approximately 5 o' clock as shown here is our preferred orientation. (**c**) Mucosal incision allowing endoscope entry into the submucosal space. Creation of a small orifice as shown here allows for better insufflation control within the tunnel and easier tunnel closure at the end of the procedure. (**d**) Submucosal tunnel dissection. Here a multifunction knife (I-Type, Hybrid knife, ERBE, Tubingen, Germany) is used that can inject saline to expand the submucosal space ahead of the dissection front in addition to its electrosurgical dissecting function. The knife is also used to coagulate small vessels as shown here (whereas a coagulation forceps—not shown—is used for larger vessels). Two small penetrating vessels are seen that can be identified as small arteries (rather than veins) based on their pale appearance and thicker wall appreciated as thin white borders. (**e**) Post coagulation appearance of the medial of the two arteries shown in image **d**. Coagulation was affected with the side of the knife using pulses of forced coagulation current. The circular muscle fibers of the muscular layer can be easily appreciated at the 5–6 o' clock position within the tunnel (consistent with a posterior POEM 5 o' clock orientation, our preferred approach). (**f**) Aberrant longitudinal muscle fibers that span a few centimeters in length and originate from and insert into the circular muscle layer represent one of the identifiers of the EGJ. (**g**) The so-called spindle veins on the surface of the muscle represent another identifier of the EGJ that is seen in the majority of cases. (**h**) The double endoscope transillumination technique permits definitive confirmation of tunnel extension into the cardia. The light of the dissecting gastroscope positioned at the tunnel terminus can be seen by a retroflexed slim endoscope inserted alongside the gastroscope and positioned in the proximal stomach thus confirming that the tunnel has been extended to the cardia. (**i**) Myotomy. A full-thickness myotomy, as demonstrated here, is our preferred technique. (**j**) Closure of the tunnel entry orifice by endoscopic suturing using the Overstitch device (Apollo Endosurgery, Austin, Texas) is our preferred closure technique as this appears to be a more secure type of closure and is also cost-effective in regard to clip closure based on US pricing and our relative closure times. (A more detailed discussion of such comparative closure technique data is beyond the scope of this general review but can be found elsewhere [10]). We suture in a transverse rather than longitudinal direction to minimize luminal narrowing. Furthermore, in this patient, due to the unusually small caliber of the esophagus, three interrupted sutures were used to further minimize narrowing of the lumen (rather than our customary single-running-suture technique used in the majority of POEM patients that have a dilated esophagus). (**k**) Post-POEM patulous EGJ appearance confirming successful myotomy (compared to pre-POEM "puckered" appearance in image **a**)

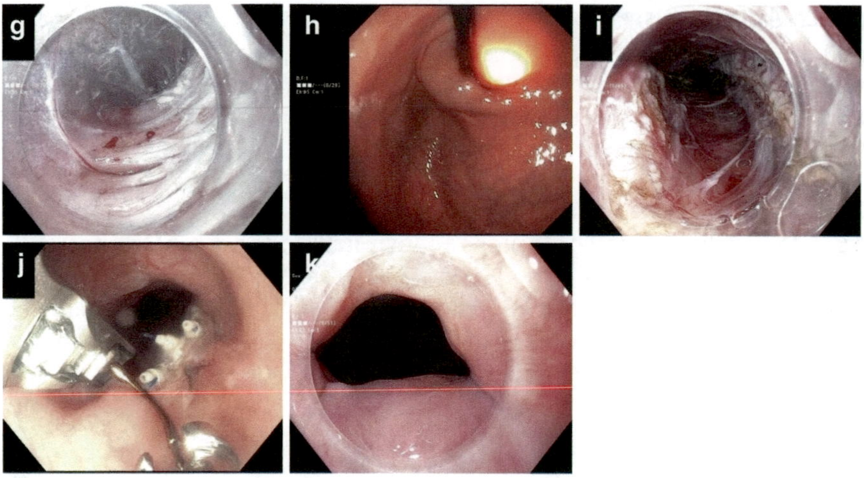

Fig. 17.1 (continued)

Chicago Classification [18], there are three subtypes of achalasia, characterized by distinctive esophageal body motility patterns (type I—absent contractility; type II—pan-esophageal pressurization; type III—spastic contraction). We now know that type III achalasia responds to treatment quite differently from type I and II [19–21], and a longer myotomy is often needed to achieve satisfactory symptom relief [22, 23], possibly by cutting the long spastic muscle segment in the distal esophagus. For type I and II achalasia, in contrast, many investigators now believe a short myotomy (4–5 cm) on the esophageal side is sufficient for most patients [24, 25]. This conjecture is based on the manometry finding that the LES itself is rather short (around ~3 to 4 cm) [26] and in type I or II patient there is no hypercontractile or obstructive segment above the LES. It is also backed by the fact that dilation, which disrupts only the LES, has a markedly higher success rate in type II and type I patients than in type III patients (96% and 75% for type II and type I, respectively, vs. 48% for type III patients after 5 years according to the recent European achalasia trial [20]). Three ongoing randomized controlled trials (RCT) from India (NCT03186248), Italy (NCT03450928), and China (NCT03012854) are investigating short vs. long myotomy (6 vs. 3 cm on the esophageal side in the Indian study, 9 vs. 4 cm in the Italian study, >5 vs. <5 cm in the Chinese study). The former two studies chose 3 cm gastric myotomy and the third chose 2 cm. The merits of a short myotomy are obvious: faster operation, less trauma, and less disruption to the wall of the non-obstructive portion of the esophagus which will minimize the risk of luminal dilation, formation of diverticula and potential abrogation of any regained peristaltic activity which is often observed after the functional obstruction is relieved [27]. There is no trial comparing short (1.5–2 cm) vs. long (3 cm) myotomy on the gastric side currently, which may be an important consideration as POEM practitioners are attempting to decrease the rate of post-POEM reflux while not sacrificing POEM efficacy.

17.2.2 Anterior vs. Posterior Myotomy

Orientation of myotomy is another hotly debated area in POEM. Anterior myotomy at 2 o'clock toward the lesser curvature was used by Inoue in the first POEM publication [8]. Fourteen out of the 16 pioneer centers surveyed by IPOEMS followed suit and favored anterior myotomy (between 11 and 3 o'clock). Only two centers (Zhongshan from Shanghai and Winthrop from Mineola) favored posterior myotomy at 5 o'clock at that time [11]. Various theoretical pros and cons have been proposed for each approach. Anterior myotomy avoids cutting the sling fibers, a natural barrier for reflux, and thus has the theoretical benefit of causing less reflux. However, it is technically more cumbersome because of the acute tip angulation required to hook the muscle fibers during the myotomy and the unstable endoscope positioning [28]. Proximity to the pericardium probably adds to the risk of anterior myotomy, and three cases of pericardial injury leading to shock, cardiac arrest, and/or leakage into the pericardium have been reported [29–31]. Pneumopericardium not leading to hemodynamic compromise but requiring temporary arrest of the procedure in a high volume center that does POEM under fluoroscopy has also been reported, indicating that pneumopericardium occurs more frequently than is appreciated [32]. Posterior myotomy avoids dissection near the pericardium and allows more stable endoscope positioning. In addition, the spine acts as a useful landmark for orientation especially in patients with severe esophageal tortuosity. It should be noted that in certain situations the choice of the site of myotomy is limited by prior surgical changes, scars, diverticula, mucosal ulcers, or severe esophageal angulation. A recent study surveyed 34 POEM practitioners from Asia, Europe, USA, and south America, and showed that there is still a lack of global consensus, with posterior myotomy being the preferred technique for approximately half of the practitioners surveyed [33]. Inoue's group appears to have become a posterior myotomy convert in their recent practice [28]. Four RCTs have been conducted comparing outcomes of anterior vs. posterior myotomy. In the smallest study from India (30 patients in each arm), anterior myotomy was related to a similar rate of GERD symptoms and esophagitis but fewer positive pH study findings (total acid exposure 3% vs 14%; DeMeester score > 14.7 in 16% vs. 37% patients) [34]. These substantial differences in pH metrics that were observed despite the small sample size of this study were not replicated by the other three studies, namely one single-center study from China with also a small sample size of 31 anterior vs. 32 posterior POEM [35], one international multicenter study on 73 anterior vs 77 posterior POEM [36] and one single-center study from the USA on 101 anterior vs. 114 posterior POEM (preliminary results, NCT03228758) [37]. None of the studies identified a difference between the two arms on technical or clinical success rates or clinically significant adverse event (csAE) rates. The largest study (from our center, Winthrop University Hospital) did find anterior myotomy to have a slower myotomy and closure and more accidental mucosotomies (39.6% vs. 17.5%) which is consistent with a less stable endoscope position and a shorter distance of the knife from the mucosa at the EGJ. The slower closure and increased mucosotomies in anterior POEM were also confirmed in the study from India. The largest study from

Winthrop also found less postoperative pain requiring narcotics in anterior POEM (25.7% vs. 50%). In short, current evidence in the literature does not show clear superiority of either approach, but our group views this evidence as favorable for a posterior approach, which is our preferred approach.

17.2.3 Full vs. Partial-Thickness Myotomy

In the recent international survey of 34 practitioners, 13 out of 34 practitioners use full-thickness myotomy [33], compared to only 2 out of 16 centers surveyed in 2012 [11]. The distinction between the two approaches is somewhat artificial since the longitudinal muscle layer of the esophagus is thin and often splits under insufflation or endoscope manipulation, while at the EGJ and cardia the different muscle layers (oblique, circular, and longitudinal) are more intertwined, and it is difficult to preserve any of the outer layers without sacrificing completeness of the myotomy. Proponents of partial myotomy are concerned of exposing the mediastinum and thus causing bacterial translocation or damage to extraluminal structures. In addition, they point to some limited, unconfirmed, low-quality evidence suggesting somewhat less postoperative reflux in patients receiving only circular myotomy [38]. Only two retrospective studies have been done to directly compare full vs. partial thickness myotomy [38, 39]. Li et al. compared 103 full and 131 partial-thickness myotomy and found mean operation time to be shorter for the full-thickness group (41.7 vs. 48.9 min, $p = 0.02$). There was no significant difference in reflux, defined as either GERD symptom or esophagitis on endoscopy (21.2% full vs. 16.5% partial, $p = 0.38$) [39]. A smaller study by Wang et al. examined 56 patients who received both postoperative EGD and 24-h pH studies and ≥3 years follow-up (24 full vs. 32 partial myotomy) and found a higher percentage of clinically relevant GERD, defined as a >5% total reflux time (pH < 4) plus GERD symptoms and/or esophagitis, in patients receiving full-thickness myotomy (37.5% vs. 12.5%, $p = 0.03$) [38]. Neither study found a difference in clinical success or postoperative LES pressure. Proponents of full-thickness myotomy argue that there is no evidence of an increase in csAEs in full-thickness myotomy, while completeness of myotomy is essential to long-term POEM success. There is some evidence of better postoperative esophageal emptying on patients receiving full-thickness myotomy [40]. Furthermore, any concerns regarding full-thickness myotomy leading to more adverse events appear unsubstantiated. Large-scale studies published by centers that have routinely performed full-thickness myotomy since early on reported very low incidence of csAEs (3.3% by Zhongshan, Shanghai, which came down to ~1% after 3.5 years [41]; ~1% by Winthrop, Mineola [42]), in line with data from centers that routinely perform selective circular myotomy (1.7% moderate and 0.8% severe adverse events in an international survey [43]). One ongoing RCT from China (NCT03012854) is comparing both long vs. short myotomy and full vs. partial-thickness myotomy using a parallel design.

17.2.4 Confirming Adequate Dissection on the Gastric Cardia

Adequate dissection on the cardia is essential for POEM success. A variety of indicators have been used to determine extension of the tunnel onto the cardia: (1) endoscopic measurements; (2) narrowing of the submucosal space at the GEJ with resistance to endoscope insertion followed by prompt expansion of the submucosal space in the cardia; (3) slender palisading vessels along the mucosal flap, indicating the distal-most aspect of the esophagus; (4) spindle-like veins on the surface of the muscularis propria and overall increased vascularity on the gastric cardia (see Fig. 17.1g); (5) large-caliber arborizing, perforating vessels in the cardia, usually branches of the left gastric artery; (6) aberrant inner longitudinal muscle bundles at the GEJ originating from circular muscle fibers and inserting into circular muscle fibers after a short course of 2–3 cm (see Fig. 17.1f); and (7) visualization of a blue hue on intraluminal inspection of the mucosa of the cardia (due to the dye in the injection fluid) [44]. Recently Tanaka et al. proposed a novel indicator for the proper distal end of myotomy, the two penetrating vessels (TPVs) [45]. TPV is essentially the same as indicator [5] above, but the concept was much expanded under the very close observation of the authors. "*When making submucosal tunnel in the 5 o'clock direction...two vessels penetrating through the circular muscle along the edge of oblique muscle in the cardia can be exposed...The myotomy was extended until the second TPVs was exposed.*" In their publication, TPVs was found in 34 (91.2%) out of 37 patients who underwent myotomy at 5 o'clock, indicating TPVs (branches of the left gastric artery) to be a reliable landmark at the gastric cardia. Furthermore, using the double scope technique (see below), sufficient submucosal tunneling on the gastric side was confirmed, with a median gastric myotomy of 3 cm (range 2–4 cm).

Apart from these visual indicators, methods of verifying adequate gastric dissection using auxiliary techniques have been proposed [1]. The "double-scope" transillumination technique (see Fig. 17.1h). Initially described by Baldaque-Silva et al., this technique involves insertion of an ultrathin endoscope transnasally parallel to the orally inserted gastroscope. The ultrathin scope is advanced to the level of the stomach and placed in the retroflexed position with visualization of the cardia while the gastroscope is kept within the tunnel with its tip at the tunnel terminus. The light intensity of the thin endoscope is diminished, and the light from the gastroscope within the submucosal tunnel is identified, thereby confirming its position in the cardia [2, 46]. Fluoroscopy guidance. Kumbhari et al. reported placing markers (hemolip or needle on the skin) at the gastroesophageal junction (GEJ) level to accurately assess placement of the myotomy [47]. Ramchandani et al., meanwhile, used guidewire and fluoroscopy for proper orientation in patients with sigmoid esophagus [48]. Despite studies showing extension of myotomy in 34% [49] and 21% [47] of patients using the double-scope and fluoroscopy methods, respectively, the studies did not demonstrate a difference of clinical outcomes, raising questions on the utility of these auxiliary techniques in routine, uncomplicated cases.

A relatively new tool for endoscopists, impedance planimetry (EndoFLIP, Crospon Ltd., Galway, Ireland), has gained popularity in recent years. Compared to

HRM, impedance planimetry is a quick test and does not require patient cooperation, and thus can be done intraoperatively for real-time assessment of esophageal anatomy and function. Increased post-POEM GEJ distensibility comparable to those of healthy volunteers [50] and those of patients post-Heller myotomy [51] has been demonstrated, and some researchers reported using EndoFLIP guidance to achieve adequate LES ablation [52, 53]. Currently there is little evidence regarding the optimal parameter, reference range, or prognostic value for EndoFLIP, and further research is needed to understand the value of this tool in POEM and in achalasia patients [54].

17.3 Poem Outcomes

17.3.1 Therapeutic Success

With the first reported POEM series as recently as 2010, long-term outcomes for POEM are still limited, and only a few centers (Yokohama [55], Europe/US three-center [56], Hyderabad [32], Hangzhou [57], Shanghai [58], Portland [59], Prague [60], Mineola [61]) have published their outcomes beyond 2 years (Table 17.1). In the larger cohorts, the percentage of patients who were followed for over 3 years are relatively small (number of patients that were followed for 3 years: Yokohama—61, Hyderabad—51, Shanghai—237, Prague—44, Mineola—142). Loss-to-follow-up is frequent in most of the large studies from Asia. Acquiring long-term follow-up for POEM patients often proves to be difficult since achalasia is a benign disease, and

Table 17.1 POEM cohorts reporting longitudinal outcomes beyond 3 years

Center	Publication	Total cohort size	Year 1	Year 2	Year 3	Year 4	Year 5
Yokohama	Inoue, J Am Coll Surg 2015	500	91%		88.5%	NA	NA
Hamburg, Portland, Rome	Werner, Gut 2016	80	88.5%		78.5%	NA	NA
Hyderabad	Nabi, EIO 2017	408	94%	91%	90%	NA	NA
Hangzhou	He, Dig Dis Sci 2018	115	91.3%	90.3%	89.0%	83.7%	80.1%
Shanghai	Li, GIE 2018	564	94.2%	92.2%	91.1%	88.6%	87.1%
Portland	Teitelbaum, Surg Endosc 2018	36[a]	NA	NA	NA	NA	83%
Prague	Rabekova, ESGE Days 2018	223	99%	94%	93%	NA	NA
Mineola	Stavropoulos, DDW 2018	417	94%	93%	93%	92%	90%

[a]The total cohort size was not given in this publication. Number represents patients at least 5 years out of their POEM

the procedure is mostly done in highly specialized centers that are not necessarily the regular site of care for these patients or even geographically close to the patient.

Studies which presented data with "median follow-up" without success rate at specific times are not listed, nor are studies which did not take into account effect of censored data or studies which included only particular patient populations.

All centers reported a 3-year success rate at least in the high 80%, apart from the Hamburg/Portland/Rome study which reported a 3-year success rate of 78.5%. The authors attributed the more modest result to a learning curve effect since 8 out of the 17 failures occurred in the first 10 patients from each of the 3 centers [56]. Four centers have published their 5-year data, showing a success rate of 80–90%, comparable to or higher than that of Heller myotomy [62–65] and higher than that of dilation [62, 65–67]. The most recent Kaplan Meier efficacy data from our series exceeding 500 patients and spanning a 9-year period, the largest single operator POEM series in the USA are shown in Fig. 17.2. Clinical success and 95% CIs at 1, 2, 3, 4, and 5 years were 99% (98–99.97%), 98% (97–99.7%), 96% (94–99%), 94% (90–97%), and 90% (85–95%), respectively. It should be noted that unlike other large series from Asia, our lost-to-follow-up rate is very low ranging from 8 to 14% at various time points despite the long 9-year study period and the fact that 30% of our patients are from distant geographic locales (out-of-state or international). Consequently the Kaplan Meier success estimates provided are very reliable with narrow confidence intervals (CIs).

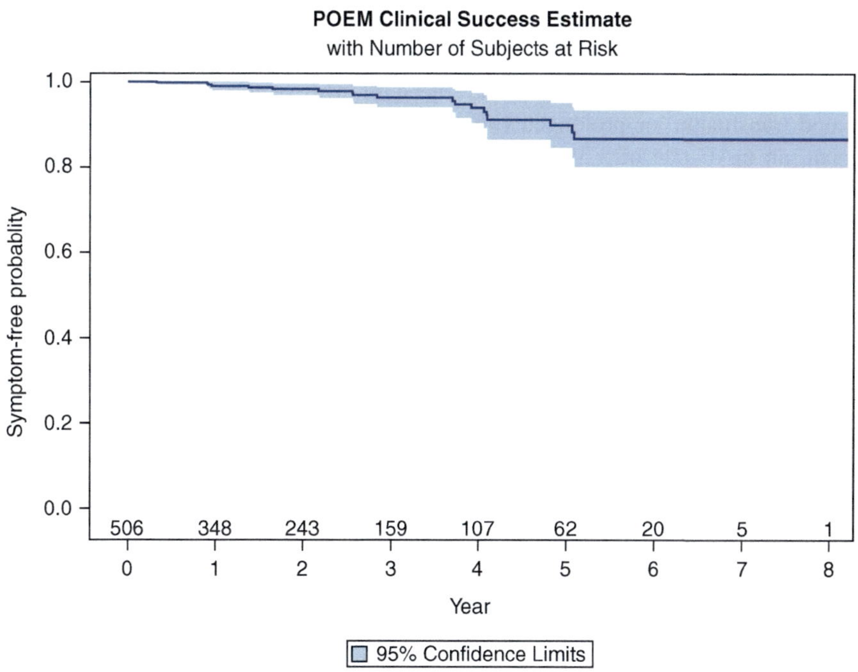

Fig. 17.2 Kaplan Meier clinical success curve of Winthrop POEM series

A trend for slow decrease in therapeutic success is seen with POEM as is the case for any other achalasia treatment including Heller myotomy [68]. However, as noted above the efficacy of POEM remains outstanding in mid-term and emerging long-term data. Admittedly these are data from high-volume centers, which tend to have better outcomes. However, the procedure itself is also evolving and improving, with a more personalized treatment approach being used which may potentially further improve outcomes in the future (e.g., longer myotomy for patients with type III achalasia [22]; new methods of identifying adequate gastric dissection [45] and preventing reflux [69]). Apart from its overall success, POEM has also demonstrated excellent efficacy in specialized groups such as achalasia patients of all ages [70–75], those with prior endoscopic and surgical interventions [42, 76–86], sigmoid esophagus [87, 88], type III achalasia [22, 23, 89] (which responds poorly to both Heller myotomy and pneumatic dilation) and spastic esophageal motility disorders [90].

17.3.2 Perioperative Adverse Events (AEs)

Procedure safety has been a major concern in the early days of POEM. The Shanghai center which used air insufflation in their early cases reported a staggering rate of gas-related AEs in the initial 119 cases, including 25.2% pneumothorax, 55.5% subcutaneous emphysema, and 49.7% pleural effusion [91]. These events later proved to be rare, mild and largely inconsequential or entirely avoidable if CO_2 insufflation is used. In their later study which focused exclusively on "major adverse events" (mAEs), defined as vital-sign instability, intensive care unit (ICU) stay, hospital readmission, conversion to surgery, need for invasive postoperative procedures, blood transfusion, or prolonged (>5 days) hospitalization for functional impairment, an mAE rate of 3.3% (55/1680 patients) including 0.8% delayed mucosa barrier failure and 0.2% delayed bleeding was reported. There were no surgical conversions or deaths [41]. The Hamburg center, meanwhile, reported three (1.2%) severe procedural-related AEs, namely one case of pneumothorax requiring intra-procedural drainage, one ischemic gastric cardia perforation requiring esophagectomy, and one hemothorax requiring surgery [92]. One study pooling data from 11 centers reported 0.5% severe, 1.7% moderate, and 6.4% mild AEs based on the ASGE lexicon [43], but given the large number of centers aggregating data that were not centrally vetted or collected via a prospective multicenter protocol, under-reporting is a significant concern. Also at issue is the reporting system used (the ASGE Lexicon) which was developed for traditional advanced endoscopic procedures rather than endo-surgical procedures. For example, five pneumothoraxes requiring chest tubes, six delayed esophageal leaks at 48 hours, and one esophageal perforation, all of which required interventions with clipping, stent, and/or vacuum therapy, were counted as "moderate AEs" in this multicenter trial. In most of the other trials discussed, these events would have been included in the "clinically significant" or "major adverse event" rate reported, given their severity and the invasiveness of the interventions that were required to treat them. The lack of widely adopted consensus on how to report AEs for POEM makes comparison between studies difficult unless one reviews the individual reported AEs themselves. Nevertheless, the data from the different centers is consistent in that clinical significant AEs are rare for POEM (including AEs that lead to severe hemodynamic/cardiopulmonary compromise, require interventional procedures to correct or cause irreversible sequelae). Only one death directly related to POEM has been reported (intraoperative PEA arrest secondary to severe coronary artery disease and pulmonary hypertension unrecognized preoperatively [60]) implying an operative mortality of ~1/5000 (0.02%) or so based on current published series reporting on AEs. In comparison, laparoscopic Heller myotomy, according to a query on 1237 procedures registered between 2005 and 2011 in the US National Surgical Quality Improvement Program database, has a major complication rate of 2.3%, reoperation rate of 2.3%, and death rate of 0.03% [93]. A systematic review on 6834 Heller myotomies reported in 48 studies showed a postoperative perforation rate to be 0.37% (akin to delayed mucosa barrier failure/leak for POEM) and 30-day mortality rate of 0.15% [94]. Overall, POEM has a csAE rate in line with that of Heller myotomy (in the order of 1–3%) [41–43, 55, 56], the most serious one probably being delayed esophageal leak. Delayed bleeding, anesthesia AEs, postoperative cardiopulmonary events (pneumonia, pulmonary embolism, arrhythmia, acute coronary syndrome, etc.), certain insufflation-related AEs requiring emergent decompression (tension pneumothorax, pneumopericardium, etc.) have all been reported, but infrequently and more often in the early cases where the operator is still within the learning curve.

17.4 Gastroesophageal Reflux After Poem

A concern with POEM is that unlike laparoscopic Heller myotomy with fundoplication, there is no concomitant anti-reflux procedure. It is now apparent that GERD is common after POEM with symptoms in 15–28%, esophagitis in 20–48%, and positive pH studies in 38–58% in western populations [61, 95–98] (Table 17.2).

Table 17.2 Major Western POEM studied with data on both follow-up endoscopy and pH study

Center	Publication	Total cohort size	GERD symptoms	Erosive esophagitis	Positive pH study
Portland	Sharata, J Gastrointesti Surg 2015	100	12/100 (15%)	20/73 (27%)	26/68 (38%)
Chicago	Hungness, Ann Surg 2016	115	31/111 (28%)	17/68 (25%)	10/22 (45%)
Rome	Familiari, Dig Endosc 2016	103	19/103 (18%)	21/103 (20%)	52/103 (50%)
Prague	Martinek, Surg Endo 2017	132	28/111 (25%)	41/109 (38%)	39/94 (42%)
Mineola	Stavropoulos, DDW 2018	417	112/414 (27%)	109/226(48%)	114/209 (55%)

Appraising GERD in achalasia patients can be complicated since GERD and achalasia can have overlapping symptoms, and there is a significant discordance between subjective symptoms and objective testing. This phenomenon is well demonstrated by the recent meta-analysis by Repici et al. [99], which showed postoperative GERD symptoms in 19% of POEM patients vs. 9% of Heller patients, but positive pH testing in 39% of POEM vs. 17% of Heller patients. When interpreting a pH study for achalasia patients, a careful visual examination of the curve is needed since prolonged modestly decreased pH plateaus can occur secondary to slow clearance, stasis, and fermentation even after a single reflux episode [100, 101], leading to a falsely high DeMeester score and total acid exposure time. Crookes et al. suggested distinguishing "a slow steady drift to pH below 4" (a marker for food fermentation) and "multiple sharp dips to pH nadirs of <3 characteristic of typical reflux." They recommended using a pH threshold of 3 rather than 4 in achalasia patients since such a threshold differentiated well true reflux from prolonged depressed pH plateaus due to poor clearance stasis and fermentation [101]. Another caveat involves assessment of erosive esophagitis in POEM patients. Solitary ulcers at the EGJ in an orientation corresponding to the POEM tunnel may be due to poor healing and/or increased susceptibility to injury of the devascularized mucosa overlying the tunnel and may not constitute evidence of erosive esophagitis secondary to pathologic acid reflux. Considering such ulcers as evidence of reflux esophagitis may overestimate GERD in POEM patients. Endoscopic assessment for GERD should be performed at least 6 months and possibly 12 months post POEM to allow maximal healing and by experienced operators familiar with post POEM tunnel ulcers.

These caveats aside, GERD post-POEM (or surgical myotomy) tends to happen in patients with more complete LES ablation and is in fact a predictor for better dysphagia relief [56]. A trade-off between some modest degree of reflux in return for better dysphagia relief might be necessary. This is also supported by data such as those from a prospective non-randomized study by the Portland group comparing 37 POEM with 64 Heller patients (42% with Toupet and 58% with Dor fundoplication) that found a trend for more abnormal acid exposure in POEM patients (39% vs. 32%, $p = 0.7$), and also superior achalasia symptom relief (dysphagia to solids, 32% vs. 62%, $p = 0.06$; Eckardt score at 6 months 1.2 vs. 1.7, $p = 0.7$) [102].

Numerous studies have been conducted comparing POEM with Heller retrospectively. Caution should be used when interpreting these studies. Some consist of systematic reviews or meta-analyses that suffer from methodological flaws such as inclusion of poor quality studies and lack of assessment of publication bias [103]. Other single-center studies compare POEM and Heller procedures done in different periods, and there is often no unified protocol for patient follow-up or outcome appraisal. For example, a recent case–control study that compared POEM and Heller patients from a single center matched for age, gender, BMI, and achalasia type showed markedly higher esophageal acid exposure in POEM patients compared to Heller patients (48.4% vs. 13.6%). A critical look at these data, however, reveals that only 47% of POEM patients versus 95% of Heller patients received pH testing, raising concerns regarding patient selection bias. One could reasonably assume that POEM patients with GERD would be much more likely to be among the less than half of the POEM patients that received pH testing, whereas such patient selection bias would not be present in Heller patients where the vast majority (95%) received pH testing. On close inspection, other issues raising concerns were also evident. One-third of patients in the POEM group had a prior Heller compared to none in the Heller group. Heller patients with recurrent or persistent symptoms are a much more complex group. Furthermore, these patients essentially received a double myotomy (anterior Heller + posterior POEM) and obviously, even if the prior Heller myotomy was not entirely adequate, as a group they would be expected to have lower LES pressures and be at a higher risk for reflux. Finally, it is notable that no dysphagia relief data were provided for either group. If one is to argue that much lower GERD is seen after Heller and fundoplication than after POEM, it is essential to provide evidence that this is not accomplished at the expense of poorer dysphagia relief because of a tight fundoplication. The presence of regurgitation in 10% of the Heller patients but none of the POEM patients in this study raises concerns in that regard [104]. In addition, it should be pointed out here that the Dor or Toupet "loose" fundoplication performed in achalasia patients might be reasonably expected to have only modest long-term efficacy. High-quality studies from expert LHM centers have shown abnormal acid exposure rates in 18–42% of patients after LHM with fundoplication [105–107], rates not too dissimilar to those after POEM, but these rates are generally determined within a year of the fundoplication. Long-term data are limited but do suggest decreasing fundoplication efficacy with time. For example, in the large European multicenter randomized study comparing laparoscopic Heller with Dor fundoplication to pneumatic dilation, the rate of positive pH studies in LHM pts. increased from 23% at 1 year to 34% at 4 years, whereas in the pneumatic dilation group, pH study positivity actually decreased slightly from 15 to 12% [20, 108]. One would expect that GERD after POEM, similarly to pneumatic dilation, would also not change significantly or even slightly improve with time as the myotomy heals and remodels. In contrast, fundoplication, especially the loose fundoplication performed in achalasia patients, would be expected to loosen with time as suggested by the increase in pH study positivity in the long-term randomized trial discussed above. In another study that assessed GERD outcomes at 6 years after Heller + Toupet fundoplication, 33/51 patients (65%) were on acid suppression at that time [109]. Therefore, any modest advantage of LHM + fundoplication over POEM with respect to GERD may be associated with somewhat inferior efficacy in dysphagia relief and may erode with time.

One may reasonably wonder why the rate of GERD after POEM is not substantially greater than that after LHM combined with a fundoplication. The explanation may lie in the lack of hiatal dissection during POEM compared to extensive dissection of the hiatus during a standard LHM. This extensive dissection disrupts important "suspensory ligaments" of the esophagus, notably the phrenoesophageal membrane, thought to contribute to the maintenance of the angle of His and to have an important anti-reflux function separate from the intrinsic esophageal "sphincter" itself [110].

17.5 Conclusion

POEM has gained rapid global adoption since its first performance in 2008. It has well-documented excellent short- to mid-term efficacy and perioperative safety data. Ongoing areas of research include long-term (5–10 years) efficacy, appraisal and prevention of postoperative reflux, prospective comparative studies versus Heller myotomy and dilation, and optimal technique refinements (e.g., orientation and length of myotomy, methods to confirm adequate myotomy including cardio-myotomy length, anti-reflux modifications).

References

1. Pandolfino JE, Gawron AJ. Achalasia: a systematic review. JAMA. 2015;313(18):1841–52.
2. Park W, Vaezi MF. Etiology and pathogenesis of achalasia: the current understanding. Am J Gastroenterol. 2005;100(6):1404.
3. Plummer HS. Cardiospasm, with a report of forty cases. J Am Med Assoc. 1908;LI(7):549–54.
4. Heller E. Extramukose Cardioplsstik beim chronischen Cardiospasmus mit Dilatation des Oesophagus. Mitt Grenzgeb Med Chir. 1913;27:141–9.
5. Ortega J, Madureri V, Perez L. Endoscopic myotomy in the treatment of achalasia. Gastrointest Endosc. 1980;26(1):8–10.
6. Sumiyama K, Gostout CJ, Rajan E, Bakken TA, Knipschield MA. Transesophageal mediastinoscopy by submucosal endoscopy with mucosal flap safety valve technique. Gastrointest Endosc. 2007;65(4):679–83.
7. Pasricha PJ, Hawari R, Ahmed I, Chen J, Cotton PB, Hawes RH, et al. Submucosal endoscopic esophageal myotomy: a novel experimental approach for the treatment of achalasia. Endoscopy. 2007;39(9):761–4.
8. Inoue H, Minami H, Kobayashi Y, Sato Y, Kaga M, Suzuki M, et al. Peroral endoscopic myotomy (POEM) for esophageal achalasia. Endoscopy. 2010;42(04):265–71.
9. Stavropoulos SN, Harris MD, Hida S, Brathwaite C, Demetriou C, Grendell J. Endoscopic submucosal myotomy for the treatment of achalasia (with video). Gastrointest Endosc. 2010;72(6):1309–11.
10. Stavropoulos SN, Modayil R, Friedel D. Current applications of endoscopic suturing. World J Gastrointest Endosc. 2015;7(8):777.
11. Stavropoulos SN, Modayil RJ, Friedel D, Savides T. The international per oral endoscopic myotomy survey (IPOEMS): a snapshot of the global POEM experience. Surg Endosc. 2013;27(9):3322–38.
12. Gockel I, Junginger T, Eckardt VF. Long-term results of conventional myotomy in patients with achalasia: a prospective 20-year analysis. J Gastrointest Surg. 2006;10(10):1400–8.
13. Costantini M, Salvador R, Capovilla G, Vallese L, Costantini A, Nicoletti L, et al. A thousand and one laparoscopic Heller myotomies for esophageal achalasia: a 25-year experience at a single tertiary center. J Gastrointest Surg. 2019;23(1):23–35.
14. Oelschlager BK, Chang L, Pellegrini CA. Improved outcome after extended gastric myotomy for achalasia. Arch Surg. 2003;138(5):490–7.
15. Wright AS, Williams CW, Pellegrini CA, Oelschlager BK. Long-term outcomes confirm the superior efficacy of extended Heller myotomy with Toupet fundoplication for achalasia. Surg Endosc. 2007;21(5):713–8.
16. Zaninotto G, Costantini M, Portale G, Battaglia G, Molena D, Carta A, et al. Etiology, diagnosis, and treatment of failures after laparoscopic Heller myotomy for achalasia. Ann Surg. 2002;235(2):186–92.

17. Pandolfino JE, Kwiatek MA, Nealis T, Bulsiewicz W, Post J, Kahrilas PJ. Achalasia: a new clinically relevant classification by high-resolution manometry. Gastroenterology. 2008;135(5):1526–33.
18. Kahrilas PJ, Bredenoord A, Fox M, Gyawali C, Roman S, Smout A, et al. The Chicago classification of esophageal motility disorders, v3. 0. Neurogastroenterol Motil. 2015;27(2):160–74.
19. Salvador R, Costantini M, Zaninotto G, Morbin T, Rizzetto C, Zanatta L, et al. The preoperative manometric pattern predicts the outcome of surgical treatment for esophageal achalasia. J Gastrointest Surg. 2010;14(11):1635–45.
20. Moonen A, Annese V, Belmans A, Bredenoord AJ, Bruley des Varannes S, Costantini M, et al. Long-term results of the European achalasia trial: a multicentre randomised controlled trial comparing pneumatic dilation versus laparoscopic Heller myotomy. Gut. 2016;65(5):732–9.
21. Ou YH, Nie XM, Li LF, Wei ZJ, Jiang B. High-resolution manometric subtypes as a predictive factor for the treatment of achalasia: a meta-analysis and systematic review. J Dig Dis. 2016;17(4):222–35.
22. Kane ED, Budhraja V, Desilets DJ, Romanelli JR. Myotomy length informed by high-resolution esophageal manometry (HREM) results in improved per-oral endoscopic myotomy (POEM) outcomes for type III achalasia. Surg Endosc. 2019;33(3):886–94.
23. Kumbhari V, Tieu AH, Onimaru M, El Zein MH, Teitelbaum EN, Ujiki MB, et al. Peroral endoscopic myotomy (POEM) vs laparoscopic Heller myotomy (LHM) for the treatment of Type III achalasia in 75 patients: a multicenter comparative study. Endosc Int Open. 2015;3(3):E195.
24. Stavropoulos SN, Modayil R, Friedel D. Per-oral endoscopic myotomy. NOTES and endoluminal surgery. Springer; 2017. p. 71–85.
25. Li L, Chai N, Linghu E, Li Z, Du C, Zhang W, et al. Safety and efficacy of using a short tunnel versus a standard tunnel for peroral endoscopic myotomy for Ling type IIc and III achalasia: a retrospective study. Surg Endosc. 2019;33(5):1394–402.
26. Pandolfino JE, Ghosh SK, Zhang Q, Jarosz A, Shah N, Kahrilas PJ. Quantifying EGJ morphology and relaxation with high-resolution manometry: a study of 75 asymptomatic volunteers. Am J Physiol Gastrointest Liver Physiol. 2006;290(5):G1033–G40.
27. Roman S, Kahrilas PJ, Mion F, et al. Partial recovery of peristalsis after myotomy for achalasia: more the rule than the exception. JAMA Surg. 2013;148(2):157–64.
28. Bechara R, Onimaru M, Ikeda H, Inoue H. Per-oral endoscopic myotomy, 1000 cases later: pearls, pitfalls, and practical considerations. Gastrointest Endosc. 2016;84(2):330–8.
29. Maher SZ, Chintanaboina J, Kim DE, Mathew A. Pneumopericardium complicating per-oral endoscopic myotomy due to inadvertent use of air instead of carbon dioxide. ACG Case Rep J. 2018;5:e59.
30. Banks-Venegoni AL, Desilets DJ, Romanelli JR, Earle DB. Tension capnopericardium and cardiac arrest as an unexpected adverse event of peroral endoscopic myotomy (with video). Gastrointest Endosc. 2015;82(6):1137–9.
31. Lourdusamy D, Patel S, Thyagarajan B, Gorcey S, Kramer V. Pneumopericardium due to delayed esophageal leak after per oral endoscopic myotomy (POEM). Chest. 2016;150(4):671A.
32. Nabi Z, Ramchandani M, Chavan R, Kalapala R, Darisetty S, Rao GV, et al. Per-oral endoscopic myotomy for achalasia cardia: outcomes in over 400 consecutive patients. Endosc Int Open. 2017;5(5):E331–9.
33. Kaplan JH, Ansari N, Stavropoulos SN, Khashab MA, Duvvur NR, Bapaye A, et al. Tu1162 esophageal peroral endoscopic myotomy: a worldwide survey on institutional practice. Gastrointest Endosc. 2018;87(6, Suppl):AB548–9.
34. Ramchandani M, Nabi Z, Reddy DN, Talele R, Darisetty S, Kotla R, et al. Outcomes of anterior myotomy versus posterior myotomy during POEM: a randomized pilot study. Endosc Int Open. 2018;6(2):E190–8.
35. Tan Y, Lv L, Wang X, Zhu H, Chu Y, Luo M, et al. Efficacy of anterior versus posterior per-oral endoscopic myotomy for treating achalasia: a randomized, prospective study. Gastrointest Endosc. 2018;88(1):46–54.

36. Khashab MA, Sanaei O, Ponchon T, Eleftheriadis N, Yan W, Chiu PW, Shiwaku H, et al. 837 peroral endoscopic myotomy (POEM): anterior versus posterior approach, a randomized single-blinded clinical trial. Gastrointest Endosc. 2018;87(6, Supplement):AB119.
37. Stavropoulos SN, Modayil RJ, Zhang X, Khodorskiy DO, Taylor SI, Kollarus MM, et al. 841 is there a difference in outcomes between anterior and posterior peroral endoscopic myotomy (POEM)? a randomized study from an experienced high-volume operator. Gastrointest Endosc. 2018;87(6):AB121–2.
38. Wang XH, Tan YY, Zhu HY, Li CJ, Liu DL. Full-thickness myotomy is associated with higher rate of postoperative gastroesophageal reflux disease. World J Gastroenterol. 2016;22(42):9419–26.
39. Li Q-L, Chen W-F, Zhou P-H, Yao L-Q, Xu M-D, Hu J-W, et al. Peroral endoscopic myotomy for the treatment of achalasia: a clinical comparative study of endoscopic full-thickness and circular muscle myotomy. J Am Coll Surg. 2013;217(3):442–51.
40. von Renteln D, Inoue H, Minami H, Werner YB, Pace A, Kersten JF, et al. Peroral endoscopic myotomy for the treatment of achalasia: a prospective single center study. Am J Gastroenterol. 2012;107(3):411–7.
41. Zhang XC, Li QL, Xu MD, Chen SY, Zhong YS, Zhang YQ, et al. Major perioperative adverse events of peroral endoscopic myotomy: a systematic 5-year analysis. Endoscopy. 2016;48(11):967–78.
42. Zhang X, Modayil RJ, Friedel D, Gurram KC, Brathwaite CE, Taylor SI, et al. Per-oral endoscopic myotomy in patients with or without prior Heller's myotomy: comparing long-term outcomes in a large U.S. single-center cohort (with videos). Gastrointest Endosc. 2018;87(4):972–85.
43. Haito-Chavez Y, Inoue H, Beard KW, Draganov PV, Ujiki M, Rahden BHA, et al. Comprehensive analysis of adverse events associated with per oral endoscopic myotomy in 1826 patients: an international multicenter study. Am J Gastroenterol. 2017;112:1267.
44. Stavropoulos SN, Desilets DJ, Fuchs K-H, Gostout CJ, Haber G, Inoue H, et al. Per-oral endoscopic myotomy white paper summary. Surg Endosc. 2014;28(7):2005–19.
45. Tanaka S, Kawara F, Toyonaga T, Inoue H, Bechara R, Hoshi N, et al. Two penetrating vessels as a novel indicator of the appropriate distal end of peroral endoscopic myotomy. Dig Endosc. 2018;30(2):206–11.
46. Baldaque-Silva F, Marques M, Vilas-Boas F, Maia JD, Sá F, Macedo G. New transillumination auxiliary technique for peroral endoscopic myotomy. Gastrointest Endosc. 2014;79(4):544–5.
47. Kumbhari V, Besharati S, Abdelgelil A, Tieu AH, Saxena P, El-Zein MH, et al. Intraprocedural fluoroscopy to determine the extent of the cardiomyotomy during per-oral endoscopic myotomy (with video). Gastrointest Endosc. 2015;81(6):1451–6.
48. Ramchandani M, Reddy DN, Darisetty S, Kotla R, Chavan R, Kalpala R, et al. Peroral endoscopic myotomy for achalasia cardia: Treatment analysis and follow up of over 200 consecutive patients at a single center. Dig Endosc. 2016;28(1):19–26.
49. Grimes KL, Inoue H, Onimaru M, Ikeda H, Tansawet A, Bechara R, et al. Double-scope per oral endoscopic myotomy (POEM): a prospective randomized controlled trial. Surg Endosc. 2016;30(4):1344–51.
50. Rieder E, Swanström LL, Perretta S, Lenglinger J, Riegler M, Dunst CM. Intraoperative assessment of esophagogastric junction distensibility during per oral endoscopic myotomy (POEM) for esophageal motility disorders. Surg Endosc. 2013;27(2):400–5.
51. Teitelbaum EN, Boris L, Arafat FO, Nicodème F, Lin Z, Kahrilas PJ, et al. Comparison of esophagogastric junction distensibility changes during POEM and Heller myotomy using intraoperative FLIP. Surg Endosc. 2013;27(12):4547–55.
52. Familiari P, Gigante G, Marchese M, Boskoski I, Bove V, Tringali A, et al. EndoFLIP system for the intraoperative evaluation of peroral endoscopic myotomy. United European Gastroenterol J. 2014;2(2):77–83.

53. Teitelbaum EN, Sternbach JM, El Khoury R, Soper NJ, Pandolfino JE, Kahrilas PJ, et al. The effect of incremental distal gastric myotomy lengths on EGJ distensibility during POEM for achalasia. Surg Endosc. 2016;30(2):745–50.
54. Hirano I, Pandolfino JE, Boeckxstaens GE. Functional lumen imaging probe for the management of esophageal disorders: expert review from the clinical practice updates committee of the AGA institute. Clin Gastroenterol Hepatol. 2017;15(3):325–34.
55. Inoue H, Sato H, Ikeda H, Onimaru M, Sato C, Minami H, et al. Per-oral endoscopic myotomy: a series of 500 patients. J Am Coll Surg. 2015;221(2):256–64.
56. Werner YB, Costamagna G, Swanstrom LL, von Renteln D, Familiari P, Sharata AM, et al. Clinical response to peroral endoscopic myotomy in patients with idiopathic achalasia at a minimum follow-up of 2 years. Gut. 2016;65(6):899–906.
57. He C, Li M, Lu B, Ying X, Gao C, Wang S, et al. Long-term efficacy of peroral endoscopic myotomy for patients with achalasia: outcomes with a median follow-up of 36 months. Dig Dis Sci. 2019;64(3):803–10.
58. Li Q-L, Wu Q-N, Zhang X-C, Xu M-D, Zhang W, Chen S-Y, et al. Outcomes of per-oral endoscopic myotomy for treatment of esophageal achalasia with a median follow-up of 49 months. Gastrointest Endosc. 2018;87(6):1405–12.e3.
59. Teitelbaum EN, Dunst CM, Reavis KM, Sharata AM, Ward MA, DeMeester SR, et al. Clinical outcomes five years after POEM for treatment of primary esophageal motility disorders. Surg Endosc. 2018;32(1):421–7.
60. Rábeková Z, Vacková Z, Lanska V, Spicak J, Hucl T, Štirand P, et al. Long–term results of peroral endoscopic myotomy (POEM) for achalasia. Endoscopy. 2018;50(4):OP129.
61. Stavropoulos SN, Modayil RJ, Zhang X, Khodorskiy DO, Taylor SI, Kollarus MM, et al. Tu1146 per oral endoscopic myotomy (POEM) for achalasia: long term outcomes from a large prospective single-center us series. Gastrointest Endosc. 2018;87(6):AB540–1.
62. Vela MF, Richter JE, Khandwala F, Blackstone EH, Wachsberger D, Baker ME, et al. The long-term efficacy of pneumatic dilatation and Heller myotomy for the treatment of achalasia. Clin Gastroenterol Hepatol. 2006;4(5):580–7.
63. Zaninotto G, Costantini M, Molena D, Buin F, Carta A, Nicoletti L, et al. Treatment of esophageal achalasia with laparoscopic Heller myotomy and Dor partial anterior fundoplication: prospective evaluation of 100 consecutive patients. J Gastrointest Surg. 2000;4(3):282–9.
64. Kilic A, Schuchert MJ, Pennathur A, Gilbert S, Landreneau RJ, Luketich JD. Long-term outcomes of laparoscopic Heller myotomy for achalasia. Surgery. 2009;146(4):826–33.
65. Weber CE, Davis CS, Kramer HJ, Gibbs JT, Robles L, Fisichella PM. Medium and long-term outcomes after pneumatic dilation or laparoscopic Heller myotomy for achalasia: a meta-analysis. Surg Laparosc Endosc Percutan Tech. 2012;22(4):289–96.
66. West R, Hirsch D, Bartelsman J, de Borst J, Ferwerda G, Tytgat G, et al. Long term results of pneumatic dilation in achalasia followed for more than 5 years. Am J Gastroenterol. 2002;97(6):1346.
67. Karamanolis G, Sgouros S, Karatzias G, Papadopoulou E, Vasiliadis K, Stefanidis G, et al. Long-term outcome of pneumatic dilation in the treatment of achalasia. Am J Gastroenterol. 2005;100:270.
68. Vaezi MF, Pandolfino JE, Vela MF. ACG clinical guideline: diagnosis and management of achalasia. Am J Gastroenterol. 2013;108:1238.
69. Tanaka S, Kawara F, Abe H, Ariyoshi R, Watanabe D, Hoshi N, et al. 839 significant reduction of post-operative gastroesophageal reflux development by the posterior myotomy using two penetrating vessels (TPVS) in peroral endoscopic myotomy (POEM). Gastrointest Endosc. 2018;87(6):AB120–1.
70. Miao S, Wu J, Lu J, Wang Y, Tang Z, Zhou Y, et al. Peroral endoscopic myotomy in children with achalasia: a relatively long-term single-center study. J Pediatr Gastroenterol Nutr. 2018;66(2):257–62.
71. Nabi Z, Ramchandani M, Reddy DN, Darisetty S, Kotla R, Kalapala R, et al. Per oral endoscopic myotomy in children with achalasia cardia. J Neurogastroenterol Motil. 2016;22(4):613.

72. Tan Y, Zhu H, Li C, Chu Y, Huo J, Liu D. Comparison of peroral endoscopic myotomy and endoscopic balloon dilation for primary treatment of pediatric achalasia. J Pediatr Surg. 2016;51(10):1613–8.
73. Stavropoulos SN, Sosulski AB, Modayil RJ, Gurram KC, Brathwaite CE, Coren CV, et al. Sa2075 use of peroral endoscopic myotomy (POEM) in pediatric patients as a primary or rescue therapy for achalasia. Gastrointest Endosc. 2017;85(5):AB285–6.
74. Chen W-F, Li Q-L, Zhou P-H, Yao L-Q, Xu M-D, Zhang Y-Q, et al. Long-term outcomes of peroral endoscopic myotomy for achalasia in pediatric patients: a prospective, single-center study. Gastrointest Endosc. 2015;81(1):91–100.
75. Chen Y-I, Inoue H, Ujiki M, Draganov PV, Colavita P, Mion F, et al. An international multicenter study evaluating the clinical efficacy and safety of per-oral endoscopic myotomy in octogenarians. Gastrointest Endosc. 2018;87(4):956–61.
76. Fumagalli U, Rosati R, De Pascale S, Porta M, Carlani E, Pestalozza A, et al. Repeated surgical or endoscopic myotomy for recurrent dysphagia in patients after previous myotomy for achalasia. J Gastrointest Surg. 2016;20(3):494–9.
77. Ngamruengphong S, Inoue H, Ujiki MB, Patel LY, Bapaye A, Desai PN, et al. Efficacy and safety of peroral endoscopic myotomy for treatment of achalasia after failed Heller myotomy. Clin Gastroenterol Hepatol. 2017;15(10):1531–7.e3.
78. Kristensen HØ, Kirkegård J, Kjær DW, Mortensen FV, Kunda R, Bjerregaard NC. Long-term outcome of peroral endoscopic myotomy for esophageal achalasia in patients with previous Heller myotomy. Surg Endosc. 2017;31(6):2596–601.
79. Tyberg A, Sharaiha RZ, Familiari P, Costamagna G, Casas F, Kumta NA, et al. Peroral endoscopic myotomy as salvation technique post-Heller: international experience. Dig Endosc. 2018;30(1):52–6.
80. Nabi Z, Ramchandani M, Chavan R, Tandan M, Kalapala R, Darisetty S, et al. Peroral endoscopic myotomy in treatment-naive achalasia patients versus prior treatment failure cases. Endoscopy. 2018;50(4):358–70.
81. Jones EL, Meara MP, Pittman MR, Hazey JW, Perry KA. Prior treatment does not influence the performance or early outcome of per-oral endoscopic myotomy for achalasia. Surg Endosc. 2016;30(4):1282–6.
82. Orenstein SB, Raigani S, Wu YV, Pauli EM, Phillips MS, Ponsky JL, et al. Peroral endoscopic myotomy (POEM) leads to similar results in patients with and without prior endoscopic or surgical therapy. Surg Endosc. 2015;29(5):1064–70.
83. Louie BE, Schneider AM, Schembre DB, Aye RW. Impact of prior interventions on outcomes during per oral endoscopic myotomy. Surg Endosc. 2017;31(4):1841–8.
84. Sharata A, Kurian AA, Dunst CM, Bhayani NH, Reavis KM, Swanstrom LL. Peroral endoscopic myotomy (POEM) is safe and effective in the setting of prior endoscopic intervention. J Gastrointest Surg. 2013;17(7):1188–92.
85. Liu Z-Q, Li Q-L, Chen W-F, Zhang X-C, Wu Q-N, Cai M-Y, et al. The effect of prior treatment on clinical outcomes in patients with achalasia undergoing peroral endoscopic myotomy. Endoscopy. 2019;51(4):307–16.
86. Onimaru M, Inoue H, Ikeda H, Yoshida A, Santi EG, Sato H, et al. Peroral endoscopic myotomy is a viable option for failed surgical esophagocardiomyotomy instead of redo surgical Heller myotomy: a single center prospective study. J Am Coll Surg. 2013;217(4):598–605.
87. Hu J-W, Li Q-L, Zhou P-H, Yao L-Q, Xu M-D, Zhang Y-Q, et al. Peroral endoscopic myotomy for advanced achalasia with sigmoid-shaped esophagus: long-term outcomes from a prospective, single-center study. Surg Endosc. 2015;29(9):2841–50.
88. Lv L, Liu J, Tan Y, Liu D. Peroral endoscopic full-thickness myotomy for the treatment of sigmoid-type achalasia: outcomes with a minimum follow-up of 12 months. Eur J Gastroenterol Hepatol. 2016;28(1):30–6.
89. Zhang W, Linghu E-Q. Peroral endoscopic myotomy for type III achalasia of Chicago classification: outcomes with a minimum follow-up of 24 months. J Gastrointest Surg. 2017;21(5):785–91.

90. Khashab MA, Messallam AA, Onimaru M, Teitelbaum EN, Ujiki MB, Gitelis ME, et al. International multicenter experience with peroral endoscopic myotomy for the treatment of spastic esophageal disorders refractory to medical therapy (with video). Gastrointest Endosc. 2015;81(5):1170–7.
91. Ren Z, Zhong Y, Zhou P, Xu M, Cai M, Li L, et al. Perioperative management and treatment for complications during and after peroral endoscopic myotomy (POEM) for esophageal achalasia (EA) (data from 119 cases). Surg Endosc. 2012;26(11):3267–72.
92. Werner YB, von Renteln D, Noder T, Schachschal G, Denzer UW, Groth S, et al. Early adverse events of per-oral endoscopic myotomy. Gastrointest Endosc. 2017;85(4):708–18.e2.
93. Ross SW, Oommen B, Wormer BA, Walters AL, Matthews BD, Heniford BT, et al. National outcomes of laparoscopic Heller myotomy: operative complications and risk factors for adverse events. Surg Endosc. 2015;29(11):3097–105.
94. Lynch KL, Pandolfino JE, Howden CW, Kahrilas PJ. Major complications of pneumatic dilation and Heller myotomy for achalasia: single-center experience and systematic review of the literature. Am J Gastroenterol. 2012;107(12):1817–25.
95. Hungness ES, Sternbach JM, Teitelbaum EN, Kahrilas PJ, Pandolfino JE, Soper NJ. Per-oral endoscopic myotomy (POEM) after the learning curve: durable long-term results with a low complication rate. Ann Surg. 2016;264(3):508–17.
96. Sharata AM, Dunst CM, Pescarus R, Shlomovitz E, Wille AJ, Reavis KM, et al. Peroral endoscopic myotomy (POEM) for esophageal primary motility disorders: analysis of 100 consecutive patients. J Gastrointest Surg. 2015;19(1):161–70; discussion 70
97. Familiari P, Greco S, Gigante G, Calì A, Boškoski I, Onder G, et al. Gastroesophageal reflux disease after peroral endoscopic myotomy: analysis of clinical, procedural and functional factors, associated with gastroesophageal reflux disease and esophagitis. Dig Endosc. 2016;28(1):33–41.
98. Kumbhari V, Familiari P, Bjerregaard NC, Pioche M, Jones E, Ko WJ, et al. Gastroesophageal reflux after peroral endoscopic myotomy: a multicenter case-control study. Endoscopy. 2017;49(7):634–42.
99. Repici A, Fuccio L, Maselli R, Mazza F, Correale L, Mandolesi D, et al. GERD after per-oral endoscopic myotomy as compared with Heller's myotomy with fundoplication: a systematic review with meta-analysis. Gastrointest Endosc. 2018;87(4):934–43.e18.
100. Demeester TR, Johnson LF, Joseph GJ, Toscano MS, Hall AW, Skinner DB. Patterns of gastroesophageal reflux in health and disease. Ann Surg. 1976;184(4):459.
101. Crookes PF, Corkill S, DeMeester TR. Gastroesophageal reflux in achalasia. When is reflux really reflux? Dig Dis Sci. 1997;42(7):1354–61.
102. Bhayani NH, Kurian AA, Dunst CM, Sharata AM, Rieder E, Swanstrom LL. A comparative study on comprehensive, objective outcomes of laparoscopic Heller myotomy with per-oral endoscopic myotomy (POEM) for achalasia. Ann Surg. 2014;259(6):1098–103.
103. Schlottmann F, Luckett DJ, Fine J, Shaheen NJ, Patti MG. Laparoscopic Heller myotomy versus peroral endoscopic myotomy (POEM) for achalasia: a systematic review and meta-analysis. Ann Surg. 2018;267(3):451–60.
104. Sanaka MR, Thota PN, Parikh MP, Hayat U, Gupta NM, Gabbard S, et al. Peroral endoscopic myotomy leads to higher rates of abnormal esophageal acid exposure than laparoscopic Heller myotomy in achalasia. Surg Endosc. 2019;33(7):2284–92.
105. Kumagai K, Kjellin A, Tsai JA, Thorell A, Granqvist S, Lundell L, et al. Toupet versus Dor as a procedure to prevent reflux after cardiomyotomy for achalasia: results of a randomised clinical trial. Int J Surg. 2014;12(7):673–80.
106. Rawlings A, Soper NJ, Oelschlager B, Swanstrom L, Matthews BD, Pellegrini C, et al. Laparoscopic Dor versus Toupet fundoplication following Heller myotomy for achalasia: results of a multicenter, prospective, randomized-controlled trial. Surg Endosc. 2012;26(1):18–26.
107. Khajanchee YS, Kanneganti S, Leatherwood AE, Hansen PD, Swanstrom LL. Laparoscopic Heller myotomy with Toupet fundoplication: outcomes predictors in 121 consecutive patients. Arch Surg. 2005;140(9):827–33; discussion 33–4

108. Boeckxstaens GE, Annese V, des Varannes SB, Chaussade S, Costantini M, Cuttitta A, et al. Pneumatic dilation versus laparoscopic Heller's myotomy for idiopathic achalasia. N Engl J Med. 2011;364(19):1807–16.
109. Popoff AM, Myers JA, Zelhart M, Maroulis B, Mesleh M, Millikan K, et al. Long-term symptom relief and patient satisfaction after Heller myotomy and Toupet fundoplication for achalasia. Am J Surg. 2012;203(3):339–42; discussion 42
110. Stavropoulos SN, Modayil R, Friedel D. Achalasia. Gastrointest Endosc Clin. 2013;23(1):53–75.

GPSR Compliance

The European Union's (EU) General Product Safety Regulation (GPSR) is a set of rules that requires consumer products to be safe and our obligations to ensure this.

If you have any concerns about our products, you can contact us on ProductSafety@springernature.com

In case Publisher is established outside the EU, the EU authorized representative is:

Springer Nature Customer Service Center GmbH
Europaplatz 3
69115 Heidelberg, Germany

Batch number: 10732090

Printed by Printforce, the Netherlands